Cultural Competencies for Nurses

Impact on Health and Illness

Linda Dayer-Berenson, MSN, CRNP, APRN, BC
Clinical Assistant Professor
College of Nursing and Health Professions
Drexel University
Philadelphia, Pennsylvania
Assistant Professor
Department of Physical Medicine and Rehabilitation
School of Osteopathic Medicine
University Pain Center
University of Medicine and Dentistry of New Jersey
Stratford, New Jersey

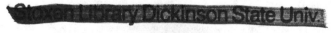

JONES AND BARTLETT PUBLISHERS
Sudbury, Massachusetts
BOSTON   TORONTO   LONDON   SINGAPORE

World Headquarters
Jones and Bartlett Publishers
40 Tall Pine Drive
Sudbury, MA 01776
978-443-5000
info@jbpub.com
www.jbpub.com

Jones and Bartlett Publishers
Canada
6339 Ormindale Way
Mississauga, Ontario L5V 1J2
Canada

Jones and Bartlett Publishers
International
Barb House, Barb Mews
London W6 7PA
United Kingdom

Jones and Bartlett's books and products are available through most bookstores and online booksellers. To contact Jones and Bartlett Publishers directly, call 800-832-0034, fax 978-443-8000, or visit our website, www.jbpub.com.

Substantial discounts on bulk quantities of Jones and Bartlett's publications are available to corporations, professional associations, and other qualified organizations. For details and specific discount information, contact the special sales department at Jones and Bartlett via the above contact information or send an email to specialsales@jbpub.com.

The authors, editors, and publisher have made every effort to provide accurate information. However, they are not responsible for errors, omissions, or for any outcomes related to the use of the contents of this book and take no responsibility for the use of the products and procedures described. Treatments and side effects described in this book may not be applicable to all people; likewise, some people may require a dose or experience a side effect that is not described herein. Drugs and medical devices are discussed that may have limited availability controlled by the Food and Drug Administration (FDA) for use only in a research study or clinical trial. Research, clinical practice, and government regulations often change the accepted standard in this field. When consideration is being given to use of any drug in the clinical setting, the health care provider or reader is responsible for determining FDA status of the drug, reading the package insert, and reviewing prescribing information for the most up-to-date recommendations on dose, precautions, and contraindications, and determining the appropriate usage for the product. This is especially important in the case of drugs that are new or seldom used.

Production Credits

Publisher: Kevin Sullivan
Acquisitions Editor: Amy Sibley
Associate Editor: Patricia Donnelly
Editorial Assistant: Rachel Shuster
Production Editor: Amanda Clerkin
Marketing Manager: Rebecca Wasley

V.P., Manufacturing and Inventory Control: Therese Connell
Composition: DDC/ASI
Cover Design: Scott Moden
Cover Image Credit: © Wiret/ShutterStock, Inc.
Printing and Binding: Malloy, Inc.
Cover Printing: Malloy, Inc.

Library of Congress Cataloging-in-Publication Data
Dayer-Berenson, Linda.
Cultural competencies for nurses : impact on health and illness / Linda Dayer-Berenson.
   p. ; cm.
Includes bibliographical references and index.
ISBN-13: 978-0-7637-5650-5 (alk. paper)
ISBN-10: 0-7637-5650-4 (alk. paper)
1. Transcultural nursing. 2. Cross-cultural studies. 3. Nurse and patient. I. Title.
[DNLM: 1. Transcultural Nursing—methods. 2. Cross-Cultural Comparison. 3. Cultural Competency.
   4. Nurse-Patient Relations. 5. Nursing Care—methods. WY 107 D275c 2011]
RA418.5.T73D39 2011
362.17'3—dc22
                                        2009033395
6048

Printed in the United States of America
14 13 12 11   10 9 8 7 6 5 4

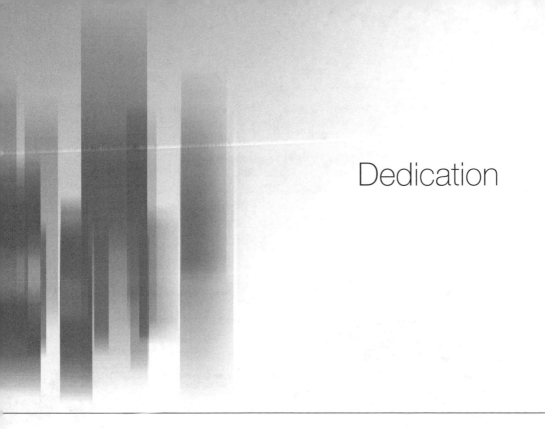

Dedication

To My Family

This book is dedicated to my husband Richard and our sons, Justin and Jarret, with whom all things are possible.

To My Parents

Robert and Mary Ellen Dayer, who always encouraged my pursuit of education and the importance of being a caring member of society.

To My Nursing Colleagues

To all present and future nurses who desire to provide nursing care in a culturally appropriate manner; this book is for all of you.

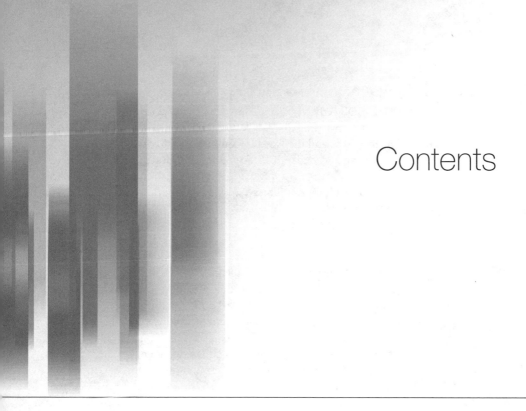

Contents

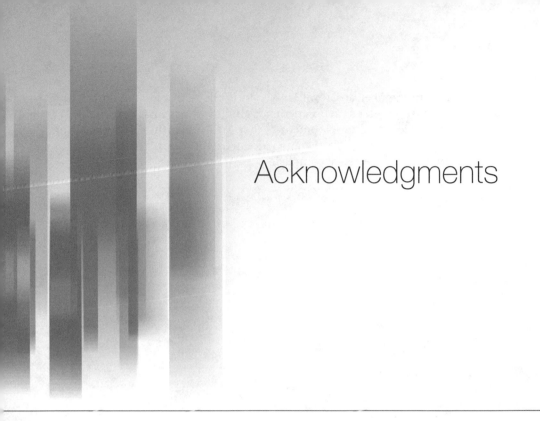

Acknowledgments

I would like to acknowledge and thank the members of my dissertation committee. Their commitment and passion for the topic of cultural competency has been contagious and has resulted not only in a dissertation, but also this textbook. Dr. Robin Eubanks, who is the chair of my dissertation, is an Associate Professor in the Department of Interdisciplinary Studies at the University of Medicine and Dentistry of New Jersey (UMDNJ), School of Health Related Professions, in Newark, New Jersey. Her expertise in cultural competency has been invaluable during my doctoral work at UMDNJ, School of Health Related Professions. Dr. Richard Jermyn, a physiatrist/pain management specialist, is an Associate Professor at the UMDNJ School of Osteopathic Medicine in Stratford, New Jersey. Dr. Jermyn, in addition to serving on my committee, is also the collaborating physician for my pain management nurse practitioner practice at the UMDNJ, School of Osteopathic Medicine, Comprehensive Pain Center. Dr. Linda Wilson, an Assistant Professor at Drexel University, College of Nursing and Health Professions in Philadelphia, Pennsylvania, is the final dissertation committee member. She is also a nursing colleague and fellow faculty member at Drexel University, College of Nursing and Health Professions. All of their experience and knowledge has contributed to my professional development as they are wonderful role models and demonstrate through their practice what the provision of culturally competent care can accomplish.

Preface

With each passing year, the United States is becoming more racially, ethnically, and culturally diverse. This growth in diversity is not occurring in our population of healthcare professionals and this lack of parallel growth often results in the provision of culturally discordant care. While it is not in our power to change the demographic characteristics of our licensed nursing personnel, we can educate nurses to be able to negotiate across cultural divides that may occur during our interactions with a patient whose cultural background is different from our own. It is from this perspective that my personal journey of striving to achieve cultural competency was born, and it is the motivating factor for writing this book. While there are several textbooks available on this topic, I have not found one book that can serve as a stand-alone resource for student nurses, practicing nurses, and advanced practice nurses. This book strives to be that stand-alone resource. By reading this book, nurses from all educational levels and backgrounds will be able to determine how to interact effectively and to provide care for patients whose ethnic and/or cultural background differs from their own.

An overview of the major transcultural and cultural competency models are provided in Unit One. The model that guides my nursing practice, Giger and Davidhizar's *Transcultural Nursing: Assessment and Intervention* (2004), provides the theoretical foundation for this textbook. The five chapters of Unit Two on specific cultural groups are organized so that the six cultural phenomena that shape care, as identified by Giger and Davidhizar, are incorporated in such a way so the nurse will know how to proceed in situations where these phenomena provide a barrier to patient care delivery. Overall, the emphasis of the book is for the nurse to strive toward providing individualized care that considers and incorporates the cultural uniqueness of any given patient—a task that can be complicated by today's fast-paced, highly technical healthcare environment with its emphasis on excessive documentation that takes time away from actual patient interactions and delivery of care. If the nurse can understand the patient's or family's motivation behind certain requests and behaviors, and if the nurse can feel comfortable that the inclusion of these requests or beliefs will not be harmful to the patient, then there can be no reason why the plan of care cannot be mutually defined in order to achieve our mutually established objectives for the patient encounter. As nurses, we are used to working with our patients to establish goals for nursing care; it should not require much of a stretch to extend this thinking, and spirit of inclusion, to also pertain to the actual care delivery as well.

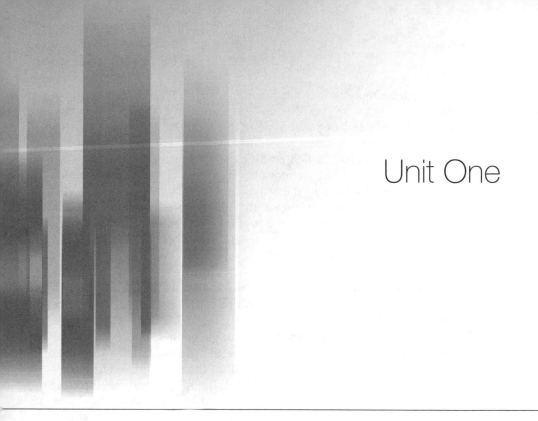

Unit One

Overview of Cultural Foundations, Cultural Competency, and Transcultural Nursing/Health Care

This textbook is intended to be a resource for both student nurses (diploma, Associate's degree [AA], Bachelor of Science in Nursing [BSN]) and graduate student nurses (Master of Science in Nursing [MSN] and Doctor of Nursing Practice [DNP]) on cultural competency and its impact on health and illness. There has been an explosion in the allied health and nursing literature on cultural competency in the last few years, and a textbook of this kind is necessary to help the nurse, at all levels, navigate through the obstacles that culture can place on the patient experience. The textbook will provide a "one stop shop" so the nurse can find the history and theory behind cultural competency in nursing as well as a resource for "pearls" regarding health beliefs and the impact of culture on health and illness.

The textbook is intended for all students of nursing, basic (diploma and AA), professional (BSN), and graduate (MSN, postmaster's, and DNP), as well as a resource for the practicing nursing professional. It is hoped that this textbook will be the reference that all nurses use when they need to learn more about cultural competency and health/illness beliefs of patients. Although providing information is an extremely important consideration, ideally, education is not just about information—it is also about knowledge. In order for information to become knowledge, it requires added context and interactivity. It is the intent that this textbook will transcend just being an information source to provide a framework and structure that permits the acquisition of knowledge by the reader truly possible. It is for this reason that this textbook will have the following pedagogic features: at the beginning of each chapter, objectives will be provided; inside each chapter that describes a particular racial/ ethnic or cultural group there will be one to two case studies that reinforce and highlight the essential facts regarding each group; key terms will be highlighted and definitions provided at the beginning of each chapter; pertinent research studies will be placed as a boxed article (this will be done for important or landmark research studies or findings); and review questions to help students to gauge their understanding of the key concepts will be provided at the end of each chapter. Unit One will provide the cultural foundation; all of the existing models related to cultural competence will be included. The history and development of transcultural nursing will be included and will begin with Madeline Leininger to the present. Unit One is entitled, "Overview of Cultural Foundations, Cultural Competency, and Transcultural Nursing/Health Care" and will consist of four chapters. The outline for each of the four chapters is as follows:

Chapter 1—Birth of Transcultural Nursing to Current Theories and Conceptual Models for Cultural Diversity

Madeline Leininger—founder of the field of transcultural Nursing in the mid-1960s; her Sunrise Model developed in response to nurses increased exposure to diverse groups of patients because of the changing demographics in the United States. Additionally, because of our global relationships, and the United States' leadership in the area of healthcare delivery, many people from other countries come to America for medical care. As a result, US nurses are often called upon to assess clinically, in a short period of time, individuals who, in many cases, are very different culturally, racially, and ethnically from themselves. *Culture Care Diversity and Universality* has been studied, praised, and criticized since it was first published in 1970.

Giger and Davidhizar's Model (1991)

Campinha-Bacote's Model (1991)

Purnell and Paulanka Model (1998)

Chapter 2—Culture

Appropriate terms defined: culture, ethnicity, acculturation, assimilation, health, health belief model, illness, sick role, healing, ethnocentrism, cultural diversity, cultural awareness, cultural sensitivity, cultural competency, stereotyping, generalizations

Chapter 3—Global Diversity

Multicultural populations

Census data

Cultural groupings/health disparities

Chapter 4—Organization of Healthcare Delivery in the 21st Century

Interdisciplinary healthcare delivery

Standards of Care: Institute of Medicine reports on unequal treatment

National Standards for Culturally and Linguistically Appropriate

Services in Health Care, The Joint Commission

Shift from medical model (Western medicine) to health belief model

Barriers (communication issues, lack of access to preventive care, history of discrimination and abuse in some cultures, distrust of healthcare providers, noncompliance and/or refusal to enter the healthcare system at all).

Impact on Provision of Primary Care by nurse practitioners—The integration of cultural competency into primary care practice has been clarified in the National Organization of Nurse Practitioner Faculties document on cultural competency. It states that the nurse practitioner demonstrates cultural competence when she/he shows respect for the inherent dignity of every human being, whatever their age, gender, religion, socioeconomic class, sexual orientation, and ethnic or cultural group; accepts the rights of individuals to choose their care provider, participate in care, and refuse care; acknowledges personal biases and prevents these from interfering with the delivery of quality care to persons of other cultures; recognizes cultural issues and interacts with clients from other cultures in culturally sensitive ways and incorporates cultural preferences, health beliefs, and behaviors and traditional practices into the management plan; develops client-appropriate educational materials that address the language and cultural beliefs of the client and accesses culturally appropriate resources to deliver care to clients from other cultures; and lastly, assists clients to access quality care within a dominant culture.

Certification opportunities—Cultural Competence Certification for Clinicians is offered by the Center for Professional Development at the School of Nursing, University of Pennsylvania.

Unit Two will consist of chapters for different ethnic groups with an emphasis of the impact of health and illness on each group.

I do realize that it would be unreasonable to expect that any single textbook could satisfy all of the needs of a student/learner and that the same needs exist in all students/learners. This would dispute the importance of individuality which lies at the heart of the cultural competency movement. While writing this textbook, an attempt was made to consider the many different reasons, aims, and needs a student/learner has that led them on the journey of acquiring knowledge about cultural competency while also recognizing that different people with the same learning goal do have different needs in this learning process. Each of us has individual learning styles, habits, abilities, as well as life and work circumstances. As a framing reference, this textbook will attempt to introduce cultural competency as a theoretical foundation; to explain the why and how when caring for patients from cultures that differ from our own; to teach the nurse how to use, implement, and utilize this new knowledge; to verify that this new knowledge has been acquired; and finally, to assist the nurse with the every day application of this newly gained knowledge. To provide safe and effective nursing "care" in the 21st century, the nurse must not only have knowledge about our diverse society and the science of nursing, but also focus on the art of nursing care. This requires a global focus from the nurse given the extensive cultural diversity that exists in the United States.

Unit One Objectives

1. Differentiate among the various theories of cultural competency to select the model that will best support your nursing care delivery in the 21st century.

2. Know the history of the transcultural nursing movement from its birth (Dr. Madeline Leininger) to its present.

3. Distinguish among various ethnic/cultural groups as well as the primary and secondary characteristics of culture.

4. Describe the impact of global diversity on healthcare delivery in the United States.

5. Develop proficiency in cultural concepts and race categories and provide definitions for essential terminology.

6. Commit to providing cultural competent care to all patients.

Unit One provides the nurse with the theoretical foundation of the cultural competency movement. Various important cultural competency theories are described as well as the impact of diversity on cross-cultural exchanges and the impact that the Western biomedical model has on healthcare delivery in the United States. The Western Biomedical Model—with its emphasis on patient autonomy—often is in conflict with the health beliefs of many different racial and ethnic groups who enter the healthcare system and who require nursing care. In order to provide culturally aware nursing care, the nurse must not only understand where he/she comes from but also needs at a minimum a basic working understanding of the cultures of the patients for whom he or she delivers nursing care. This requires the nurse to be able to answer two questions: what is my culture, and what do I know/understand about my patient's culture? The overriding goal is for the nurse to develop a respect for cultural differences that will allow the nurse to demonstrate a genuine appreciation of different cultural values and views wherever they are encountered. Often, what we do not understand is viewed negatively. Cultural assessment is integral to understanding the meaning of patient behaviors so this does not occur. Nurses need to consider that each patient experience is likely to vary in many ways beyond just its medical presentation. The nurse needs to ask questions in an attempt to determine the likely response so that the appropriate interventions can be offered. For example, the nurse needs to consider if this is a patient who would respond to touch positively. Also, how should physical assessment be adjusted to provide for modesty or to determine oxygen status of the tissues in a dark-skinned patient? The questions are many, but the answers likely to be determined when the nurse possesses a foundation of cultural awareness and has demonstrated a willingness to learn about, recognize, and most importantly, appreciate the differences that make up the individuality of each and every patient in our care.

Unit Two provides cultural information on selected population groups in detail with a focus on traditional health and illness beliefs so that the nurse can determine if these beliefs are impacting on the current healthcare issues. It is not possible to fully define or describe a cultural group, but the information provided can serve as a foundation for the nurse to inform and sensitize the nurse as to the needs and beliefs of various cultural groups. The material is presented in a sensitive manner and is not intended to be viewed as stereotypical but to serve as a starting point for the nurse to seek clarification from the patient so that individual variation can be taken into account so that truly individualized patient care can be provided.

The journey begins by knowing ourselves and accepting our values; we possess the framework to accept the existence of values that differ from our own. This realization, and ultimately acceptance, of these differing values and needs will permit the nurse to work collaboratively with patients in the provision of safe professional nursing care.

The book will also provide tips for effective cross-cultural communication as well as specific information to increase the chance that a cross-cultural patient encounter will be viewed as successful by both the patient and the nurse. Strategies on how to effectively use interpreters, for communicating with patients with limited or no English speaking ability, and for integrating every patient's cultural beliefs and traditional health practices (whenever possible considering safety) into the treatment plan will also be included.

Disclaimer

Membership in a particular culture does not mean that the person will necessarily reflect all of the customs, traditions, and beliefs that are associated with the culture. There are many other variables that impact all of us and contribute to who we are as people. These factors, including our place of birth, family background, socioeconomic status, educational level, urban versus rural geography, and level of acculturation attained, will also impact the degree to which we subscribe to the health and illness beliefs associated with that culture and our approach and preferences for health care. The material provided is meant as a guide; it is not a rule book. It provides information that the nurse can refer to and consider when providing individualized patient care and evaluating its response. The labels used in the book to classify or categorize various cultural groups are broad; it is important to remember that each group is comprised of different cultures, nationalities, histories, and heritages and that the nurse must remember that individuals are unique and not all of the material will be pertinent to every person. Every effort was made to be as culturally sensitive in writing this book, but I do recognize that the information (that is based on an extensive review of the literature) may be interpreted differently from my intent, and offense may be taken by readers who are members of the cultural groups described in this book. Please know that the intent was to present factual information that is evidence-based and a true desire to improve nursing care delivery in the 21st century to be the best that it can be. Our patients do better when their needs are met and beliefs are understood.

Knowing about our patients' cultures and individual beliefs is as important as knowing about their physical problems, functional limitations, and response to illness to provide safe, competent, and comprehensive nursing care. Given the increasing diversity of patients and nurses, as well as other members of the healthcare team, cultural competence is an absolute necessity. It is hoped that this book will assist the nurse and nurse practitioner to provide the best nursing care possible and to confidently practice when in a cross-cultural patient encounter.

Birth of Transcultural Nursing to Current Theories and Conceptual Models for Cultural Diversity

Chapter Objectives

Upon completion of this chapter, the nurse will be able to:

1. Provide a definition for transcultural nursing and select a theoretical model that is complementary to the reader's nursing philosophy of patient care.

2. Identify various areas of diversity that the nurse should assess for and be aware of in order to provide culturally competent care.

3. Describe three nursing theories that promote the delivery of competent nursing care to culturally diverse patients.

Key Terms

➤ Campinha-Bacote's The Process of Cultural Competency in the Delivery of Healthcare Services

➤ Cultural competency

➤ Giger and Davidhizar Transcultural Assessment Model

➤ Leininger's Sunrise Model

➤ Purnell and Paulanka Model of Cultural Competence

Introduction

Whether a nursing student in the clinical setting, a seasoned nurse, or nurse practitioner, you observe diversity within your patient population on a daily basis. Our patients come from many different races and ethnic groups which means they often do not look, feel, or respond like we do. Helping you to develop a plan for proceeding in the face of a cultural mismatch is the guiding force behind this textbook. The Office of Minority Health states unequivocally that all healthcare providers must "promote and support the attitudes, behaviors, knowledge, and skills necessary for staff to work respectfully and effectively with patients and each other in a culturally diverse work environment" (Office of Minority Health, 2000, p. 7). The Office of Minority Health has recommended 14 national standards for culturally and linguistically appropriate services in health care to achieve this goal. These standards are called CLAS for short. CLAS will be described and discussed in more detail in Chapter 4 of this book.

How have we come to this point where the federal government has mandated standards? It would appear that we need to do a better job. The CLAS standards were developed with input from national leaders (including the American Nurses Association [ANA]) and are based on an analysis of current standards in use that are deemed essential and appropriate.

The members of the expert panel on cultural competence of the American Academy of Nursing (AAN) have developed recommendations (Box 1-1) to ensure that measurable outcomes be achieved to reduce or eliminate health disparities commonly found among racial, ethnic, uninsured, underserved, and underrepresented populations residing throughout the United States.

Achieving cultural competence suggests possession of the ability to respond effectively to the cultural needs of our patients. This view would be too narrow, however. We must recognize that diversity exists among patients but also within the members of the healthcare team (nurses, physicians, and other allied health professionals). As we continue to struggle with a nursing shortage, one solution will be for large numbers of immigrant nurses to continue to enter and work within the American healthcare system. Not only will the immigrant nurses have the challenge of adapting to our healthcare delivery system, but often their ethnocultural background may be different than that of the dominant culture and of the patient to whom they are to deliver nursing care. This not only will impact on the nursing care they provide, but also may negatively affect the ability of the immigrant nurse to assimilate to the healthcare team of which the nurse is an essential member. The growing diversity that has been seen and which continues to widen in the US population has not been seen within the population of healthcare professionals. This lack of parallel growth in the diversity among healthcare professionals

Box 1-1

Twelve Recommendations of the Expert Panel on Cultural Competence of the American Academy of Nursing

1. The AAN, through its publications, mission statements, and yearly conferences, must make an explicit commitment to quality, culturally competent care that is equitable and accessible by targeting four groups: healthcare customers, healthcare providers, healthcare systems, and communities.

2. The AAN will collaborate with other organizations and communities in developing guidelines.

3. The AAN shall develop mechanisms to synthesize existing theoretical and research knowledge concerning nursing care of ethnic/minorities and other vulnerable populations.

4. The AAN, through its expert panels and commissions, must create an interdisciplinary knowledge base that reflects healthcare practices within various cultural groups, along with human communication strategies that transcend interdisciplinary boundaries to provide a foundation for education, research, and action.

5. The AAN, through its expert panels and commissions, must identify, describe, and examine methods, theories, and frameworks appropriate for utilization in the development of knowledge related to health care of minority, stigmatized, and vulnerable populations.

6. The AAN shall seek resources to develop and sponsor studies to describe and identify principles used by organization magnets that provide an environment that enhances knowledge development related to cross-cultural, ethnic minority/stigmatized populations, and attract and retain minority and other vulnerable students, faculty, and clinicians.

7. The AAN, through its various structures, must identify healthcare system delivery models that are the most effective in the delivery of culturally competent care to vulnerable populations and develop mechanisms to promote the necessary changes in the United States healthcare delivery system toward the identified models.

8. The AAN must collaborate with other organizations in establishing ways to teach and guide faculty and nursing students to provide culturally competent nursing care practices to clients in diverse clinical settings in local, regional, national, and international settings.

9. The AAN must collaborate with racial/ethnic nursing organizations to develop models of recruitment, education, and retention of nurses from racial/ethnic minority groups.

10. The AAN will collaborate with other organizations in promoting the development of a document to support the regulation of content reflecting diversity in nursing curricula. In addressing regulations, specific attention needs to be given to the National Council Licensure Examinations, continuing education, and undergraduate curricula.

11. The AAN must take the lead in promulgating support of research funding for investigation with emphasis on interventions aimed at eliminating health disparities in culturally and racially diverse groups and other vulnerable populations in an effort to improve health outcomes. The AAN must take a more proactive stance to encourage policy makers to create policies that address the elimination of health disparities and ultimately improve health outcomes.

12. The AAN must encourage funding agencies' requests to solicit proposals focusing on culturally competent interventions designed to eliminate health disparities.

Source: Giger, J., Davidhizar, R. E., Purnell, L., Harden, J. I., Phillips, J., & Strickland, O. (2007). American Academy of Nursing Expert Panel Report: Developing cultural competence to eliminate health disparities in ethnic minorities and other vulnerable populations. *Journal of Transcultural Nursing, 18,* 2, 95–102.

impacts healthcare delivery and suggests that many patients are receiving culturally discordant care. Culturally discordant care arises from unaddressed cultural differences between healthcare providers and patients. Research has shown that significant disparities in health status, treatment, and medical outcomes between groups of patients who differ on the basis of gender, race, and/or ethnicity exist. Unconscious bias suggests that a provider's unconscious bias about a particular race, ethnicity, or culture and/or lack of effective cross-cultural communication skills may contribute to discordant medical care and health disparities. This suggests that all healthcare providers should know how to interact effectively with and provide care for patients whose ethnic and/or cultural background differs from their own.

Health and illness are defined and interpreted by our personal experiences and the context of our world view. Our own culture provides the framework for how we strive to obtain and attain health, how we recognize when we are ill, and how we act in the "sick" role. The impact or meaning that is attached to the alteration in health is also culture bound. This means that the impact and meaning ascribed to an illness by a patient could be in conflict with the meaning ascribed to the illness by the nurse. This different view can result in cultural misunderstandings that can negatively impact the process and outcome for the patient. This is why all nurses must develop at a minimum cultural sensitivity: so that the nurse can be the bridge between the patient and the healthcare system.

Population Growth

There has been an explosion in population growth. Between the years of 1980 and 1995, the Caucasian population has grown 12%, the African American population has grown 24%, the Native American population has grown by 57%, the Hispanic American groups have exploded with a growth of 83%, and Asian Americans have grown by 160% (Cohen, Bloom, Simpson, & Parsons, 1997). Today, the total minority population of the United States is 100.7 million which means one in three US residents is a member of a minority group (US Department of Commerce, 2007). According to the most recent census, our country continues toward diversity, as demonstrated by significant increases in the numbers and proportion of populations such as Hispanics, Asians, and Pacific Islanders (US Department of Commerce, 2000).

Bicultural/Multicultural

Another important consideration is that in contemporary US society, many individuals, probably the majority, are bicultural (McGrath, 1998). Membership in more than one culture is not the same as being biracial or multiracial. A person may self-identify with more than one cultural group, and that bicultural person sees both sides and can function in both worlds.

In today's increasingly diverse and mobile world, growing numbers of individuals have internalized more than one culture and can be described as bicultural or multicultural. In fact, one out of every four individuals residing in the United States has lived in another country before moving to the United States and presumably has internalized more than one culture (US Census, 2002). We must also consider that US-born ethnic and cultural minorities (descendants of immigrants) identify with their ethnic culture and the mainstream culture of the United States. It is a process for the bicultural or multicultural person to navigate between these different cultural identities.

Biculturalism can be associated with feelings of pride, uniqueness, and a rich sense of community and history, while also bringing to mind identity confusion, dual expectations, and value clashes (Benet-Martínez & Haritatos, 2005).

Acculturation

Acculturating immigrants and ethnic minorities have to deal with two central issues. The first issue is the extent to which they are motivated or permitted to retain their identification with their culture of origin (their ethnic culture), and the second is the extent to which they are motivated or are permitted to identify with the dominant mainstream American culture. The dominant mainstream American culture is usually defined as having a Northern European cultural tradition while utilizing the English language. As the immigrant wrestles and negotiates with this, he or she can end up in one of four identified acculturation positions. According to Berry (1990), the four distinct acculturation positions are: assimilation (identification mostly with the dominant culture), integration (high identification with both cultures), separation (identification largely with the ethnic culture), or marginalization (low identification with both cultures). Acculturation is not a linear process—one does not move forward in a direct line from one position to the next. This is why individuals can simultaneously hold two or even more cultural orientations. People who are biculturals can move easily between their two cultural identities by engaging in cultural frame switching (Hong, Morris, Chiu, & Benet-Martínez, 2000). Cultural frame switching occurs in response to cultural cues. The important point is the individual response. There will be individual variation in the way the bicultural identity is negotiated and organized. Some biculturals will find both cultural identities are compatible, integrated, and easy to negotiate. Others may struggle if they find the two cultures are oppositional or difficult to integrate or negotiate. Various terms for the acculturation process of biculturals have been developed by different theorists. Some examples of these terms are "fusion" (Chuang, 1999), "blendedness" (Padilla, 1994), and "alternating biculturalism" (Phinney & Devich-Navarro, 1997).

Other Areas of Diversity

Although racial diversity is becoming more known, it is not the only potential area of diversity encountered by healthcare providers. Other areas include culture, religion, mental or physical abilities, heritage, age, gender, and sexual orientation. Healthcare providers have to increasingly care for and communicate with patients of varying backgrounds, preferences, and cultures. Diversity may even impact on treatment response. Some researchers suggest that there may be subtle differences in the way that members of different racial and ethnic groups respond to treatment, particularly with regard to some pharmaceutical interventions, suggesting that variations in some forms of treatment may be justified on the basis of patient race or ethnicity. And finally, diversity may also impact on rejection of treatment recommendations by patients. As an example, it was cited in the Institute of Medicine (IOM) report (2003) that a number of studies concluded that African Americans are slightly more likely to reject medical recommendations for some treatments, but these differences in refusal rates are generally small (African Americans are only 3–6% more likely to reject recommended treatments, according to these studies). The IOM report recommends that more research is needed to fully understand the reason(s) for the refusal of treatment as this may lead to the development of different strategies to help patients make informed treatment decisions. The IOM report hypothesizes that stereotypes, bias, and clinical uncertainty may influence clinicians' diagnostic and treatment decisions; education may be one of the most important tools as part of an overall strategy to eliminate healthcare disparities. Clearly, there is much to consider, and we have much more that we need to learn.

Overview of Conceptual Models for Cultural Diversity

For more than five decades, nurses have recognized cultural diversity as an important variable and have attempted to provide culturally specific and appropriate care to a population that is continuing to become even more racially and ethnically diverse. This desire to provide appropriate care was based on the knowledge that people belonging to different cultures have different kinds of demands and needs in terms of health and illness. People having different cultural values should be respected, and the health care offered and provided should be inclusive of the patient's cultural values whenever possible. Transcultural nursing models provide the nurse with the foundation to become knowledgeable about the various cultures seen in their practice setting. Nurse scholars continue to develop and refine a vast number of cultural theories, models, and assessment guides that are used internationally. Dr. Madeline Leininger has provided the basic foundation for cultural competency in nursing practice. Today, arguably the most well-known and commonly used nursing cultural competency models are by Leininger (1991), Purnell and Paulanka (1998), Giger and Davidhizar (2004), and Campinha-Bacote (2007). Each of these four theories/models will be discussed in greater detail in this chapter because it is essential for the nurse to utilize the knowledge gained from these models to deliver culturally appropriate care. In today's diverse world, our nursing care must be grounded in the knowledge and science of transcultural nursing. Through these theories, nursing has made an important contribution to the provision of all health care by all types of practitioners.

Because of our global relationships and the leadership in the area of healthcare delivery in the United States, many people from other countries come to America for medical care. As a result, US nurses are often called upon to assess clinically, in a short period of time, individuals who, in many cases, are very different culturally, racially, and ethnically from themselves. An area of formal study and practice developed in response to this fact; the knowledge and understanding of different cultures is called transcultural nursing (Leininger, 1995). Transcultural nursing is a learned branch of nursing that focuses on the comparative study and analysis of cultures as they apply to nursing and health–illness practices, beliefs, and values. Transcultural nursing was developed in the mid-1960s by Madeline Leininger, a nurse anthropologist. In the 1960s, the field received financial support for nurses who wished to obtain doctoral degrees and become nurse anthropologists. These nursing pioneers were convinced that an understanding of cultural diversity relative to health and illness was an essential component of nursing knowledge. The essential foundation of transcultural nursing is that cultures exhibit both diversity and universality.

The first course in transcultural nursing was offered by Dr. Leininger in 1966 at the University of Colorado (1 year after she earned her PhD in anthropology from the University of Seattle). Dr. Leininger stated that transcultural nursing developed in response to nurses having increased exposure to diverse groups of patients. This increased exposure to diversity in nursing care delivery was because of the changing demographics in the United States as well as the leadership of the United States in healthcare delivery resulting in many people from other countries coming to America for medical care. Dr. Leininger, as well as other transcultural nursing scholars, refer to care as a universal phenomenon that transcends cultural boundaries. It is critical for nurses, because we provide direct patient care, to understand how to work effectively within a diverse cultural atmosphere.

Transcultural nursing, as defined by Leininger (1984), is a humanistic and scientific area of formal study and practice in nursing, which is focused on the comparative study of cultures with regard to differences and similarities in care, health, and illness patterns based on cultural values, beliefs, and practices of different cultures in the world, and the use of knowledge to provide culturally specific and/or universal nursing care to people. The goal of transcultural nursing is to provide care that is congruent with cultural values, beliefs, and practices, which is culturally specific care (Leininger, 1984). Today, transcultural nursing concepts are found in the curricula for nursing programs in the United States and Canada. This theory has provided the basic foundation for transcultural nursing practice.

The Transcultural Nursing Society was founded in 1974. It publishes a monthly journal (*The Journal of Transcultural Nursing*) and provides a certification process for transcultural nursing to nurses in the United States and Canada.

Although the importance of the work done by Dr. Leininger cannot be denied, there have been some problems identified in her transcultural nursing framework by nurse scholars. The major flaw, according to Tripp-Reimer and Fox (1990), is that it has been based on the anthropological theory of functionalism. Dr. Leininger did, after all, receive her doctorate in anthropology. Functionalism in anthropology stresses understanding culture by stressing specific customs, folkways, and patterns such as diet preferences, religious practices, communication styles, and health beliefs and practices (Tripp-Reimer & Fox, 1990). Critics (Brink, 1990; Browning & Woods, 1993; Sprott, 1993; Tripp-Reimer & Fox, 1990) feel that this "narrow view" of people results in stereotyping. This is by no means a small concern. The fear of stereotyping is often cited as the major criticism of the cultural competency movement. It is important that this process of identifying the characteristics that may be associated with certain cultural groups be done with an extremely open mind and for the nurse to realize that, just like in anything, exceptions can be found. It is important that we do not proceed with blinders on as the nurse must continually assess for affirmation or for exceptions.

Although the concern about stereotyping is an important one, there are other nurse scholars who argue that a reliance on generalizations about race, ethnicity, and culture are necessary to expand a nurse's knowledge about a particular patient population (Giger & Davidhizar, 2004; McGoldrick, 1993; Valente, 1989). Looking at the situation from both sides, it is clear that it is important for the nurse to be cautious and to use these generalizations as a flexible guide that permits individualization of patient care at all times.

All of nursing's largest professional organizations, the ANA in 1991, the National League for Nursing in 1993, and the American Association of Colleges of Nursing in 1998, have cited the need for nurses to practice cultural competence.

The ANA established the AAN in 1973. Its purpose is to advance health policy and practice and is often referred to as the "think tank" of nursing. The AAN has a number of expert panels including the Expert Panel on Cultural Competence. This expert panel developed its most recent position paper in 2007 to help serve as a catalyst for substantive nursing action to promote outcomes that reduce or eliminate health disparities commonly found among racial, ethnic, uninsured, underserved, and underrepresented populations residing throughout the United States. From 1991 to 1992 the Expert Panel on Cultural Competence proposed 10 recommendations in an attempt to address health disparities. While some progress has been made, much more remains, and this was the impetus for the most recent recommendations in 2007 by the expert panel.

Membership on any of the expert panels within the AAN are by invitation only to fellows of the AAN. Fellowship in the AAN is considered to be one of the highest honors a nurse can achieve. The members consist of major nursing theorists and scholars.

The Expert Panel on Cultural Competence developed and published its most recent position paper (2007) that provides a comprehensive list of 12 recommendations (see Box 1-1) that can serve as a starting point for all health professionals who seek to address the problem of health disparities in the United States through cultural competency with the hope that measurable outcomes be achieved to reduce or eliminate health disparities commonly found among the minority and vulnerable populations in the United States (Giger et al., 2007).

Nurses are ideally suited to strive toward cultural competence. When nurses consider the race, ethnicity, culture, and cultural heritage of their patients, they become more sensitive to each patient's individual needs. This is by no means an easy feat as evidenced by the vast number of cultures and subcultures that exist on our planet (estimated as more than 2500 by Leininger) but a highly complex issue that requires a lifelong commitment (McGee, 2001).

It is important to learn from our mistakes as with each cultural gaffe comes the opportunity to learn, improve, and to grow professionally. We must also realize that the practice of nursing should never be done by using a "cookbook approach." There is much variation within certain races, cultures, or ethnic groups as there is across cultural groups. The informed nurse is being asked to consider the significance of culture to ensure that patients are then approached and cared for from a more informed perspective—this is the crux of transcultural nursing care delivery.

Nonnursing Models for Cultural Assessment

There are both nonnursing and nursing models for cultural assessment from which to choose. Arguably, the two most well-known nonnursing models are the *Outline of Cultural Materials* by Murdock (1971) and Brownlee's (1978) *Community, Culture and Care: A Cross-Cultural Guide for Health Workers*. The Murdock tool was designed for use by anthropologists and as such does not utilize the nursing process. The Brownlee tool is considered difficult by some and also is not a nursing tool. This lack of nursing focus has been a driving point behind the development of nursing specific cultural assessment models.

Selected Nursing Models for Cultural Assessment

Culture Care, Diversity, and Universality: A Theory of Nursing

The first nursing cultural assessment model was by developed over 40 years ago by Dr. Madeline Leininger. She developed her theory, Culture Care, Diversity, and Universality, from both anthropology and nursing principles. She first published her theory in *Nursing Science Quarterly* in 1985. In 1988, the theory was further described in the same journal, and in 1991, she published her textbook: *Culture Care, Diversity and Universality: A Theory of Nursing*. The theory states that nurses must take into account the cultural beliefs, caring behaviors, and values of individuals, families, and groups to provide effective, satisfying, and culturally congruent nursing care (Leininger, 1991). The purpose of the theory is to explicate transcultural nursing knowledge and practice, and the goal is to identify ways to provide culturally congruent nursing care to people of diverse or similar cultures. The foundation of the theory is that cultures exhibit both diversity and universality. Leininger (1985) defined diversity as perceiving, knowing, and practicing care in different ways and universality as commonalities of care.

To fully understand any nursing theory or nursing care model, one must understand the operational definitions for key terms. Traditionally nursing has four metaparadigms: the concepts of person, environment, health, and nursing. Leininger feels that the paradigm of nursing is too limited in its definition, so that construct was replaced by caring. Caring, according to Leininger, has a better ability to explain nursing. She feels that the concept of "person" is too limiting and culture bound to explain nursing because the concept of person does not exist in every culture. The term *person* is often used globally to refer to families, groups, and communities. Leininger also views the paradigm health as belonging to many other healthcare disciplines and as such is not unique to nursing. The fourth paradigm is environment which Leininger has replaced with environmental context. Environmental context includes events with meanings and interpretations given to them in particular physical, ecological, sociopolitical, and/or cultural settings (Leininger, 1995).

Leininger (1985) defines culture as a group's values, beliefs, norms, and life practices that are learned, shared, and handed down. Culture guides thinking, decision making, and our actions in specific ways. Culture is the framework people use to solve human problems. In that sense, culture is universal yet also diverse. Cultural values are usually long-term and are very stable. Caring is defined by Leininger (1985) as assisting, supporting, or enabling behaviors that ease or improve a patient's condition. Leininger (1985) states that the essence of nursing is caring; caring is unique to nursing. It is essential to life, survival, and human development. It is through caring that people can deal with life's events. Caring is the verb counterpart to the noun care and is a feeling of compassion, interest, and concern for people. Caring has different meanings in different cultures. Individual cultural definitions of caring can be discovered by examining the cultural group's view of the world, social structure, and language (Leininger, 1985). Culture care refers to the values and beliefs that assist, support, or enable another person or group to maintain well-being, improve personal condition, or face death or disability. Culture care, according to Leininger (1985), is universal but the actions, expressions, patterns, lifestyles, and meanings of care may be different. A nurse cannot provide appropriate cultural care without having a knowledge and understanding of cultural diversity. Worldview is defined as the outlook a group or person has based on their view of the world or universe. Worldview consists of both a social structure and environmental context. The social structure provides an organization to a culture, and it can come from religion, education, or economics. The environmental context is any event or situation that gives meaning to human expressions. Folk health or well-being systems are care practices that have a special meaning within the culture. These practices are used to heal or assist people in their homes or within the community at large. Folk or well-being systems have the potential to supplement traditional healthcare delivery systems. Person is defined as a human being that is capable of being concerned about others. A key construct of all nursing theory is environment. Leininger did not specifically define environment in her theory other than providing an operational definition for environmental context. Health is viewed as a state of well-being. Most importantly though, health is culturally defined, valued, and practiced. Health is viewed as a universal concept across all cultures, but is defined differently by each to reflect its specific values and beliefs. Nursing is defined as a learned humanistic art and science that focuses on personalized behaviors, functions, processes to promote and maintain health, or recovery from illness. According to Leininger (1985), nursing uses three modes of action to deliver care: culture care preservation or maintenance, culture care accommodation or negotiation, or culture care restructuring or repatterning.

Leininger's Sunrise Model (1991) illustrates the major components and interrelationships of the culture care, diversity, and universality. Nurses can use the Sunrise Model when caring for patients to ensure that nursing actions are culture specific. It requires that the nurse understand the values, beliefs, and practices of the patient's culture. The Sunrise Model symbolizes the rising of the sun (the sun represents care). The model depicts a full sun with four foci. Within the circle in the upper portion of the model are components of the social structure and worldview factors that influence care and health.

When applying Leininger's model, it is important for the nurse to consider if there is a cultural mismatch present. A cultural mismatch is what occurs when people violate each other's cultural expectations. The healthcare provider needs to develop awareness into his or her personal style of interaction because he or she may have a personal style of interaction that does not match the patient. An example of a cultural mismatch would be the healthcare provider, attempting to keep to a tight schedule, interrupting the prayer session of a devoutly Muslim patient (Leininger, 1995). This interruption would definitely result in a cultural mismatch, but it could also result in causing cultural pain to the Muslim patient which is a much more serious situation. Leininger (1997) states cultural pain occurs when hurtful, offensive, or inappropriate words are spoken to an individual or group. These spoken words are experienced by the receiver as being insulting, discomforting, or stressful. Cultural pain occurs because of a lack of awareness, sensitivity, and understanding by the offender of differences in the cultural values, beliefs, and meanings of the offended persons. When these types of events occur during a patient–provider encounter, they can result in significant consequences. It is essential that if a cultural mismatch or the infliction of cultural pain does occur, it be recognized or else we risk the development of consequences; one of which would be the inability to establish a therapeutic alliance with the patient. It is best, if a cultural mismatch or mistake is made, for the healthcare provider to attempt to recover quickly from the mistake and to avoid becoming defensive. If the provider suspects that the mismatch has been serious enough to have caused "cultural pain" (as evidenced by seeing a sudden negative change in attitude), the health professional must act on this feeling and ask if they did or said anything offensive. Cultural pain occurs if the clinician inadvertently ignores an important cultural obligation or violates a cultural taboo. Making this type of adjustment requires cultural flexibility—this is only possible in those healthcare providers who have taken the time to develop self-awareness and who have examined their own cultural background and biases.

The importance of Leininger's model is substantial as it has served as the prototype for the development of other culturally specific nursing models. In 1984, Tripp-Reimer, Brink, and Saunders analyzed selected culturally appropriate models and tools to determine if significant differences existed among the models. They concluded that most cultural assessment guides are similar because they all seek to identify major cultural domains that are important variables if culturally appropriate care is to be rendered. Nine culturally appropriate models were analyzed (Aamodt, 1978; Bloch, 1983; Branch & Paxton, 1976; Brownlee, 1978; Kay, 1977; Leininger 1977; Orque, 1983; Rund & Krause, 1978; Tripp-Reimer et al., 1984). Tripp-Reimer et al. (1984) concluded that two limitations existed in each guide. The first was a tendency to include too much cultural content, and the second was that it is often impossible to separate client specific data from normative data. It was clear that more refinement was required which guided the development of the more recent models that followed Leininger's pioneering work.

Giger and Davidhizar Transcultural Assessment Model

Giger and Davidhizar's (2004) model provides a framework for assessment that focuses on the six cultural phenomena that they believe shapes care: communication, space, social organization, time, environmental control, and biologic variations. They also systematically explore the variations that exist in caregivers' response and recipients' perspectives relative to the cultural diversity that is present in the United States. The model serves as a resource for healthcare professionals when they are called upon to provide culturally discordant care. The model was first developed in 1988 to help undergraduate nursing students assess and provide care for patients that were culturally diverse. Giger and Davidhizar (2004) state that although all cultures are not the same, they share the same basic organizational factors: environmental control, biologic variations, social organization, communication, space, and time orientation. In its present form, the model provides a framework to systematically assess the role of culture on health and illness and has been used extensively in a variety of settings and by diverse disciplines. In 1993, Spector combined this model with the Cultural Heritage Model which appears in the *Potter and Perry Fundamentals of Nursing* textbook. Spector (1993) used the model's six phenomena but placed them in a different hierarchical arrangement, and then used it as a guide for cultural assessment of people from a variety of racial and cultural groups. The model has been utilized in other healthcare disciplines such as medical imaging, dentistry, education, and administration. The model has also been the theoretical framework for dissertations and other research studies.

Giger and Davidhizar (2004) offer the following definition of culture:

> culture is a patterned behavioral response that develops over time as a result of imprinting the mind through social and religious structures and intellectual and artistic manifestations. Culture is also the result of acquired mechanisms that may have innate influences but are primarily affected by internal and external environmental stimuli. Culture is shaped by values, beliefs, norms and practices that are shared by members of the same ethnic group. Culture guides our thinking, doing and being and becomes patterned expressions of who we are. These patterned expressions are passed down from one generation to the next. (p. 3)

The model postulates that every individual is culturally unique and should be assessed according to the six identified phenomena. It is important to emphasize that the model does not presuppose that every person within an ethnic or cultural group will act or behave in a similar manner. In fact, Giger and Davidhizar (2004) inform that a culturally appropriate model must recognize differences in groups while also avoiding stereotypical approaches to client care. In addition, the six cultural phenomena described are not mutually exclusive but are related and are often interacting. Whereas the phenomena vary with application across cultural groups, the six concepts of the model are evident in every cultural group. The six cultural phenomena will be discussed individually.

The Phenomena

Communication
The first phenomenon is communication. Communication embraces the entire world of human interaction and behavior. Communication is the way by which culture is transmitted and preserved. It is a continuous and complex process as it can be transmitted through written or oral language and nonverbal behaviors, such as gestures, facial expressions, body language, or the use of space. Effective communication is essential for effective healthcare delivery because it motivates both the patient and the nurse to work together to manage the patient's health because the patient is better informed and empowered to participate more fully. Motivating our patients to take action on behalf of their own health is one of the tenets of Healthy People 2010.

Communication can present a barrier between the nurse and the patient, as well as the patient's family, especially when the nurse and the patient are from different cultural backgrounds. This feeling of alienation or powerlessness can occur if the language spoken is the same or if it is different. Impaired communication can result in a poor outcome. There are many different types of communication differences that the nurse may experience. Even when the language is shared between patient and nurse, misunderstandings can occur because of cultural orientation. Even though people may speak the same language, word meanings may differ between the sender and the receiver. This is because vocabulary words have both a connotative and denotative meaning. A denotative meaning is the meaning that is used by most people who share that common language, but the connotative meaning comes from the person's personal experience. Differences in the meaning of words can cause numerous conflicts among various cultural groups. Overcoming language differences is probably the most difficult hurdle to overcome when attempting to provide cross-cultural health care. Clear and effective communication is essential. Nurses often become frustrated and find it difficult to overcome when faced with a language difference between patient and nurse. All parts of nursing process are impacted negatively when we are unable to speak with our patients. When verbal communication is not possible, then we must rely instead on interpretation of the patient's nonverbal language. When patient's feel they cannot communicate with us, they may withdraw or become hostile or uncooperative.

Both verbal and nonverbal communication is learned within one's culture. Communication and culture are intertwined. Our culture determines how our feelings are expressed and what is and what is not appropriate. It is felt that cultural patterns of communication are firmly a part of us as early as age 5. Communication is essential to human interaction—it discloses information or provides a message. Through communication, we become aware of how another is feeling. Often, communication issues cause the most significant problems when working with people from a different culture. One of the most common barriers to communication is overcoming ethnocentrism (viewing one's culture as superior to another), particularly when assessing patients. An example of how to ensure that a patient's communication needs for patient education are met would be to provide oral instructions if the patient feels less comfortable with written materials. In contrast, when educating the Asian population, it would be helpful to realize that the majority of Asians prefer written materials over oral instructions.

Language differences need to be overcome with the use of competent interpreters. When caring for a patient who does not speak the dominant language, an interpreter is a must. The Office of Minority Health recommends against the use of a patient's friends or family members as interpreters. One reason for this is that the patient may not be comfortable disclosing certain symptoms of behaviors to their friends or family. Other important considerations for the effective use of interpreters will appear later in the book.

Differences between patient and provider influence communication and clinical decision making. There is strong evidence that provider–patient communication is directly linked to patient satisfaction. When these differences are not acknowledged or explored, they result in poor patient satisfaction, poor adherence, and most alarmingly, a poor outcome (Betancourt, Green, Carrillo, Emilio, & Ananeh-Firempong, 2003). Failure to recognize the uniqueness of all can result in stereotyping and biased and discriminatory treatment.

Space

The second of the six phenomena is space. Space refers to the distance between people when they interact. Personal space is the area that surrounds the body. All communication occurs within the context of space. Rules concerning personal distance vary from culture to culture; therefore, views of appropriate spatial distance will vary between persons of different cultures. European North Americans are aware of the zones associated with personal space: the intimate zone, personal distance, social distance, and public distance. Other cultures may not be aware of these distinctions. Humans are similar to felines in that we wish to establish territoriality and become uncomfortable when our territory is encroached upon. How large our territorial space is depends on individual and cultural preferences. Encroachment into one's intimate zone by another can cause many different types of reactions. One possible outcome is embarrassment and modesty. Modesty may pose a significant barrier that may be difficult to overcome when it is time to examine the patient.

Giger and Davidhizar (2004) identified four aspects of behavior patterns related to space that must be assessed to promote a healthy interaction: (1) proximity to others, (2) attachment with objects in the environment, (3) body posture, and (4) movement in the setting. These four concepts are particularly important during periods when family members are experiencing emotional chaos, such as during the grieving process. Although the desired degree of physical proximity between the client and provider is based on the degree of intimacy and the trust that has been mutually established, as a general rule, Hispanics and Asians tend to stand closer to each other than do Euro-Americans.

Social Organization

The third phenomenon is social organization. Social organization refers to the manner in which a cultural group organizes itself around the family group. Family structure and organization, religious values and beliefs, and role assignments, all relate to ethnicity and culture. Where we grow up and choose to live in adulthood plays an essential role in our socialization process. There is a strong need among many cultural groups to maintain social congruency. This need can impact health care negatively. Access to healthcare providers does not necessarily translate into positive lifestyle behaviors or risk-reduction activities as prescribed by the dominant society. People from some cultures may verbally agree with a treatment plan out of respect to the provider but then defer to folk remedies or alternative health practices upon discharge. Social organization consists of the family unit and the social organizations in which one may have membership. Social organizations are structured in a variety of groups, including family, religious, ethnic, racial, as well as special interest groupings. Membership in groups, except for ethnic or racial groups, is voluntary. Social barriers also exist and can impact access to health care as was pointed out in the IOM (2003) report. These social barriers include unemployment, socioeconomic status, and lack of health insurance.

Time Orientation
The fourth phenomenon of the Giger and Davidhizar model (2004) is time. While it may not be readily apparent on the surface, time is an important aspect of interpersonal communication. The concept of time is not only based on clock hours and social influences (e.g., meals and holidays) but is perceived differently by persons in various cultures. Clock time is frequently more highly valued by the majority of Western cultures, where appointments tend to be kept at the prescribed time. In a culture in which places and persons are more important than social time, activities start when a previous social event has been completed, and to be dominated by adherence to clock time is often considered rude. Persons in different cultures tend to have a time orientation that may focus on either the past, present, or future. This can impact tremendously on preventative health care because a patient must have at least a small degree of future time orientation to be motivated by a future situated reward (improved health down the road or a longer life).

Time orientation (past, present, or future) also is culture bound. People who are future-oriented are more likely to embrace preventive health measures as they are concerned about the onset of illness in the future. People who are present-oriented arc often late for medical appointments or may skip them entirely. Recognizing our patient's time orientation has value for the nurse. Considering the time, orientation can provide a bridge to increase compliance with a medication regimen or with recommended health screenings.

Environmental Control
The fifth phenomenon is the environment and locus of control and refers to the ability of the person to control nature and to plan and direct factors in the environment that may affect them. Many Americans believe they have internal control over nature which impacts the decision to seek out health care. If the patient comes from a culture in which

there is less belief in internal control and more in external control, there may be a fatalistic view in which seeking health care is viewed as useless. Human attempts to control nature and the environment are as old as recorded history. At its most basic level, locus of control is a significant variable in how people react within the American healthcare system. In general, the willingness to accept responsibility for one's health is considered an internal locus of control. Persons who have an external locus of control believe the healthcare delivery system exists to provide essential care and can become especially frustrated with the complexities of health care in America and the myriad of options available.

The environment also encompasses a person's health and illness beliefs and whether they expand health delivery from that provided only from Western medicine with those of complementary or alternative practitioners. Understanding the patient's perspective on alternative therapies is essential when developing an optimal plan of care for our patients.

Biological Variations

The last of the six phenomena is biologic variations (Giger & Davidhizar, 2004). Biologic differences, especially genetic variations, exist between individuals in different ethnic groups. Although there is as much difference within cultural and ethnic groups as there is across and among cultural and racial groups, knowledge of general baseline data relative to the specific cultural group is an excellent starting point to provide culturally appropriate care. This is also an important area when it comes to racial differences in how pharmaceuticals are metabolized and utilized (ethnopharmacology).

Ethnopharmacologic research has revealed that ethnicity significantly affects drug response. Genetic or cultural factors, or both, may influence a given drug's pharmacokinetics (its absorption, metabolism, distribution, and elimination) and pharmacodynamics (its mechanism of action and effects at the target site), as well as patient adherence and education. In addition, the tremendous variation within each of the broader racial and ethnic categories defined by the US Census Bureau (categories often used by researchers) must be considered. For example, some researchers use the terms race, ethnicity, and culture synonymously, even though they each have distinct and unique definitions. Improper labeling can result in inaccuracies with data collection and the nurse should consider that when critically evaluating ethnopharmacologic research findings. In addition, most clinical drug trials are conducted on White men with the results then generalized to all patients who might be prescribed and administered the drugs. Despite the growing evidence that ethnicity influences drug response, many nurses and healthcare providers still remain largely unaware of this. Research has shown that genetic variations in certain enzymes may cause differing drug responses (although the precise mechanism is unknown); also, certain ethnic groups have more of these variations than others do. Individual factors, such as diet and alcohol and tobacco usage, can also influence gene expression, and therefore drug metabolism (Munoz & Hilgenberg, 2005).

Nurses need to become knowledgeable about drugs that are likely to elicit varied responses in people with different ethnic backgrounds, as well as the potential for adverse effects. The existing ethnopharmacologic research focuses primarily on psychotropic and antihypertensive agents (Munoz & Hilgenberg, 2005). The nurse should utilize caution and consider the possibility of biologic variations when administering antihypertensives and/or psychotropic drugs to culturally diverse patients. Some patients will have a therapeutic response at a lower dose than those typically recommended for a particular agent. The nurse must carefully monitor the patient to help prevent unnecessary increases in dosage which will increase the likelihood of adverse events.

The nurse must also be on guard in the event a therapeutic substitution is required. Sometimes this is done to contain costs or because a drug is not on an institution's formulary. Drugs may vary in how they are metabolized, and it is more clinically risky for patients from non-White racial and ethnic groups. While individual differences exist and should be considered, the nurse would be wise to be extra vigilant when drug substitutions occur in their non-White patients.

Healthcare providers must understand the biologic differences and susceptibility that exist in persons from different cultures; for example, African Americans have a higher prevalence of cardiovascular disease, cancer, and diabetes than others. Cultural differences can also contribute to either noncompliance or poor compliance with therapy. Unfortunately, in many cases, lack of knowledge limits the ability of healthcare professionals to differentiate environmental, familial, and genetic predisposition to disease states. Although research is being conducted on biologic differences relating to ethnic groups, it lags behind the knowledge available regarding other cultural phenomena. An important example of this is that the development of pain measurement instruments remains culturally centered, even though significant differences exist among members of different cultural groups in their perception and response to pain management.

There are several ways that people from one cultural group differ biologically from members of a different cultural group. These differences are called biologic variants. They can include stature or size, skin color, genetic differences, disease susceptibility, and nutritional variants. Asians traditionally are smaller in stature than other racial or ethnic groups. Skin color differences among races also impacts hair and nail texture. Genetic differences can result in enzyme deficiencies such as a lack of lactase, causing lactose intolerance. Certain ethnic groups, such as Hispanics and African Americans, have higher morbidity rates than other groups because of differences in disease susceptibility. Even the diets that are followed by our patients can be culture bound, such as keeping a Kosher diet by a Jewish patient or balancing hot and cold foods that is common in many Hispanic homes.

Clinical Application of the Model

It is essential for all healthcare professionals to be aware that not all patients with the same medical diagnosis are likely to have the same experience. The performance of a cultural assessment by the nurse is integral to understanding the meaning of behaviors that might, if not understood within the context of ethnic values, be regarded as puzzling or even negative. It is not meant to be stereotypical. If we are careful to listen and observe closely and question appropriately, the nurse should be able to discover the health traditions or beliefs that belong to that individual patient. The recognition of the importance of providing culturally appropriate clinical approaches has developed in response to the easily discernible fact that the United States is rapidly becoming a multicultural, heterogeneous, pluralistic society. As the demographics of the population of the United States continues to expand, and especially when the demographics of the healthcare professional and the patient do not match, it is essential, the healthcare professional has embarked on the journey to develop sensitivity and ultimately cultural competence in order to provide safe and effective care. This can be achieved by performing cultural assessment according to the guidelines established by any transcultural nursing model.

See Box 1-2 for some cultural gaffes that can occur within the Giger and Davidhizar Model.

Purnell and Paulanka Model

One of the unique components of the Purnell and Paulanka (1998) model is that it has applicability and can be used by all healthcare team members. Nurses who are members of interdisciplinary teams may wish to use this model for this reason. Not only can this model be used by all team members, but it is also unique in that it includes the recognition of biocultural ecology and workforce issues and the impact of this on the culturally diverse patient. Often, team members can be from various cultures and this model can be helpful when trying to forge a greater understanding of what is similar and different among the various cultures that make up the healthcare team. Purnell and Paulanka (1998) identify many benefits to the use of their model. First, the model provides a framework for all healthcare providers to utilize when learning about the inherent concepts and characteristics of new cultures. The model provides a link between historical perspectives and its impact on one's cultural worldview. It also provides a link for the central relationships of culture so that congruence can occur and to facilitate the delivery of consciously competent care.

Box 1-2

Six Phenomena of the Giger and Davidhizar Model and Examples of Cultural Gaffes

Phenomena	Event	Response
Time	Visiting hours are not being respected.	Explain institution's time expectations.
Space	Poor eye contact on the part of your patient.	Make sure you are aware of the customs regarding contact, such as eye contact and touch, for many different cultural groups (optimally all that you will come in contact with in practice). Poor eye contact is a sign of respect in some cultures (Vietnamese Americans, American Indian, Appalachians); excessive eye contact may be perceived as rude by Chinese Americans.
Communication	Family member is using a lot of hand gesturing when communicating.	Gestures do not have universal meaning, what is acceptable to one group may be taboo to another.
Social Organization	Prayer sessions in a hospital room by patient and family members.	Be aware of the expected rituals and how religious services are conducted for many different groups.
Biologic Variations	Family members repeatedly bring in-home prepared meals for the patient with foods that are in violation of the prescribed diet plan.	Look for foods that are not in violation of the prescribed diet and encourage the family to only bring in foods from the approved list.
Environmental Control	Family members wish to bring in a folk medicine healer as a member of the health team.	Advocate for the patient for inclusion of the complementary provider as a member of the team.

Source: Giger, J. N., & Davidhizar, R. E. (2004). *Transcultural nursing: Assessment and Intervention* (4th ed.). Philadelphia: Mosby.

Consciously competent care is an important concept because when we are conscious of the care we provide, we ensure that it is culturally competent and we can replicate that care delivery for this patient and for other patients in the future. The model also provides a framework that allows the nurse to reflect on and consider each patient's unique human characteristics such as motivation, intentionality, and meaning when planning for and providing patient care. The model provides a structure for analyzing cultural data, and it permits the nurse to view the individual, family, or group within its own unique and ethno-cultural environment. The model encourages the nurse to consider communication strategies to overcome identified barriers. Effective communication depends not only on verbal language skills that include the dominant language, dialects, and the contextual use of the language but also other important factors such as the paralanguage variations of voice volume, tone, intonations, reflections, as well as the openness of the patient or willingness to share their thoughts and feelings. Another important component is nonverbal communication. The varied and numerous components of nonverbal communication must also be considered. The nurse must engage in the use of eye contact or to avoid it depending on the cultural norms of the patient. This consideration must also be given to the type of facial expressions to utilize as not all facial expressions will be acceptable to all patients. If or when to touch a patient is also culturally dependent as is our use of and interpretation of the patient's body language. Even how close we are to our patients communicates information about us. Nurses must become aware of the spatial distancing practices and acceptable greetings associated with the various cultural groups who come under their care. The nurse's worldview in terms of whether the nurse or the patient utilizes a past, present, or future orientation must be considered and planned for. Does the patient place a focus on clock time (as is the case with the western biomedical model) or is the focus on social time? Even consideration must be given on how to address our patient. Miscalculating the degree of formality in the use of names that a patient requires can result in breaking trust or blocking the establishment of a therapeutic alliance between nurse and patient. Communication styles may vary between insiders (family and close friends) and outsiders (strangers and unknown healthcare providers). Purnell and Paulanka (1998) remind us that in regard to verbal and nonverbal communication, there is indeed much to consider.

The Purnell and Paulanka (1998) model has an organizing framework of 12 domains that are common to all cultures. The 12 domains are interconnected. The 12 domains considered essential for assessing the ethnocultural attributes of an individual, family, or group are overview, inhabited localities, and topography; communication; family roles and organization; workforce issues; biocultural ecology; high-risk health behaviors; nutrition; pregnancy and childbearing practices; death rituals; spirituality; and healthcare practices and healthcare practitioners.

An important consideration for the nurse to keep in mind that is mentioned by Purnell and Paulanka (1998) is the higher level of regard or esteem that nurses are given in the United States compared to what is given to nurses in other parts of the world. They believe this higher regard may be because of the amount of educational preparation required and the need to pass a licensing examination to become a nurse in the United States. In some ethnic or cultural groups, however, folk healers or other nonlicensed healthcare providers (e.g., shamans, medicine men, lay midwives) are held in higher regard than nurses who are educationally prepared and who practice within the western biomedical model. When providing care to patients from a culture where this may be an issue, the nurse should spend time establishing a good interpersonal relationship in order to bridge the cultural gap and to improve the patient's outcome as well as the overall healthcare experience of the patient.

Campinha-Bacote Model: The Process of Cultural Competency in the Delivery of Healthcare Services

In 1991, Campinha-Bacote developed the model Culturally Competent Model of Care, which was based on four constructs: cultural awareness, cultural knowledge, cultural skill, and cultural encounters. In 1998, the model was revised to make cultural competency more of a process and to highlight the interdependence of the constructs. At that time, a fifth construct was added, cultural desire, and the model name changed to The Process of Cultural Competency in the Delivery of Healthcare Services. Cultural competence is viewed as a process, not an end point. The nurse must continually strive to achieve the ability to work effectively with individuals, families, and the community of diverse cultural groups. In 2002, the model was further refined by Campinha-Bacote to symbolically resemble a volcano because of the dynamic changes in the field. The focus of this model is on the process of cultural competence, not on being culturally competent utilizing the five constructs. Cultural awareness is defined as the process of conducting self-examination of one's own biases toward other cultures and the in-depth exploration of one's cultural and professional background. Cultural awareness also involves being aware of the existence of documented racism and other "isms" in healthcare delivery. Cultural knowledge is defined as the process in which the healthcare professional seeks and obtains a sound information base regarding the worldviews of different cultural and ethnic groups as well as biologic variations, diseases and health conditions, and variations in drug metabolism found among ethnic groups (biocultural ecology). Cultural skill is the ability to conduct a cultural assessment to collect relevant cultural data regarding the client's presenting problem as well as accurately conducting a culturally based physical assessment. Cultural encounter is the process that encourages the healthcare professional to directly engage in face-to-face cultural interactions and other types of encounters with clients from culturally diverse backgrounds in order to modify existing beliefs about a cultural group and to prevent possible stereotyping. Cultural desire is the motivation of the healthcare professional to "want to" engage in the process of becoming culturally aware, culturally knowledgeable, and culturally skillful by seeking cultural encounters, not by "having to." The important point is the nurse wants to do this, and that the nurse does not feel that they have to develop this skill. Despite being the last construct identified, Campinha-Bacote feels it is pivotal construct as it provides the foundation for one's journey toward cultural competence. It is only once the nurse possesses cultural desire that the nurse will feel required to be available to provide care for patients, even when there may be a natural instinct to remove oneself from the patient encounter (Campinha-Bacote, 1999). Campinha-Bacote has chosen the symbol of a volcano because it is the release of cultural desire that stimulates the process of cultural competence. It is felt that when cultural desire erupts, it motivates the desire to enter into the process of becoming culturally competent through the seeking out of cultural encounters, obtaining cultural knowledge, conducting culturally sensitive assessments, and the process of developing cultural awareness.

To help the nurse to begin or continue the cultural competency journey, Campinha-Bacote (2002) advocates asking the question, "Have I ASKED myself the right questions?" The mnemonic ASKED was developed by Campinha-Bacote in 2002 and provides a reminder for the questions that the nurse must ask to determine where they are in terms of their awareness, skills, knowledge, and desire to move toward cultural competency.

A = Awareness. Am I aware of any biases or prejudices that I possess toward others?

S = Skill. Do I have the skill to conduct a sensitive cultural assessment?

K = Knowledge. Am I knowledgeable about other cultural groups?

E = Encounters. Do I seek out encounters with those who are different from me?

D = Desire. Do I really want to be culturally competent? (Campinha-Bacote, 2002)

Summary

By now, it should be clear that it is impossible to practice high-quality nursing to our culturally diverse patient population unless we gain knowledge in transcultural health care and cultural competency models. See Table 1-1 for more information on cultural factors and Table 1-2 for a process to follow to develop cultural competence. It is not enough to just gain this knowledge, however. In order to deliver high-quality culturally diverse nursing care, nurses need to utilize this unique nursing knowledge. It is not enough just to know, but we must also attempt to do. Utilizing any of the described nursing models allows the nurse to gain the knowledge and to deliver culturally appropriate care. The use of transcultural models is beneficial for nurses to become knowledgeable about and for evaluating society in terms of culture, to find the cultural data in a more systematic and standardized way, and to improve the field of transcultural nursing. Having a greater knowledge of the cultures served by the nurse will play an important role in improving the quality of health care. It is well known that the meaning of health and illness is different for various cultural

Table 1-1

Cultural Factors

Family structure and characteristics
Education levels
Family assets
Family in the community
Communication style
Health beliefs and practice
Help-seeking style
View of professional and family roles
View of early intervention
Knowledge of health and education system
Time orientation
Socioeconomic status

groups. Nurses who utilize transcultural theories are in an ideal position to demonstrate how the provision of culturally competent care will shape health care in the future. Each and every one of these models provides a starting point for assessment of patients who are culturally diverse from us. The nurse just need to select the one that fits him or her the best. The key is to remember that patients' cultural behaviors are relevant to health assessment and should be considered when planning care for all patients. Nurses can be guided in this process by selecting and following one of the available nursing models. A description of four of these models was provided in this chapter: Leininger's Sunrise Model, Giger and Davidhizar's Transcultural Model, Purnell and Paulanka's model, and Campinha-Bacote's model to help you select the model that is best for you. You are now ready to begin to develop your transcultural nursing practice.

Table 1-2

Process for Attaining Cultural Competence

Develop awareness of own cultural biases
Understand facets of culture
Acknowledge and honor range of diversity in families' values and beliefs
Develop cultural sensitivity
Develop collaborative partnerships with families
Develop methods of cross-cultural communication
Learn to collaborate with interpreters
Minimize cultural bias in assessments
Identify and address barriers to assessment and intervention

Pertinent Research Studies of Selected Medical Disorders and Cultural Competency

TUBERCULOSIS: Many studies have found that patients who stopped treatment worldwide for tuberculosis did so because they felt better, their symptoms abated, and/or they thought that they were cured.

VIETNAMESE PATIENTS: Johannson, E., Long, N. H., Diwan, V. K., & Winkvist, A. (1999). Attitudes to compliance with tuberculosis treatment among women and men in Vietnam. *International Journal Tuberculosis and Lung Disease*, 3, 862–868.

ASIAN INDIAN PATIENTS: Singh, V., Jaiswal, A., Porter, J.D.H., Ogden, J.A., Sarin, R., et al. (2002). TB control, poverty and vulnerability in Delhi, India. *Tropical Medicine International Health*, 7, 693–700.

GAMBIA PATIENTS: Harper, M., Ahmadu, F. A., Ogend, J. A., McAdam, K. P., & Lienhardt, C. (2003). Identifying the determinants of tuberculosis control in resource poor countries: Insight from a qualitative study in The Gambia. *Transactions of the Royal Society of Tropical Medicine and Hygiene*, 97, 506–510.

DIABETES PATIENTS: According to the Centers for Disease Control, there are 900,000 new cases of diabetes mellitus (DM) annually, which translates to more than 2600 new cases each and every day. The worst-case scenario results when a strong genetic predisposition is combined with a poor lifestyle. When this occurs repeatedly, it results in escalating rates of type 2 diabetes. It is believed that this is one of the primary reasons why minority populations are experiencing such a high type 2 diabetes incidence. This is a worldwide problem since the burden of diabetes is growing even more rapidly in other countries than it is growing in the United States. This will result in a huge economic burden to some countries that are not in a financial position to handle it. Type 2 DM is becoming epidemic in areas with higher proportions of at risk ethnic groups. In these areas, a child as young as 12 years old is more likely to have type 2 DM than type 1 DM (sometimes still referred to as juvenile diabetes).

It is felt that the recognition that poor diabetes outcomes may be related to inadequate cultural competency will result in a reduction or elimination of these poor outcomes in these high-risk ethnic groups. These poor outcomes can be eliminated or reduced by enhanced awareness and improved skills in cross-cultural encounters. This understanding needs to extend to the complications that can be associated with DM in minorities as well. The following contributing factors have been identified to explain the high incidence of long-term complications of diabetes in ethnic minorities: high prevalence rate of DM, earlier age of onset that results in a longer duration of diabetes, poor glycemic control, delayed diagnosis, limited access to health care, less intense or comprehensive healthcare encounters, and a genetic susceptibility to complications (IOM, 2002).

Type 2 diabetes affects different populations in different ways. The prevalence is significantly higher in minority groups in comparison to the White population. This important disparity is beginning to be shared with the public through public service announcements. The American Diabetes Association has used the public service campaign of "Diabetes Favors Minorities." These facts were included in that public service announcement: diabetes strikes 1 out of 3 Native American Indians, 1 out of 7 Hispanics, and 1 out of 14 Blacks.

The Translating Research Into Action for Diabetes (TRIAD) study was published in *Medical Care* in December 2006 by the authors Duru et al. (Triad Study Group). TRIAD's overall goal is to understand and influence the quality of care (both processes and outcomes of care) for patients with diabetes in managed care settings. TRIAD is a 10-year project funded by the Centers for Disease Control and Prevention and the National Institute of Diabetes and Digestive and Kidney Diseases, and is a six-center prospective study of managed care and diabetes quality of care, costs, and outcomes in the United States.

The goal of this study was to see if the utilization of clinical care strategies (diabetes registry, physician feedback, and physician reminders) in managed care is associated with attenuation of known racial/ethnic disparities in diabetic care. The study did not support the goal in that it was found that for the most part, high-intensity implementation of a diabetes registry, physician feedback, or physician reminders, three clinical care strategies similar to those strategies that are used in many healthcare settings, are not associated with an attenuation of known disparities of diabetes care in managed care. The authors also reported that disparities in care do exist, particularly among the African American population.

References

Aamodt, A. (1978). The care component in a health and healing system. In E. E. Bauwens (Ed.), *Anthropology and health* (pp. 34–45). St. Louis: Mosby.

Benet-Martinez, V., & Haritatos, J. (2005). Bicultural Identity Integration (BII): components and psychosocial antecedents. University of California Postprints. Paper 967. Retrieved April 14, 2009, from http://repositories.cdlib.org/cgi/viewcontent.cgi?article=3021&context=postprints

Berry, J. W. (1990). Psychology of acculturation. In N. R. Goldberger, & J. B. Veroff (Eds.), *The culture and psychology reader* (pp. 457–488). New York: New York University Press. (Reprinted from Nebraska symposium on motivation: Berman, J. J. [Ed.] [1989]. *Cross-cultural perspectives.* Lincoln: University of Nebraska Press).

Betancourt, J. R., Green, A. R., Carrillo, J., Emilio, J., & Ananeh-Firempong, O. (2003). Defining cultural competence: a practical framework for addressing racial ethnic disparities in health and health care. *Public Health Reports,* 118, 4, 293–302.

Bloch, B. (1983). Bloch's assessment guide for ethnic/cultural variations. In M. S. Orque, B. Bloch, & L. S. A. Monrroy (Eds.), *Ethnic nursing care: A multicultural approach* (pp. 49–75). St. Louis: Mosby.

Branch, M. F., & Paxton, P. P. (Eds.). (1976). *Providing safe nursing care for ethnic people of color.* Englewood Cliffs, NJ: Prentice-Hall.

Brink, P. J. (1990). *Transcultural nursing: A book of readings.* Prospect Heights, IL: Waveland Press.

Browning, M. A., & Woods, J. H. (1993). Cross-cultural family nurse partnerships. In S. I. Feetham, S. B. Meister, & J. M. Bell (Eds.), *The nursing of families: Theories, research, education, and practice.* Newbury Park, CA: Sage.

Brownlee, A.T. (1978). *Community, culture, and care: A cross-cultural guide for health workers.* St. Louis: Mosby.

Campinha-Bacote, J. (2007). *The process of cultural competence in the delivery of healthcare services: a culturally competent model of care* (5th ed.). Cincinnati: Transcultural C.A.R.E. Associates.

Campinha-Bacote, J. (2002). The process of cultural competence in the delivery of healthcare services: A model of care. *Journal of Transcultural Nursing,* 13,3, 181–184.

Campinha-Bacote, J. (1999). A model and instrument for addressing cultural competence in health care. *Journal of Nursing Education,* 38, 5, 203–207.

Campinha-Bacote, J. (1991). *The process of cultural competence: A culturally competent model of care* (2nd ed.). Wyoming, OH: Transcultural C.A.R.E.

Chuang, Y. (1999). *Fusion: The primary model of bicultural competence and bicultural identity development in a Taiwanese-American family lineage.* Unpublished doctoral dissertation.

Cohen, R. A., Bloom, B., Simpson, G., & Parsons, P. E. (1997). Access to health care. Part 3: Older adults. *Vital Health Statistics,* 10,1–39.

Duru, O. K., Mangione, C. M., Steers, N. W., Herman, W. H., Karter, A. J., Kountz, D., et al. (2006). The association between clinical care strategies and the attenuation of racial/ethnic disparities in diabetes care: the Translating Research Into Action for Diabetes (TRIAD) study. *Medical Care,* 44, 12, 1121–1128.

Giger, J. N., & Davidhizar, R. E. (2004). *Transcultural nursing: Assessment and intervention.* (4th ed.) Philadelphia: Mosby.

Giger, J., Davidhizar, R. E., Purnell, L., Harden, J. T., Phillips, J., et al (2007). American Academy of Nursing Expert Panel Report: Developing Cultural Competence to Eliminate Health Disparities in Ethnic Minorities and Other Vulnerable Populations. *Journal of Transcultural Nursing,* 18, 2, 93–102.

Hong Y Y, Morris, M., Chiu, C. Y., & Benet- Martínez, V. (2000). Multicultural minds: A dynamic constructivist approach to culture and cognition. *American Psychologist,* 55, 709–720.

The Institute of Medicine. (2003). *Patient safety: Achieving a new standard of care.* Washington, DC: The National Academies Press.

The Institute of Medicine. (2002). *Exploring the biological contributions to human health: Does sex matter?* Washington, DC: The National Academies Press.

Kay, M. A. (1977). Health and illness in a Mexican American barrio. In E. H. Spicer (Ed.), *Ethnic medicine in the Southwest* (pp. 99–169). Tucson: The University of Arizona Press.

Leininger, M. M. (1997). Understanding cultural pain for improved health care. *Journal of Transcultural Nursing,* 9, 1, 32–35.

Leininger, M. M. (1995). *Transcultural nursing: Concepts, theories, research and practices.* (2nd ed.) New York: McGraw-Hill.

Leininger, M. M. (1991). *Culture care diversity and universality: A theory of nursing.* New York: National League for Nursing Press.

Leininger, M. M. (1985). *Transcultural care, diversity, and universality: A theory of nursing.* Nursing and Health Care, 6, 4, 209–212.

Leininger, M. M. (1984). Transcultural nursing: An overview. *Nursing Outlook,* 32, 2, 72–73.

Leininger, M. (1977). Transcultural nursing: A promising subfield of study for nurse educators and practitioners. In A. Reinhardt & M. D. Quinn (Eds.), *Current practice in family centered community nursing.* St. Louis: Mosby.

McGee, C. (2001). When the golden rule does not apply: Starting nurses on the journey toward cultural competence. *Journal for Nurses in Staff Development,* 17, 3, 105–112.

McGoldrick, M. (1993). *Ethnicity, cultural diversity and normality.* New York: Guilford Press.

McGrath, B. (1998). Illness as a problem of meaning: Moving culture from the classroom to the clinic. *Advanced Nursing Science,* 21, 2, 17–29.

Munoz, C., & Hilgenberg, C. (2005). Ethnopharmacology: Understanding how ethnicity can affect drug response is essential to providing culturally competent care. *American Journal of Nursing,* 105, 8, 40–48.

Murdock, G. P. (1971). Ethnographic atlas. *Ethnology World Cultures,* 19, 1, 24–136.

Office of Minority Health. (2000). *Assuring cultural competence in health care: Recommendations for national standards and an outcomes-focused research agenda.* Washington, DC: US Department of Health and Human Services.

Orque, M. S. (1983). Orque's ethnic/cultural system: A framework for ethnic nursing care. In M. S. Orque, B. Bloch, & Monrroy, L. S. A. (Eds.), *Ethnic nursing care: A multicultural approach* (pp. 5–48). St. Louis: Mosby.

Padilla, A. M. (1994). Bicultural development: A theoretical and empirical examination. In Malgady, R., & Rodriguez, O. (Eds.), *Theoretical and conceptual issues in Hispanic mental health* (pp. 20–51). Melbourne, FL: Krieger Publishing Co., Inc.

Phinney, J. S., & Devich-Navarro, M. (1997). Variations in bicultural identification among African American and Mexican American adolescents. *Journal of Research on Adolescence,* 7, 3–32.

Purnell, L., & Paulanka, B. (1998). *Transcultural health care: A culturally competent approach.* Philadelphia: F. A. Davis.

Rund, N., & Krause, L. (1978). Health attitudes and your health programs. In E. E. Bauwens (Ed.), *The anthropology of health* (pp. 73–78). St. Louis: Mosby.

Spector, R. (1993). Culture, ethnicity and nursing. In P. Potter, & A. Perry (Eds.), *Fundamentals of nursing: Concepts, process and practice*. St. Louis: Mosby.

Sprott, J. E. (1993). The Black box in family assessment: Cultural diversity. In S. L. Feetham, S. B. Meister, J. M. Bell, & C. L. Gilliss (Eds.), *The nursing of families: Theory, research, education, & practice*. Thousand Oaks, CA: Sage.

Tripp-Reimer, T., & Fox, S. (1990). *Beyond the concept of culture*. St. Louis: Mosby.

Tripp-Reimer, T., Brink, P. & Saunders, J. (1984). Cultural assessment: content and process. *Nursing Outlook,* 32, 2, 78–82.

US Census. (2002). Retrieved August 27, 2009, from http://factfinder.census.gov/home/saff/main.html?_lang=en

US Department of Commerce, Bureau of the Census. (2000). Census data. Retrieved October 3, 2009, from http://www.census.gov/population/www/socdemo/race/ppl-146.html.

US Department of Commerce, Bureau of the Census. (2007). Census data. Retrieved October 3, 2009, from http://www.census.gov.

Valente, S. M. (1989). Overcoming cultural barriers. *California Nurses*, 85, 8, 4–5.

Review Questions

Review Question 1:

Differentiate the terms culture, cultural assessment, and cultural competency.

Review Question 2:

List the six cultural phenomena of the Giger and Davidhizar model.

Review Question 3:

Purnell and Paulanka identify the 12 domains of culture in their model. What are the similarities and differences between those 12 domains and the 6 cultural phenomena that are in the Giger and Davidhizar model?

Review Question 4:

Provide two nursing implications for a nurse administering antihypertensives or psychotropics to the non-White patient (ethnopharmacology principles).

Review Question 5:

What does the ASKED (Campinha-Bacote, 2002) mnemonic stand for? How can it help the nurse provide culturally appropriate care?

Review Question 6:

Describe the process to attain cultural competency.

Chapter 2

Culture

Chapter Objectives

Upon completion of this chapter, the nurse will be able to:

1. Provide a definition for culture and cultural competency that is complementary to the reader's nursing philosophy of patient care.

2. Describe the impact of culture and subculture on healthcare delivery in the United States.

3. Define and distinguish health and illness within the Western biomedical model and within a health–illness continuum model.

4. Identify sociocultural events and the potential impact these events may have on a patient's life or health status.

5. Consider the impact of gender on cultural beliefs and response to illness.

Key Terms

- ➤ Acculturation
- ➤ Assimilation
- ➤ Bicultural
- ➤ Collectivism
- ➤ Cultural awareness
- ➤ Cultural competency
- ➤ Cultural discordant care
- ➤ Cultural diversity
- ➤ Cultural humility
- ➤ Cultural mismatch
- ➤ Culturally competent care
- ➤ Culture
- ➤ Diversity

- ➤ Ethnic group
- ➤ Ethnicity
- ➤ Ethnocentrism
- ➤ Health
- ➤ Health Belief Model
- ➤ Illness
- ➤ LEARN
- ➤ National Standards for Culturally and Linguistically Appropriate Services in Health Care (CLAS)
- ➤ Sick role
- ➤ Stereotyping
- ➤ US Biomedical Health Belief Model

Introduction

Our patients come from many different races and ethnic groups which means they often do not look, feel, or respond like we do. According to the US Census Bureau (2000), African Americans, Hispanics, Asian Americans, Pacific Islanders, and Native Americans currently account for 29% of the US population; but this proportion is expected to increase to 36% by the year 2020. Clearly, the color of America is changing. There is and will continue to be an explosion in population growth in the United States and globally. Nurses and other healthcare providers have to increasingly care for and communicate with patients of varying backgrounds, preferences, and cultures. This change has resulted in cross-cultural encounters and the development of the cultural competency movement. The cultural competency movement is here to stay, so as nurses, we need to get on board the train so that we have a say in the destination and how we plan to get there.

No single definition of cultural competency is universally accepted, yet all of the definitions share the requirement that healthcare professionals adjust and recognize their own culture in order to understand the culture of the patient (Johnson et al., 2004). So what is culture? Culture, according to Locke (1992), is "socially acquired and socially transmitted by means of symbols, including customs, techniques, beliefs, institutions and material objects" (p. 3). According to this definition, culture is learned, not predetermined or genetic. It is important to remember that members of a particular racial group may not share the same cultural experiences. It is for this reason that one must assess for variances from the group's norm in each individual's experiences. This is an extremely important point that must be recognized.

Many definitions exist for culture. In essence, our culture sets the guidelines and standards for existing in society. Not everyone in society agrees with or follows the same guidelines and standards, and this is true for culture. It would be incorrect to believe or even to expect that all members of a cultural group follow the expected guidelines and standards ascribed by the majority. People from a given racial group may, but do not necessarily, share a common culture. Culture also can be influenced by the context or the setting we find ourselves in and must also be considered. Culture is not something that the individual is often consciously aware of despite its powerful influence on our health and response to illness. How symptoms are described and perceived is also impacted by the culture of the patient. This can have a tremendous impact on disease processes or conditions (such as chronic pain) in which patient history is the primary means of diagnosis. Culture shapes the ways in which patients express, experience, and cope with their feelings of distress and, therefore, how they describe and explain their symptoms. Social and cultural factors include the ease with taking on the sick role, the consistency of the individual's beliefs with the main cultural environment, and the consistency of the individual's beliefs with those of the healthcare provider in determining which symptoms will be reported and the expectations for treatment.

Culture influences people's health status and it shapes our concept of health, illness, and our health practices. This is a dynamic process for, as we grow and develop, we become exposed to more cultural variables. In childhood, we are molded very much by our family and community. Our family and community is influenced by history, ethnicity, religion, and socioeconomic situation. As we leave childhood and enter adulthood, we become more educated, we may change our geographic location and political perspectives, and we may even change how we define family as we begin to build our own family. These cultural variables influence our understanding of how to maintain health and health behaviors related to the development of illness in ourselves and in our loved ones.

The Sick Role and the Need for Cultural Sensitivity

Our culture provides the framework for how we strive to obtain and attain health, how we recognize when we are ill, and how we act the "sick" role because health and illness are defined and interpreted by our personal experiences and the context of our worldview. The impact or meaning that is attached to the alteration in health is also culture bound. This means that the impact and meaning ascribed to an illness by a patient could be in conflict with the meaning ascribed to the illness by the nurse. This different view can result in cultural misunderstandings that can negatively impact the process and outcome for the patient. This is why all nurses must develop a minimum of cultural sensitivity, so that the nurse can be the bridge between the patient and the healthcare system. To determine if a cross-cultural encounter was culturally sensitive, look for signs that the patient has the feeling of being understood, the feeling of being respected, and the feeling of being supported.

The decision of if or when to enter the healthcare system as a patient also has cultural implications. With the onset of illness or when an alteration in health occurs, the individual asks himself or herself many questions such as, what is the meaning of this? Is it serious? Does it require medical attention? They may seek assistance from their family or community to aid in the decision process. How each of these questions is answered and how the patient chooses to proceed is based on the person's cultural beliefs, values, practices, as well as social factors (e.g., money, employment, availability of health insurance). The decision of if or when to enter the healthcare system is also culturally determined. Many people with medical illness or health problems never enter the healthcare delivery system; or if they do, they are often nonadherent to the recommendations provided. The decision of when or if to seek medical care is a complex one with social- and symptom-related determinants. Culturally different populations have varying determinants of when, or if, the transition from person to patient occurs (e.g., the decision to seek medical care for their symptoms). The consequence of this is serious in that patients from racial and ethnic minority groups use fewer healthcare services and are less satisfied with their care than patients from the majority White population (Saha, Komaromy, Koepsell, & Bindman, 1999).

Primary and Secondary Characteristics of Culture

Culture can be further defined and described by its characteristics. The primary characteristics of culture are generally unchangeable and shape one's worldview from a very early age. The primary characteristics are what one normally thinks of when considering culture: nationality, race, color, gender, age, and religious affiliation (this is the only characteristic that has the potential for change). The secondary characteristics of culture come from life circumstance and life experience and, as such, can change over time. There are many secondary characteristics including educational level, socioeconomic status, occupation, political

Box 2-1	

Primary and Secondary Characteristics of Culture

Primary Characteristics	Secondary Characteristics
Nationality	Educational status
Race	Socioeconomic status
Color	Occupation
Gender	Military experience
Age	Political beliefs
Religious affiliation (potential to be changed)	Place of residence (urban vs. rural)
	Marital/parental status
	Physical characteristics
	Sexual orientation
	Gender issues
	Reason for migration to the United States
	Length of time away from country of origin

Source: Purnell, L., & Paulanka, B. (Eds.). (2003). *Transcultural health care: a culturally competent approach* (2nd ed.). Philadelphia: F. A. Davis.

beliefs, and marital/parental status to name a few. See Box 2-1 for more secondary characteristics. It is the secondary characteristics that change over time, which lead to variations within one's culture. Members of a culture who share secondary characteristics form a subculture that shares the same worldview, whereas members of a cultural group with differing secondary characteristics would have a very different worldview.

People belonging to a specific racial group may, but do not necessarily, share a common culture. There is great confusion among definitions for many terms such as race and ethnicity.

Subcultures

As mentioned previously, not all members of a cultural group may hold all of the same values forming a subculture. Subcultures have different experiences than those of the dominant culture. A subculture differs from the dominant group. An example of a subculture that holds differing views than the dominant culture would be second-generation Asian-Indian immigrants compared to first-generation (recent) immigrants to the United States. Although both groups share the primary characteristic of culture of nationality, they differ in time away from the country of origin (a secondary characteristic of culture).

Subcultures are groups of people who have experiences different than the dominant culture and as such may not hold all of the values held by the culture. Members of subcultures are often unified by commonalities.

The Professional Subculture and the US Biomedical Model of Health

All nurses, as well as other members of the healthcare team belong to the professional subculture. As we become educated as health professionals, we are socialized into a professional subculture (Helman, 2000). This professional subculture not only has its own unique vocabulary but it also possesses perspective on health and illness (the US biomedical model of health care or western medicine) with its emphasis on patient autonomy. This can also result in a block or barrier when the philosophy of the healthcare professional and the patient are not congruent. A common mistake made by Western-trained healthcare providers is the assumption that the US Biomedical Health Belief Model for diagnosis, healing, and prevention is common to all cultures, which is not the case. We must always strive to remember that as nurses, when we interact with patients, we come to the encounter with two cultures: our personal culture and our professional subculture.

Even when a nurse has the same culture as her patient, there can be cultural gaffes because the nurse belongs to the professional subculture. This can be even more complicated when the nurse is also a member of another different culture from the patient. According to the 2004 national sample survey of registered professional nurses, there are 2.9 million registered nurses (RNs) in the United States. There are 367,901 nurses with masters or doctoral degrees (HRSA, 2004). The vast majority of RNs are White (81.8%); male nurses only account for 5.8% of all RNs (HRSA, 2004). The likelihood of a patient of color being cared for by a White nurse is extremely high. While the population of African Americans in the United States is in the double digits, this is not true of the nursing workforce. As of 2004, Black/African American nurses were only 4.2% of the nursing workforce. For other cultural groups, the numbers of RNs are even lower. Asians make up 2.9%, Hispanic/Latinos are 1.7%, American Indians/Alaska Natives are 0.3%, and Native Hawaiian/Pacific Islanders are 0.2% of the RN workforce (HRSA, 2004).

Impact of Culture and Ethics

In addition to our professional culture being based on the US Biomedical Health Belief Model, it is also based on Western ethical principles. These ethical principles, such as do no harm, patient autonomy, self-determination, are not shared by all. In fact, in following the law, the nurse can result in a cultural gaffe. Advance directives are based on the ethical principle of patient self-determination but in some cultures,

Table 2-1	
Characteristics of Individualistic Cultural Values Versus Collectivistic Cultural Values	
Individualism—The Individual	**Collectivism—The Group**
Privacy	Company
Time over human interaction	Human interaction over time
Precise time	Loose time
Future oriented	Past oriented
Task related	Nontask related
Appreciates competition	Appreciates cooperation
Human equality	Hierarchy/rank/status
Autonomy	The group
Independence	Interdependence
Assigns individual credit and blame	Group shares credit and blame
Common sense and change	Order and tradition

especially those from a collectivist society; expect that those decisions are not patient-determined but family-determined. In a collectivist society, groups or the government take priority over individuals. (See Table 2-1 for characteristics of individualistic cultural values versus collectivistic cultural values.) An individual must be subjugated to the group and do what is good for the "common good." When dealing with patients from collectivist societies, such as Asian Indians, the nurse practitioner (NP) should consider including the family when discussing advance directives or do not resuscitate (DNR) with the patient. To be respectful of culture and ethics, the NP may wish to permit the both the patient and a family member to sign informed consents for any procedures the patient requires. For Japanese patients, the selected family member may be the eldest son instead of a spouse.

Culture and Mental Health

Mental health concerns human behavior and interaction; cultural understanding is especially important. Culture determines the behaviors that are considered normal or abnormal, the beliefs and values deemed important, and the rules that direct human interaction. Not only are behaviors important, but so are their situational contexts, along with a host of other practices, such as personal hygiene, dress, hairstyle, and religious beliefs and values. When caring for patients, nurses need to be aware of cultural variations in what is deemed appropriate or inappropriate, as well as understand how patients from particular cultures may display mental distress. See Box 2-2 for information on culture-bound syndromes.

Box 2-2

Culture-Bound Syndromes

Culture-bound syndromes are "folk" conceptualizations of patterns of mental disorders. They usually do not conform to conventional diagnostic syndromes, yet they have cultural validity in the societies in which they occur. They are thought of as culturally symbolic idioms of distress, which means responding to stress or showing distress in a style that makes sense in a particular society. The best studies of culture bound syndromes that may be seen by the nurse in clinical practice are included in the *Diagnostic and Statistical Manual of Mental Disorders (DSM)-IV*. All culture bound syndromes listed in *DSM-IV* can be found at the following Web site: http://rjg42.tripod.com/culturebound_syndromes.htm. Some of the more prevalent culture-bound syndromes have been placed here.

Amok (Malaysia) Cafard or Cathard (Laos, Polynesia, The Philippines) Mal de pelea (Puerto Rico) Iich'aa (Navajo)	The origin of the English phrase "running amok," this is a dissociative episode featuring a period of brooding followed by an outburst of aggressive, violent or homicidal behavior aimed at people and objects. It seems to occur only among males, and is often precipitated by a perceived slight or insult. It is often accompanied by persecutory ideas, automatism, amnesia, or exhaustion, following which the individual returns to their premorbid state. The victim, who is almost always a male between 20 and 45 years of age, has often experienced a loss of social status or a major life change. It is now rare, and occurs primarily in rural regions.
Ataque de nervios (Latin America, Latin Mediterranean, Caribbean)	Symptoms commonly include uncontrollable shouting, attacks of crying, trembling, heat in the chest rising into the head, and verbal and physical aggression. Some prominently feature dissociative episodes, seizure-like or fainting episodes, and suicidal gestures, while others lack those features entirely. A key feature is a sense of being out of control, and it is usually triggered by a stressful event within the family. It is commonly thought to be a result of a chronic build up of anger over time. People may not remember what they did during the ataque, and usually return to normal following the incident.
Bilis or cólera or muina (Latinos)	The cause of this disorder is seen to be a strongly expressed anger or rage, which disrupts the balance of both emotional and physical humors. Symptoms may include acute nervous tension, headache, trembling, screaming, stomach disturbances such as nausea, vomiting, or diarrhea, and even loss of consciousness. Chronic fatigue may result from an acute episode.
Ghost Sickness (Navajo)	Symptoms include weakness, bad dreams, feelings of danger, confusion, feelings of futility, loss of appetite, feelings of suffocation, fainting, dizziness, hallucinations, and loss of consciousness. The victim may become preoccupied with death or with someone who died.
Rootwork (southern United States, Caribbean) Mal puesto or brujeria (Latino societies)	The conviction that illnesses are brought about by supernatural means, such as witchcraft, voodoo, or evil influence. Symptoms include anxiety, gastrointestinal complaints, and fear of being poisoned or killed.
Hwa-byung or ul-hwa-byeong or wool-hwa-byung (Korea)	Literally translated as "fire illness," this is a fairly common disorder experienced in traditional Korean culture and is diagnosed and treated by Korean psychiatrists. Insomnia, fatigue, panic, fear of impending death, lack of appetite, "bad" mood, heart palpitations, and generalized aches and pains are its main symptoms. Patients complain of feeling a mass in the stomach. From the traditional Korean perspective, this condition is seen as an imbalance in the relationship between basic elements of life. Anger is a manifestation of lack of harmony and most often occurs in elderly or middle-aged women who are less educated, come from a lower socioeconomic level, and live in rural areas.
Boufée delirante (West Africa, Haiti)	A sudden outburst of agitated and aggressive behavior, marked confusion, and psychomotor excitement. It may be accompanied by visual and auditory hallucinations or paranoid ideation.

Brain fag or brain fog (West Africa) Studiation Madness (Trinidad)	This disorder typically begins after an intensive period of intellectual activity, and is usually associated with college or high school students. Symptoms may include watering or dry eyes, dizziness, blurring of vision, difficulty concentrating or remembering, pain or feelings of pressure in the head or neck, fatigue and difficulty sleeping, shaking hands, rapid heartbeat, crawling sensations under the skin, feelings of weakness, and depression.

Source: American Psychiatric Association. (1994). *Diagnostic and Statistical Manual of Mental Disorders* (4th ed.). Arlington, VA: Author.

Race and Ethnicity

Race and ethnicity are terms used internationally to define determinants of health. The roles race and ethnicity play in genetics, however, can be controversial. This controversy stems from the fact that the terms are poorly defined. Race and ethnicity have their roots in multiple venues including environmental, socioeconomic, ancestral/geographic origins, education, and socioeconomic status, which all influence health.

Emerging genetic knowledge may transform the current notions attached to race and ethnicity. Genomic researchers have found that any two human individuals are approximately 99.9% the same genetically, and it is hypothesized that the most important genetic material for human functioning is encompassed in that shared set. The 0.1% difference, although comparatively small, represents about 3 million differences between individuals' DNA. Whereas most of those differences probably have no effect on phenotype, a small fraction (perhaps about 200,000 common variants) is responsible for the genetic component of the differences in health, behavior, and other human traits. As we learn more, we can expect racial differences to better understood.

Race

Race is generally considered as genetic in origin because it includes physical characteristics (skin color, blood type, hair and eye color) as well as biologic variations such as predisposition to certain disease processes and differences in drug metabolism. The US government uses the classification of race, not ethnicity, for data collection.

The classification of the human race by race is extremely problematic. Newer research highlights the limitations and dangers inherent in biologic explanations of group differences in health and disease. An emphasis on biologic sources of "racial" variations in health obscures the social origins of disease, while reinforcing group stereotypes. The placement of human beings into racial categories is complicated even further when the person is multiracial. The inclusion of a multiracial demographic racial category would further undermine the concept of race as an irreducible difference between people while highlighting the arbitrariness of racial categorization in the first place (Taylor, 2008). There is a paradigm shift occurring in research related to the label of race. The dominant perspective in the social sciences views race as socially constructed through political, legal, economic, and scientific institutions. From this perspective, the meaning of race finds its origins in social practices and a system of social relations that signify social conflict and group interests. Race is a societal construct as it is not individuals who create racial categories, but macrolevel social processes and institutions (Taylor, 2008).

Despite its lack of usefulness as a biologic determinant, the use of race as an organizing principle is prevalent in society. Race is a major source of personal and collective identity as it is a central category of social recognition. The United States is a society where race is deeply fused with power and cultural patterns; it provides a social organization (Taylor, 2008). In striving toward cultural competency, the nurse should revise the definition of race to minimize or even exclude biology and consider race as a marker for historical, social, and cultural experiences and conditions. Consider that race informs and influences our perceptions, behaviors, and attitudes.

Ethnicity

Ethnicity is a cultural construct and refers to membership in a particular cultural group. It is defined by shared cultural practices, such as food, holidays, language, and customs. The perceived cultural distinctiveness makes the ethnic group. Eller (1999) states that ethnicity is fundamentally about symbolism, group cohesion, and personal identity. Ethnicity is a cultural process around which individuals affiliate themselves with a group. First, a person must be conscious of a difference between himself or herself and others. This difference must then be seen as being both important and relevant, and finally the difference must cause the individual to mobilize around that difference (Eller, 1999). According to Eller (1999), ethnicity is no mere reflection of culture, but a complex reworking, remembering, and reinvention of culture. While a unifying difference has to be identified resulting in affiliation for ethnic group development, any differences noted within the group must be overlooked in order to assure group cohesion. This embracing and overlooking of differences can result in ethnic group inconsistencies. For example, the Hispanic ethnic group is distinguished by a tremendous variation among its people (Puerto Rican, Cuban, Mexican, etc.) unified by a common language and geography from which they or their ancestors descend. Ethnicity requires a consensus of group belonging and a differentiation from others that has its roots in a shared past and a perceived future interest. Unifying differences of ethnicity include religion, socioeconomic class, geographic background of the family, and cultural experiences.

Limitations Associated with the Labels of Race and Ethnicity

It is clear that there are limitations associated with the labels of race and ethnicity.

The current use of federal definitions for race may not adequately address the individual's ancestry of origin/ethnicity. The National Healthcare Disparities report (US Department of Health and Human Services, 2008) defines race as White, Black, American Indian, Asian, Native Hawaiian, or Pacific Islander, and ethnicity is limited to only two categories: "Hispanic" or "not Hispanic" origin. It is also important

---

Table 2-2

Cultural Variations and Associated Nursing Implications

Cultural Groups	Cultural Variations	Nursing Implications
African Americans	Language—slang terms may have opposite meanings. Example: "bad" actually means "good."	Ensure understanding through careful questioning and seeking clarification.
Mexican Americans	Touch—when interacting with or admiring children, it is important to touch the child. Not doing so is giving the "evil eye." The male head of the family is the healthcare decision maker.	During encounters with children, it is important to associate touch. The nurse should include the entire family, both immediate and extended, in all aspects of nursing care delivery. Ultimately, it is the male head of the family who will make healthcare decision.
Vietnamese Americans	The head is considered sacred and should not be touched. An upturned palm is an offensive gesture.	The nurse should only touch the head if it is-absolutely essential to do so. If it is essential, then the nurse should explain the reasons for the need to touch the head and to seek permission before proceeding. The nurse should be aware of nonverbal communication and should avoid hand gesturing in order to prevent a cultural gaffe.
American Eskimos	It is not considered polite to disagree publicly.	The nurse should always clarify patient intent. A patient may nod their head yes to be polite and to avoid public disagreement, even though they actually mean no.
Orthodox Jewish Americans	Excessive touching by members of the opposite sex is offensive.	Consider ways to minimize touching the patient and only do so if absolutely necessary and only after permission from the patient has been received. If possible, male nurses should be assigned to male Orthodox patients and female nurses to female Orthodox patients.

Source: Giger, J. N., & Davidhizar, R. E. (2004). *Transcultural nursing: Assessment and intervention.* Philadelphia: Elsevier and Purnell, L., & Paulanka, B. (2003). *Transcultural health care: A culturally competent approach* (2nd ed.). Philadelphia: F. A. Davis.

to remember that terms such as "African American" are census terms and may not be considered appropriately descriptive of many Blacks in America who hail from other areas throughout the world and who have maintained their unique cultural heritage and, in some cases, their specific genotypes from their original geographical location (e.g., immigrants from Haiti, Jamaica, and Uganda).

Ethnocentrism

Ethnocentrism can be a barrier to the delivery of culturally competent nursing care. Dividing the word ethnocentrism can lead to its definition. Ethnic refers to cultural heritage and centrism refers to a central starting point. Therefore, ethnocentrism refers to judging other groups from our own cultural point of view. We are all ethnocentric—how can we not be? We need to recognize this fact because problems occur when we are placed in a situation where we have limited (or no) information about another group. This can result in the nurse making a false assumption or assumptions based on limited experience. The root of the issue and the inherent danger is that we do not know what we do not know or understand what we do not understand. An ethnocentric nurse feels that those whose beliefs are different from their own are strange or bizarre, or most alarmingly, totally wrong. Unfortunately, ethnocentrism is a universal tendency of all human beings to think that their way of thinking, acting, and believing is the only right, proper, and natural way. The nurse must avoid being ethnocentric and recognize that patients and their families feel that their values and principles are just as valid as the nurse feels her own values and principles are.

In an attempt to avoid being ethnocentric in nursing practice, we must learn more about the cultures of the patients for whom we provide care. Even learning about cultural competency in and of itself does not guarantee success or smooth sailing. There are inherent barriers, some that are obvious and visible and others yet to be identified or viewed. One barrier that is known is the impact of whether verb tenses exist or not in the language spoken. The English language does have verb tenses which result in a time orientation (the importance of time is highly valued and demonstrated by statements such as "time is money," "it is important to be punctual," or "if it was important you would make the time"). The Algonquian Indian language, in contrast, does not have tenses but has an animate or inanimate verb forms. If a Native American who speaks the Algonquian language (e.g., Chippewa tribe) does not show or is late for a medical appointment, the nurse may make the assumption that the patient has a "present time" orientation (a concept frequently highlighted in the cultural competency literature).

Cultural groups are often identified as having a present or future time orientation. This would be an incorrect assumption in this particular situation because the nurse would be imposing a time frame where none exists.

Assumptions can result in either false-negative or false-positive judgments. An example of a false-negative judgment would be the nurse who views the taking of a siesta by the Mexican American patient as being "lazy." Because western culture (and the professional healthcare subculture) values being industrious, being lazy is a very negative attribute. This view does not permit the nurse to recognize the positive impact a rest or a nap can have on the health of the patient. An example of a false-positive judgment would be for the nurse who, as a member of an industrial society, views an Amish patient living in Lancaster County, PA, as being free of the stress of a modern society. In reality, the patient may be experiencing a significant amount of stress caused by bad weather that is impacting the ability to work the land or harvest the crops. The nurse needs to be on guard and recognize that our limited experience will result in the making of false assumptions. What we have already experienced is the basis for our reality. Our perceptions on all things, such as time orientation, social roles, and even life and the universe, work for us, or else we would not have those perceptions. These perceptions help us to organize our life experience and to provide meaning to events as we live our daily lives. Our experiences provide the basis for interpreting others' behaviors. This ethnocentric view can lead to misunderstanding because we see their ways in terms of our life experiences, not their context. An ethnocentric view causes us to not understand that the ways of others have their own meanings and functions, just as our ways have for us. Carrying on in an ethnocentric manner can have serious consequences. We can unintentionally offend others, generate ill will, and even contribute to a harmful situation—the last thing that an ethical nurse would ever wish to occur. So, what should we do? We need to remove the blinders and recognize that we are all ethnocentric (we can never experience every life situation of everyone in the world). When we are being ethnocentric, we need to identify that we are, attempt to control for any bias, and strive to develop a better understanding of the other person and the situation at hand. We should strive for a grounded understanding that can only occur from the recognition and control of bias. We need to open ourselves up to the reactions or cues from our patients and ourselves that let us know that our assumptions are wrong or are not working. When we experience a negative reaction to a situation (such as feeling offended or confused), this is a clue that our assumptions are not working in this situation. Also, recognizing that our patient is not responding in the way that we would is also an important clue that again our assumptions are not working in this situation. Once we realize that we do not understand the patient or the situation, we can be in a better position to control any biases and to strive to develop a more valid understanding of the patient and the situation. Ask questions and seek information. Ask for an explanation, in a respectful manner, for what they say or do. An open "can you help me understand this better?" will often result in willingness for the other person to help us in our understanding. Avoid asking questions that impose your own reality and negates their reality, and be aware that not all patients may wish to answer your question as they may feel it is personal or even sacred. Anthropologists would suggest using an emic and etic approach to questioning our patients to provide more insight into the patient's life experiences within their context. The nurse would utilize the emic approach when trying to determine the meanings about the behavior and the situation to the patient. Questioning what are the adaptive functions of the behavior and the situation utilized by the patient would be to utilize the etic approach. "What are the adaptive functions?" is the question that is generally not asked, but which could lead to the greatest insight as we come to realize that there are many valid ways in which human beings can live and experience life. The development of a functional understanding (as opposed to the development of a true and deep understanding) is possible and important for the nurse to strive for. Practice at every opportunity to develop proficiency—just like any other nursing skill. Cross-cultural patient encounters reveal more about our own perspectives and values and as such they provide us with unique opportunities to truly learn more about ourselves.

Generalizations and Stereotyping

Any generalizations made by the nurse about the behaviors of patients or large groups of people are almost certain to be an oversimplification. When faced with the overwhelming amount of diversity present in the United States, it is easier to generalize about people. A question the nurse should ask himself or herself is: Is my generalization based on the actual observed behavior seen or is it based on motives I think underlie the behavior? If you answer yes, you are probably oversimplifying.

The consequence of generalizations is stereotyping. Stereotyping is an oversimplified opinion or belief about a group of people. This is where nursing walks a fine line. Generalizations have value for nurses because they help to guide the questioning process. It provides a starting point only—it is not the ending point. The nurse gains information, compares it with the information known about the cultural group, and then makes assessments based on prior knowledge and current findings.

The nurse must not forget to consider intraethnic differences in cultural diversity. Despite the variation that exists among all cultural groups, there is the tendency to assume that all members of the group are the same. Some experts, such as Campinha-Bacote (2003), believe that there is more variation within cultural groups than across cultural groups and that no one is a stereotype of one's culture of origin but that each of us is a unique blend of the diversity found within our culture of origin, combined with the uniqueness of our life experience, as well as the degree of acculturation that has occurred during our life.

A large body of research in psychology has explored how stereotypes evolve, persist, shape expectations, and affect interpersonal interactions. Stereotyping can be defined as the process by which people use social categories (e.g., race, sex) in acquiring, processing, and recalling information about others. The beliefs (stereotypes) and general orientations (attitudes) that people bring to their interactions help organize and simplify complex or uncertain situations and give perceivers greater confidence in their ability to understand a situation and respond in efficient and effective ways. There is considerable empirical evidence that even well-intentioned Whites who are not overtly biased and who do not believe that they are prejudiced typically demonstrate unconscious implicit negative racial attitudes and stereotypes. Stereotypes significantly shape interpersonal interactions, influencing how information is recalled and guiding expectations and inferences in systematic ways. They can also produce self-fulfilling prophecies in social interaction, in that the stereotypes of the perceiver influence the interaction with others in ways that conform to stereotypical expectations. This can also be true of healthcare professionals. According to the Institute of Medicine (IOM) report on Unequal Treatment (2002), although there is no direct evidence that provider biases affect the quality of care for minority patients, research suggests that healthcare providers' diagnostic and treatment decisions, as well as their feelings about patients, are influenced by the patients' race or ethnicity. Research findings suggest that the relationship between race or ethnicity and treatment decisions is complex and can be influenced by many different factors. It may be influenced by gender of the patient or provider, the providers' perceptions and attitudes toward their patient, as well as by the patient's race or ethnicity. So subtle are these influences that often the provider is not even aware that the influence is even being exerted (IOM, 2002).

Nurses and NPs may often make stereotypes or assumptions about patients based on limited or inaccurate information. These rushed judgments are often constructed of negative biases, assumptions, and stereotypes made in the hurry to complete the clinical encounter in the required limited time constraint. This rushed approach does not permit the recognition of the inherent diversity and preferences that may be present in each individual patient. The nurse works to foster an attitude that incorporates and validates the cultures of those we treat.

Cultural Mismatch and Cultural Pain

The nurse also needs to develop awareness into his or her personal style of interaction because he or she may have a personal style of interaction that does not match the patient. A cultural mismatch is what occurs when people violate each other's cultural expectations (Leininger, 1995). An example of a cultural mismatch would be the nurse, attempting to keep to a tight schedule, interrupting the prayer session of a devoutly Muslim patient. This interruption would definitely result in a cultural mismatch, but it could also result in causing cultural pain to the Muslim patient which is a much more serious situation. Cultural pain occurs when hurtful, offensive, or inappropriate words are spoken to an individual or group. These spoken words are experienced by the receiver as being insulting, discomforting, or stressful. Cultural pain occurs because of a lack of awareness, sensitivity, and understanding by the offender of differences in the cultural values, beliefs, and meanings of the offended persons. When these types of events occur during a patient–provider encounter, they can result in significant consequences. If cultural mismatch or cultural pain occurs, it is essential that that it be recognized and corrected. If this does not occur then we risk the development of consequences; one of which would be the inability to establish a therapeutic alliance with the patient. It is recommended if a cultural mismatch or mistake is made for the healthcare provider to attempt to recover quickly from the mistake and to avoid becoming defensive. If the provider suspects that the mismatch has been serious enough to have caused "cultural pain" (as evidenced by seeing a sudden negative change in attitude), the health professional must act on this feeling and ask if they did or said anything offensive. Cultural pain occurs if the clinician inadvertently ignores an important cultural obligation or violates a cultural taboo. Making this type of adjustment requires cultural flexibility—this is only possible in those healthcare providers who have taken the time to develop self-awareness and who have examined their own cultural background and biases.

Culture and Its Impact on the Patient Role

Many people with medical illness or health problems never enter the healthcare delivery system, or if they do, they are often nonadherent to the recommendations provided. The decision of when or if to seek medical care is a complex one with social- and symptom-related determinants. Culturally different populations have varying determinants of when, or if, the transition from person to patient occurs (i.e., the decision to seek medical care for their symptoms). It has been reported that patients from racial and ethnic minority groups use fewer healthcare services and are less satisfied with their care than patients from the majority White population (Saha et al., 1999).

Cultural Formulation and Culture-Bound Syndromes

The area of psychiatry permits healthcare providers, including psychiatric NPs and clinical nurse specialists, a comprehensive means of achieving culturally competent care through the use of cultural formulations. It is essential to consider and examine the impact of cultural factors on psychiatric illness, including on symptom presentation and help-seeking behavior. To ensure that an accurate diagnosis is made across cultural boundaries and that the formulated treatment plan is acceptable to the patient, clinicians need a reliable method to determine and evaluate the cultural information discovered during the clinical encounter. The Cultural Formulation Model has been advocated as an effective model to meet this purpose (Lewis-Fernandez & Diaz, 2002). It consists of five components: assessing cultural identity, cultural explanations of the illness, cultural factors related to the psychosocial environment and levels of functioning, cultural elements of the clinician–patient relationship, and the overall impact of culture on diagnosis and care. This assessment and diagnosis of diverse individuals, the cultural formulation, has been incorporated into the *DSM-IV-Text Revision*. The cultural identity of the individual is determined for reference. Immigrant status and the degree of involvement in the host or culture of origin are evaluated. Language abilities and preferences are noted. Cultural explanation of the individual's illness is assessed to look for culture-bound syndromes (such as posttraumatic slavery syndrome), culture-specific meanings of symptoms, and how the individual interprets disease and behaves toward health and healing within and outside of his cultural reference group. Cultural factors related to psychosocial environment and level of functioning put the family and social context of the patient's functioning into perspective and examine support networks. Cultural elements of the relationship between the individual and healthcare provider are determined. Overall cultural assessment for diagnosis and care is formulated, along with consideration of how the identified factors may influence the patient's diagnosis, management, and functioning.

Cultural Differences in Mortality and Morbidity

It is also important to be aware of cultural differences because of its effect on mortality and morbidity. For example, American Indian and Alaska Native populations have patterns of mortality that differ from the general population. Mortality data reveal excess overall mortality for American Indians and Alaska Natives. American Indians and Alaska Natives have a higher incidence of accidents, diabetes, liver disease/pneumonia/influenza, suicide, homicide, and tuberculosis, whereas a relative deficit of deaths have been noted from heart disease, cancer, and human immunodeficiency virus infection.

Knowledge of distinctive mortality patterns among populations will help healthcare providers recognize the unique needs of their patients. Just as disease entities can vary from population to population, so can the response to an illness. Remission of symptoms may be considered to be a cure by people in some ethnic groups, such as Latinos. African Americans understand and subscribe to the US Biomedical Health Belief Model and, with little variation, hold mainstream cultural views about health and management of illness. Older Latinos (older than age 50) do not hold these mainstream cultural views of health and disease management; in fact, they do not perceive themselves as responsible for changing aspects of their lifestyle, such as diet and exercise, nor do they develop self-care practices. This lack of self-care can result in a serious lack of illness management when younger family members are unavailable to take on this responsibility for the patient. Mexican Americans emphasize respect, caring, understanding, and patience in healthcare encounters or a personal process in health care. Filipino Americans' views about health, while grounded in different cultural traditions, are complementary to mainstream US cultural views of health and illness. Filipino Americans ascribe to the concept of responsibility for maintaining good health; however, this is not viewed as an individual responsibility, but as a responsibility to the family and social group. Filipino Americans, like other Asians, diminish the importance of their illness and place a strong emphasis on appearing healthy and active, which in that culture is referred to as the maintenance of "face." Inquiring about the patient's preferences and practices with the goal to incorporate and negotiate acceptable approaches to healthcare delivery will serve the patient and provider best.

Impact of Gender

Culture determines our understanding and behaviors associated with our gender role. Since gender roles are determined by our role models, how a male or female functions is ingrained in us from a very early age. The value of our gender and whether one gender is considered more valuable than another is clearly known within a culture and communicated to all of its members. How a girl should act is learned by observing her female relatives, whereas boys look to the males in the family for guidance. Body image is also culturally driven and can have a tremendous impact on health. In some cultures, weight is an important consideration. In some cultures, obesity is so revered, as in the Mauritania's White Moor Arab population in Africa, that young girls are sometimes force-fed until extremely obese. Being extremely overweight or obese is considered highly valued for a female to achieve as it makes her much more attractive as a potential mate. In other cultures, such as the dominant American culture, thinness is valued, sometimes to an obsessive level that has resulted in the onslaught of eating disorders in both females and males.

In some cultures, the female is viewed by the children as the primary caretaker not only for their family but for the community. Children observe if it is the mother's role to offer treatment whether it be tea, herbal concoctions, soup, prescribed medications, or a combination of treatment modalities. They also observe who is contacted when someone is ill—do the mothers take their children to folk healers, herbalists, older members of the community, physicians, or a combination of care providers? Children soon find out if the females or males are viewed as healers by witnessing who is consulted within the community during periods of illness.

During puberty and the onset of sexual development, different cultures react in very different ways. In some cultures, the onset of menstruation (menarche) is cause for celebration (Navajo) which is not the case in other cultures. In both Iranian and Orthodox Jewish cultures, menstruation is a period of uncleanness. Iranian tradition also holds that menstrual blood can pollute the body unless discharged each month, a belief also held by many African Americans. During menstruation, Muslims are forbidden to touch any holy object or to have intercourse. Because women are considered to be in a fragile condition during menstruation, they restrict showers and strenuous exercise. Women must also undergo a period of cleansing after each menstrual period, cleansing themselves thoroughly before participating in any religious rituals (Purnell & Paulanka, 2003). Nurses must always keep in mind that adherence to any of the highlighted menstrual traditions is not consistent throughout a culture and therefore does not hold from every patient associated with a specific culture. There are many factors impacting this process including the degree of assimilation that has occurred to the dominant mainstream culture, the degree of family and religious ties, and educational level, among others, strongly influence beliefs and practices. Because of the variety of cultural traditions that surround menstruation and the social and physical activities permitted during this period, nurses need to question each patient about her personal beliefs and practices before offering any education or advice. Failure to do so may produce care based on cultural stereotypes, which can have significant negative consequences. It is important for the nurse to recognize that education may not change these beliefs and the patient and her family should be reassured that her beliefs will be respected and incorporated into the plan of care as long as they are neutral or beneficial to the patient. The nurse's duty to do no harm would need to be considered and disclosed to the patient in the event that patient education regarding a cultural belief that is deemed potentially harmful to the patient.

Culture prescribes and determines sexual conduct, including what sexual acts are allowed, type of marriage permitted (one partner or many), sexual activity outside of marriage, as well as the rules and beliefs about cleanliness and the genitalia.

The transition to motherhood is also culture bound as it impacts existence or lack of prenatal care, types of birth, and postnatal care. The decision to breastfeed or bottlefeed is also impacted by culture.

The movement through menopause also varies based on the culture of the patient. In a study by Zeserson (2001), it was determined that the menopause experience for Japanese women was different than for White women. White women complained of "hot flashes" quite frequently, whereas the Japanese women did not. The Japanese women's main complaint was of stiff necks and shoulder discomfort. One possible explanation for this difference may be diet as Japanese women ingest a diet high in soy protein. Soy has estrogenic properties (Hamilton-Reeves, Rebello, Thomas, Slaton, & Kurzer, 2007).

Culture also impacts on health promotion and screening initiatives. No matter the age or number of children, the nurse should not assume that the female patient has had a gynecological exam, a Pap smear, and/or a mammogram. Culture plays a major role in screenings for breast cancer. A study by Lannin et al. (1998) found that psychosocial, cultural, and socioeconomic variables explained the difference between late-stage presentation of breast cancer between African American and White women. Another investigation found that Hispanic women had poorer outcomes with breast cancer, despite a lower incidence; although they may have been taught breast self-examination, so women with breast tumors in this study presented later to their healthcare providers because of cultural influences (Coe et al., 1994).

In addition to changes associated with sexuality and reproductive ability, both genders experience changes associated with aging which have cultural implications. Cultural beliefs affect attitudes about whether families should care for dying women at home or whether they should be cared for in hospitals or nursing homes. Some members of Arab, African American, and Chinese cultures prefer to die in hospitals to avoid the bad luck of dying in the home. Members of other groups, such as some Southeast Asian cultures, care for dying relatives in the home because not doing so may be viewed as shirking family duty.

Culture also influences attitudes toward life support and DNR orders. People from cultures that ascribe to ancestor worship or believe that children are the reincarnation of dead ancestors may refuse to consent to turning off the life support of an infant or adult for fear of retaliation. Patient autonomy, which is an ethical principle associated with nursing and medicine, may conflict with the patient's culture. Sharing the prognosis with the patient also has cultural implications and the wishes vary by culture. In many cultures, the family does not wish to inform the patient about a negative prognosis or to discuss how to proceed in advance in the event of any mental or physical incapacity, and they do not wish to be told of an impending death (Blackhall, Murphy, Frank, Michel, & Azen, 1995).

Impact of Lesbian, Gay, Bisexual, and Transgender

The definition of culture over the years has been expanded to ensure inclusivity for all people. This expansion has resulted in the recent call for the inclusion of lesbian, gay, bisexual, and transgender (LGBT) people as a cultural group (McManus, 2008). Nurses and advance practice nurses are ethically required to provide competent and compassionate care to all members of society. This is only the minimum standard, however. There are unique challenges all LGBT patients face when seeking health care, and there can be devastating consequences if a cultural gaffe occurs. It is for this reason that all nurses must learn more about this population in order to provide appropriate, culturally competent care. There are many situations described in the literature where even the minimum ethical standard, the provision of competent and compassionate care, was not achieved. Two examples of this are dereliction of care provided. A transgender patient who ultimately expired from ovarian cancer was refused health care by 20 healthcare providers in the state of Georgia; in New Jersey, a transgender female was denied care at several emergency departments despite having a fever of 104 degrees and an eventual diagnosis of bacterial endocarditis (Jillson, 2002).

Nurses who do not recognize the qualities and beliefs of any given culture, including LGBT patients, risk losing patient trust and poor outcomes. LGBTs are at high risk for disenfranchisement from society as a whole and enter the healthcare arena with a high degree of fear and anxiety. If they experience an uncomfortable medical or nursing encounter, often it results in the patient choosing to stop seeking medical care all together (McManus, 2008).

Basic Lesbian, Gay, Bisexual, and Transgender Definitions

It is important for the nurse to be aware of the correct definitions that can be associated with this population as well as the difference between sexual identity and gender identity. Homosexuality is a type of sexual identity and refers to a sexual, affectional, or emotional attraction toward persons of the same sex (Gay and Lesbian Medical Association, 2005). The above definition is expanded to include both males and females when describing bisexuals (Gay and Lesbian Medical Association, 2005). Sexual preference is not the same as gender identity. Gender identity refers to the perception of oneself as male or female, neither, or both and, as such, may have unique associated concerns. The label transgender is used as a global term to describe people who do not conform to typical accepted gender roles and the label transsexual to people who identify with the gender that is opposite to the gender identity that was assigned at birth. The person who has sex chromosomes, genitalia, and/or secondary sex characteristics that are neither exclusively male or exclusively female are labeled intersex (Gay and Lesbian Medical Association, 2005).

Homophobia and Incidence of Discrimination

The consequence of homophobia is discrimination. Discrimination can be overt or subtle, intended or inadvertent. Nurses often contribute to subtle inadvertent incidences of discrimination unknowingly. An example of this is when the nurse or NP, while performing a history, asks the lesbian patient about the type of birth control she is using. Our workplace can be the culprit as well. Intake forms that only list the default gender identities of male and female or that only include heterosexual couplings as options (single, married, divorced) can be offensive to the LGBT population.

Many lesbian people avoid seeking health care because of past negative experiences with homophobic practitioners. These experiences have been well documented within the medical literature and may include patronizing treatment, intimidation, attempts to change the patient's sexual orientation, hostility toward the patient or her partner(s), breach of confidentiality, invasive and inappropriate personal questioning, neglect, denial of care, undue roughness in the physical exam, and even reported cases of sexual assault (Rankow, 1995). The incidence of screening for cervical cancer and breast cancer is much lower in lesbians than what is found in the general female population. Even if the lesbian female goes for routine gynecological care, the provider may be under the false impression that lesbians do not need Pap smears (Rankow, 1995). The consequences of healthcare avoidance, including health screening activities, can run the gamut from minor to lethal.

It is difficult to truly gauge the number of LGBT people in the United States because of fear of reprisal of respondents to surveys, even when anonymity is ensured. The US Census Bureau (2000) statistics states the rate of homosexuality ranges from 2.1% to 6% in men and is about 1.5% in women, which is equivalent to almost 10.5 million people who are gay or lesbian. Again, it is felt that this number is an underrepresentation of the true prevalence rate.

Often, nurses and physicians are unaware of their patient's sexuality or are in denial. A study of gynecologists conducted by Lehmann, Lehmann, and Kelly (2004) reported that half of the respondents did not believe they had ever seen a lesbian in their practice. Unfortunately, this myopic view is not just confined to physicians.

It is essential that nurses have knowledge of their patient's sexual behavior because it can alert the nurse or NP to potential conditions that may not be considered if that knowledge is lacking.

The Importance of Acceptance

The nurse must recognize the impact of attitudes on the patient interaction and on clinical judgment and strive to develop a nonhomophobic attitude when caring for patients who are LGBT. The process to achieving cultural competency with this population is the same as for any other. The nurse must first recognize that they have a knowledge deficit as they do not possess the necessary skills or information to provide competent care for this population. They should seek out opportunities to learn more and expand their knowledge base. In the case of the NP, the patient should be referred to providers who are culturally competent regarding the LGBT community. Achieving cultural competency in caring for any cultural group, including LGBT, begins first with introspection, followed by the challenging of core beliefs, followed by the making of adjustments in how these patients are approached and managed by the nurse. Once the NP feels that competency with this group has been achieved, it is recommended that a welcoming environment be created. Many LGBT respond to symbols that indicate openness on the provider's part to caring for this group. These symbols, including displaying artwork with same sex couples, pamphlets that are inclusive, or the posting of a nondiscrimination statement that is easily visible in the waiting room, have been identified by LGBT patients as effective welcoming interventions (Saulnier, 2002). The process of striving toward a nonhomophobic environment can be prolonged, but it will result in improved health outcomes for the LGBT population.

Summary

Culture consists of primary and secondary characteristics. Culture is an important component of any healthcare encounter as it impacts communication between patient and nurse, traditional health beliefs versus those of western modern medicine, and the health practices that the patient will agree to follow. Subcultures influence cultural understanding and experiences. The nurse must not only consider the patient's cultural background when planning care, but also any subculture influences that may impact the patient as well. Once cultural data are analyzed, the nurse can adopt, modify, or reject interventions and treatments in a manner that respects the patient's cultural differences. Providing this adaptation will not only improve the quality of patient care but also the patient's life. Becoming competent in this is not an easy thing but it is a rewarding and necessary endeavor. Patients do better when their needs are understood and met. Embarking on this journey requires the nurse to learn culture specific behavior. Cross-cultural patient encounters reveal more about our own perspectives and values and as such they provide us with unique opportunities to truly learn more about ourselves. Competence requires the recognition that there are exceptions to every rule and uniqueness in all people so that the best nursing care can be provided to that patient.

Box 2-3

Glossary of Additional Cultural Terms

Cultural Humility: incorporates a lifelong commitment to self evaluation and self critique, to redressing the power imbalances in the patient clinician dynamic, and to developing mutually beneficial and advocacy partnerships with communities on behalf of individuals and defined populations. Cultural humility is proposed as a goal in healthcare education (Tervalon & Murray-Garcia, 1998).

Cultural Sensitivity: experienced when neutral language, both verbal and not verbal, is used in a way that reflects sensitivity and appreciation for the diversity of another. Cultural sensitivity may be conveyed through words, phrases, and categorizations that are intentionally avoided, especially when referring to any individual who may be interpreted as impolite or offensive (American Academy of Nursing Expert Panel on Cultural Competence, 2007).

Diversity: the concept of diversity encompasses acceptance and respect. It means understanding that each individual is unique and recognizing our individual differences. These can be along the dimensions of race, ethnicity, gender, sexual orientation, socioeconomic status, age, physical abilities, religious beliefs, political beliefs, or other ideologies. It is the exploration of these differences in a safe, positive, and nurturing environment. It is about understanding each other and moving beyond simple tolerance to embracing and celebrating the rich dimensions of diversity contained within each individual. The range of human variation, including age, race, gender, disability, ethnicity, nationality, religious and spiritual beliefs, sexual orientation, political beliefs, economic status, native language, and geographical background.

Health Literacy: the degree to which individuals have the capacity to obtain, process, and understand basic health information and services needed to make appropriate health decisions (US Department of Health and Human Services, 2000)

Vulnerable Populations: refers to social groups with increased relative risk (i.e., exposure to risk factors) or susceptibility to health-related problems. The vulnerability is evidenced in higher comparative mortality rates, lower life expectancy, reduced access to care, and diminished quality of life (Center for Vulnerable Populations Research, UCLA School of Nursing, 2008).

Box 2-4

Related Web Sites for Information on Lesbian, Gay, Bisexual, and Transgender Patients

Organization	Web Site Address
Gay and Lesbian Medical Association (GLAM)—national organization. Nurse practitioners and nurses can download the publication, "Guidelines for Care of Lesbian, Gay, Bisexual and Transgender Patients" for no charge.	www.glma.org
Gay, Lesbian, Bisexual, Transgender Health Access Project— has an online store where pamphlets and stickers can be purchased to help the nurse practitioner establish a welcoming practice environment.	www.glbthealth.org
Human Rights Campaign—largest civil rights organization in the United States working to achieve equality for LGBTs.	www.hrc.org

References

American Psychiatric Association. (1994). *Diagnostic and statistical manual of mental disorders* (4th ed.). Arlington, VA: Author.

Blackhall, L. J., Murphy, S. T., Frank, G., Michel, V., & Azen, S. (1995). Ethnicity and attitudes toward patient autonomy. *JAMA, 274*, 820–825.

Campinha-Bacote, J. (2003). Many faces: Addressing diversity in health care. *Online Journal of Issues in Nursing, 8*, 1, Manuscript 2. Retrieved September 1, 2009, from http://www.nursingworld.org/MainMenuCategories/ANAMarketplace/ANAPeriodicals/OJIN/TableofContents/Volume82003/No1Jan2003/AddressingDiversityin HealthCare.aspx.

Center for Vulnerable Populations Research, UCLA School of Nursing. (2008). Retrieved October 3, 2009, from http://www.nursing.ucla.edu/orgs/cvpr/.

Coe, K., Harmon, M. P., Castro, F. G., Campbell, N., Mayer, J. A., & Elder, J. P. (1994). Breast self-examination: Knowledge and practices of Hispanic women. *Journal of Community Health, 19*, 433–448.

Eller, J. D. (1999). *From culture to ethnicity to conflict: An anthropological perspective on international ethnic conflict.* Ann Arbor, MI: University of Michigan Press.

Gay and Lesbian Medical Association (2005). *Guidelines for care of Lesbian, Gay, Bisexual and Transgender patients.* San Francisco, CA: GLMA.

Giger, J. N., & Davidhizar, R. E. (2004). *Transcultural nursing: Assessment and intervention.* Philadelphia: Elsevier.

Hamilton-Reeves, J. M., Rebello, S. A., Thomas, W., Slaton, J. W., & Kurzer, M. Z. (2007). Soy protein isolate increases urinary estrogens and the ratio of 2:16alpha-hydroxyestrone in men at high risk of prostate cancer. *Journal of Nutrition, 137*, 10, 2258–2263.

Helman, C. G. (2000). *Culture, health & illness* (4th ed.). Oxford, UK: Butterworth-Heinemann.

HRSA. (2004). Retrieved September 1, 2009, from http://www.hrsa.gov.

Institute of Medicine Committee on Quality of Health Care in America. (2002). *Unequal treatment: understanding racial and ethnic disparities in health care.* Washington, DC: National Academies Press.

Jillson, I. A. (2002). Opening closed doors: Improving access to quality health services for LGBT populations. *Clinical Research Regulatory Affairs, 19*, 2–3, 153–190.

Johnson, R. L., Roter, D., Powe, N. R., & Cooper, L. A. (2004). Patient race/ethnicity and quality of patient-physician communication during medical visits. *American Journal of Public Health, 94*, 12, 2084–2090.

Lannin, D. R., Mathews, H. F., Mitchell, J., Swanson, M. S., Swanson, F. H., & Edwards, M. S. (1998). Influence of socioeconomic and cultural factors on racial differences in late-stage presentation of breast cancer. *Journal of the American Medical Association, 279*, 22, 1801–1807.

Lehmann, J. B., Lehmann, C. U., & Kelly, P. J. (2004). Development and health care needs of lesbians. *Journal of Women's Health, 7*, 3, 379–387.

Leininger, M. (1995). *Transcultural nursing: Concepts, theories, research, and practice.* Columbus, OH: McGraw-Hill College Custom Series.

Lewis-Fernandez, R., & Diaz, N. (2002). The cultural formulation: a method for assessing cultural factors affecting the clinical encounter. *Psychiatric Quarterly, 73*, 4, 271–295.

Locke, D. C. (1992). *Increasing multicultural understanding: A comprehensive model, multicultural aspects of counseling, series 1.* Newbury Park, CA: Sage Publications.

McManus, A. J. (2008). Creating an LGBT-friendly practice: Practical implications for NPs. *The American Journal for Nurse Practitioners, 12,* 4, 29–38.

Purnell, L., & Paulanka, B. (Eds.). (2003). *Transcultural health care: A culturally competent approach* (2nd ed.). Philadelphia: F. A. Davis.

Rankow, E. J. (1995). Breast and cervical cancer among lesbians. *Women's Health Issues, 5,* 3, 123–129.

Saha, S., Komaromy, M., Koepsell, T. D., & Bindman, A. B. (1999). Patient–physician racial concordance and the perceived quality and use of health care. *Archives of Internal Medicine, 159,* 9, 997–1004.

Saulnier, C. F. (2002). Deciding who to see: Lesbians discuss their preferences in health and mental health care providers. *Social Work, 47,* 4, 355–365.

Taylor, R. L. (2008). The changing meaning of race in the social sciences: some implications for research and social policy. Keynote Address, 2nd Statewide Meeting on Health Disparities—Monitoring Health Disparities: Creating Data Collection Policies That Work. Legislative Office Building; Hartford, CT. Retrieved April 9, 2009, from: http://www.ct.gov/dph/lib/dph/hisr/pdf/taylor_remarks.pdf

Tervalon, M., & Murray-Garcia, J. (1998). Cultural humility versus cultural competence: A critical discussion in defining physician training outcomes in multicultural education. *Journal of Health Care for the Poor and Underserved, 9,* 2, 117–125.

US Department of Commerce, Bureau of the Census. (2000). 2000 Census data. Retrieved October 3, 2009, from http://www.census.gov/main/www/cen2000.html.

US Department of Health and Human Services, Agency for Healthcare Research and Quality. (2008). *2007 National healthcare disparities report.* Rockville, MD: Author. Retrieved April 7, 2009, from http://www.ahrq.gov/qual/nhdr07/nhdr07.pdf

US Department of Health and Human Services. (2000). Retrieved September 1, 2009, from http://www.hsa.gov

Zeserson, J. M. (2001). How Japanese women talk about hot flushes: Implications for menopause research. *Medical Anthropology Quarterly, 15,* 189–205.

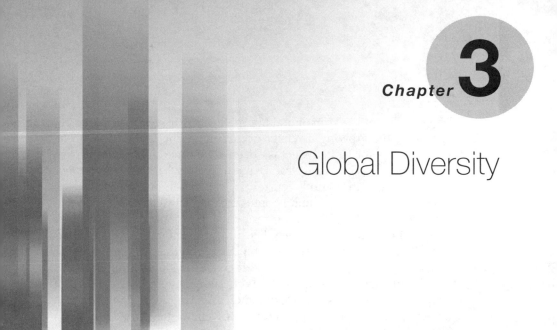

Chapter 3

Global Diversity

Chapter Objectives

Upon completion of this chapter, the nurse will be able to:

1. Define diversity.
2. Recognize that diversity is a global phenomenon.
3. Describe the impact of diversity on healthcare disparities.

Key Terms

➤ Bicultural
➤ Diversity
➤ Health disparities

Introduction

The movement toward cultural competency is in no small part a response to the growing diversity occurring in the United States. The population of the United States is extremely diverse and becoming even more so with each passing year. Depending on what Congress decides to do about immigration—curtail it, expand it, and so forth—the United States is facing a future population just 40 years away that could vary by more than 135 million residents. Our population is going to be growing in any case, largely because of immigrants who have arrived in the past few generations, but that growth could be limited to about 72 million persons (a 24.6% increase) if illegal immigration is significantly curtailed (Martin & Fogel, 2006). Alternatively, if current proposals of immigration reform, such as giving legal status to those currently here illegally, and the creation of a new guest worker program were adopted, we will likely be facing the prospect of a population in 2050 of half a billion people. That would be about 200 million more persons than today (a 67% increase) (Martin & Fogel, 2006).

What is the cultural makeup of our current and projected population? Since 1970, the Asian population has soared from 2.9 million to 10.5 million residents. During that period, 7.4 million immigrants from Asia were admitted for legal residence, accounting for virtually all of the increase in residents. During this same time period, the population identifying itself as Hispanic increased from 8.7 million to 35.3 million, surpassing the African American population as the nation's largest minority group.

In the 2000 Census, more than 13 million residents said they had arrived to live in the United States since 1990—an average increase of more than 1.3 million per year. Those who avoided being counted because they were here in violation of the law would add additional millions. Nearly 18% of those who were counted said they spoke a language other than English at home, and nearly half of them acknowledged that they spoke English "less than very well" (US Census Bureau, 2000).

In 2050, according to this Census Bureau projection, Whites (non-Hispanic) will constitute just barely over half (50.1%) of the population, Hispanics will constitute nearly one quarter (24.4%), and non-Hispanic Blacks will be half the size of the Hispanic population (12.2%), whereas Asians will be 8%, and others will constitute 5.3% (US Census Bureau, 2000).

Immigration, legal and otherwise, impacts not only the United States but also impacts the country from which the immigrants come. Mexico is the primary source of immigration into the United States today—both legal and illegal. Mexico accounted for approximately 18% of legal immigration admissions between 1993 and 2002. This rate is about two and one half times that of India. India provides the second largest source of immigrants to the United States.

Racial and ethnic minorities, especially those with low incomes and limited English proficiency, experience multiple barriers to health care, encounter lower access to and availability of health care, and experience less favorable health outcomes according to the ground-breaking Institute of Medicine report (2003). There is also evidence that stereotypes associated with sex, age, diagnosis, sexual orientation, socioeconomic status, obesity, and race/ethnicity influence providers' beliefs about and expectations of patients.

Cultural Diversity Defined

The very nature of nursing encompasses the need to be aware of cultural diversity. Campinha-Bacote (2003) contends that addressing cultural diversity goes beyond knowing the values, beliefs, practices, and customs of diverse groups. Other faces of cultural diversity include "religious affiliations, language, physical size, gender, sexual orientation, age, disability (both physical and mental), political orientation, socioeconomic status, occupational status and geographical location" (p. 1). The avoidance of ethnocentrism means that you view yourself as being different rather than the "others" as being different and to give value to each culture for its unique contributions to society and to the world at large.

Cultural Factors Impacting the Clinical Relationship

An awareness of a person's cultural frame of reference is essential to understanding of the person. Culture can be assessed according to four specific areas: cultural identity of the individual, cultural explanations of the individual, cultural factors regarding social environment, and lifestyle and cultural factors affecting relationships with others.

Unaddressed cultural differences between the nurse and the patient can result in difficulties with diagnosis, nonadherence, and mutual frustration when the patient or the nurse does not meet the implicit, culturally determined expectations of the other. There can, in some circumstances, be a benefit when there are cultural differences between nurse and patient. Patients may report symptoms and more readily accept treatment from an empathetic nurse who is not of the same culture as the patient because they may believe that confidentiality will be maintained and the stigma will be lessened (Rubi-Stipec, Hsiao-Rei Hicks, & Tsuang, 2000).

The nurse should be aware that no one, including himself or herself, is culture free in our assessments. The encounter between the patient and the nurse is an interaction between two explanatory models of illness. This is true even when both are from the same cultural background because intracultural differences in how sickness and the healthcare system are viewed can be as great as any existing intercultural differences. To avoid any misunderstandings, the nurse must be aware of his or her own belief system and take care not to stereotype or make assumptions about the patient.

The physician's model, which is the Western biomedical model, is disease-oriented, with the goal of determining the biologic or pathologic cause and executing a cure for that disease process. Nurses, by virtue of working in the healthcare system and following medical orders, often share this disease-oriented view. Many nurse practitioner programs educate using this model for diagnosis and treatment as well. Not only is the biomedical model in contrast to the illness model of the patient, it is also flawed because medicine is commonly viewed as a reductionist science. Medicine is considered to be objective and neutral: dealing only in the truth or facts. In reality, medicine is grounded in social and cultural behaviors. Therefore, the nurse, to be truly culturally sensitive, must be aware of assumptions about medical systems and recognize that other systems may be considered equally valid for patients. The patient's explanatory model will be illness-oriented. This model is culturally determined and provides the meaning of the sickness for the individual: how they decide that they are ill, what the reason for the illness is at the time may, how to cope, and when or if they decide they are no longer ill.

Although the patient's explanatory model is culturally determined, it may differ in the same individual with different illnesses or different stages of illness. Therefore, the physician must determine the model for each illness episode for each patient. For instance, a patient may have a relatively biomedical approach to a sickness episode until the stress of end-of-life issues results in a reversion to original values and traditions.

An attempt should be made to determine how culture bound the patient may be for each illness and periodically throughout a prolonged illness. The nurse should ask for an explanation, as a part of the history of present illness, as to what the patient believes caused the illness, the expected course, and expectations of treatment. Determining the patient's "explanatory model" should be a routine part of taking a patient's history (Kleinman, 1988). See Table 3-1 for questions the nurse can ask to determine the patient's explanatory model for illness.

If necessary, ask for clarifications of the patient's illness along the way. If you feel the explanation is unusual or unfamiliar, consider that it may have a cultural explanation and not immediately consider that it may be indicative of or a result of a psychiatric disorder (e.g., the African patient who feels he may have a spell cast on him). It is also

Table 3-1

Questions the Nurse Can Ask to Determine a Patient's Explanatory Model of Illness

1. What do you call this illness? Does it have a name?
2. What do you think caused it?
3. Why did it happen at this time?
4. How does the illness affect you?
5. What does it do to you?
6. How bad is it?
7. How long do you think it will last?
8. Do you think treatment will work for it?
9. What kind of treatment do you think you should have?
10. Have you tried any other treatments already?

Source: Hanson, M., Russel, L., Robb, A., & Tabak, D. (1996). *Cross-cultural interviewing: A guide for teaching and evaluation.* Toronto, Ontario: University of Toronto.

important not to automatically use culture as the sole explanation—striking a balance is the key. Culture can be a red herring, which means it is overattributed as the cause or reason for symptoms that can result in mistakes in diagnosis and treatment (Stein, 1985).

The questions associated with the patient's explanatory model of illness address the major issues of concern to the nurse and nurse practitioner: etiology, pathophysiologic alteration, usual or expected course, and treatment. Neither the medical nor the patient's model is sufficient alone. Both are needed for the provision of culturally sensitive patient-centered care. Once the nurse has a working knowledge of the patient's model, the nurse can determine if the treatments (such as herbal or alternative therapies) are previously or concurrently being used by the patient and if they are beneficial, harmful, or neutral. If a treatment is determined to be beneficial or neutral, it is recommended to incorporate the patient's intervention into the plan of care. If an intervention is deemed harmful, it requires that the nurse develop a teaching plan that is culturally competent and must ensure that the patient is fully informed as to the danger or risk for danger. The nurse's view of illness can be shared with the patient, and then negotiation must take place to achieve a shared understanding of the illness so that a treatment plan can occur.

The Importance of Striving for Understanding

The progression toward cultural understanding or ultimately to competency is vital to be an effective nurse in the multicultural 21st century. The impact of global health work can only be as strong as its cultural relevance. As much as we would like to jump in and begin the encounter, there are many various cultural nuances and ethnic differences that are not readily apparent. Success of the nursing interaction rests on the nurse's ability to work with the patient within their cultural context. The successful 21st-century nurse must be able to function in cross-cultural patient encounters. Developing this ability begins with first having the willingness to learn as much as possible, maintain cultural humility, and take the time for self-reflection to self-evaluate your progress along the way.

The degree of family involvement in patient illness is also culturally driven. Many patients come from cultures in which the family and community are very involved in the individual's illness episode much more than occur in other cultures, such as those from countries in Europe and North America. This has implications for how the nurse approaches important issues such as consent, patient confidentiality, and controversy over how to proceed with treatment and ethical dilemmas (e.g., do not resuscitate orders, transplantation, organ donation, assisted suicide, etc.) Obtaining information regarding the family structure is a good starting point. Who is the head of the family? Is this the same person who will be making the medical decisions? Is this the same person as the patient? What community resources are available, and if the patient utilizes those services, will confidentiality be maintained (this may be more of an issue in small geographic areas or if limited resources or agencies are available)? What is the patient and medical decision maker's educational background? What is the patient's health literacy level? It is important that be assessed prior to planning any educational interventions.

Language Barriers

The nurse needs to assess the patient's fluency in English if the patient is communicating without an interpreter and he or she has English as a second language. Do not automatically assume that a patient with a heavy accent is not fluent or that just because it appears a patient is fluent that they comprehend the conversation. The easiest and quickest way to assess comprehension is to ask the patient to repeat back an explanation or instruction.

Do not rely on nonverbal cues for comprehension as many patients will nod or indicate agreement out of respect or embarrassment, even when they do not understand. Even the apparent proper use of language, even in seemingly fluent individuals, can result in misunderstandings. In addition, violations in the rules of grammar may make a person seem vague and indecisive. The nurse should consciously avoid the use of idioms when speaking with patients and especially when providing patient education. The use of idiomatic expressions may baffle a person not well versed in English (e.g., quitting "cold turkey" when discussing smoking cessation).

Proper Use of Interpreters

Because it is essential that the nurse and patient be fully able to communicate effectively with each other, if it is determined that an interpreter is needed, request one. It is essential that all medical and cultural issues be fully explored, which cannot occur if there is a language barrier not bridged by the use of a qualified professional interpreter. If an interpreter is used, he or she becomes a critical component of the encounter. It is highly recommended to use only professional interpreters who are culturally competent in the patient's culture. This is so important that it is recommended that if the medical situation is not urgent, and it is safe to do so, it is preferable to postpone the interview until the services of a cultural or professional interpreter can be obtained. This is often very time-consuming and frustrating, but it will be well worth the effort because of the quality of information that will be obtained. Often, because of time constraints or other variables, this may not be possible and poor choices can be made.

The use or reliance on family members to serve as translators should be avoided unless absolutely necessary and there is absolutely no other alternative possible. This is very important to emphasize because there can be serious negative consequences if family members are used as translators/interpreters. The family member and/or the patient may editorialize extensively, and the nurse would have no way of knowing this was occurring. Editing questions and responses greatly reduces the amount and accuracy of the information transmitted from and to the patient. Role strain can be another serious consequence resulting from this practice. Both editorializing and role strain can occur if a child is asked to translate sensitive issues regarding his parents (e.g., a male child translating for his mother who is having a gynecological issue such as extensive vaginal bleeding).

Access to a professional interpreter does not mean adequate communication is guaranteed. There are some skills associated with the effective use of interpreters that the nurse should be aware of. The major points follow. Ascertain the interpreter's qualifications. If a trained professional interpreter is available, they probably need no instructions or reminders about confidentiality or the process of triadic interviewing. A professional interpreter will be capable of culturally interpreting the patient's meaning, which saves time. If there is no professional interpreter available and you must use someone who speaks the same language who is a nonprofessional, such as a hospital employee, you will need to spend time explaining the process in much more detail and emphasize the interpreter's responsibility to maintain confidentiality and not to editorialize. Brief the interpreter by informing them about the situation and the need for interpreter services. Let them know how you wish to proceed. Just because the interpreter may work in the hospital does not mean they are familiar or will be comfortable dealing with a patient encounter, especially if it is an acute or urgent situation. Let the interpreter know that you expect and need them to translate exactly what is said by both parties. Assure them that you will use brief sentences to allow the interview to proceed more quickly and to increase accuracy. Let the interpreter know that you will be looking at and speaking to the patient and that you will all three be seated in a triad during the interview process. Be alert for signs that all of the information is not being translated accurately (e.g., a long conversation in the patient's language, followed by a short translation to you or vice versa).

Cultural Humility

A nurse who possesses cultural humility recognizes the limitations of his or her cultural perspective and works toward overcoming this perspective in order to provide better nursing care to all patients. It is an acknowledgment that you are aware of the inherent barriers that exist from your own culture—that indeed your own perspective is limited. Having this focus makes it much easier for the nurse to be reflective and proactive about any prejudices or assumptions that are possessed so that they are less likely to have an impact on a cross-cultural nursing interaction. This is not the whole description, however. The nurse must also not assume that all members of a certain culture conform to a certain stereotype and that each patient is a unique individual and deserves to be treated as such.

The nurse who has cultural humility will be less likely to act in an authoritarian way or assume a power position over the patient. Cultural humility is seen as an important step in redressing power imbalance between provider and patient because the nurse who recognizes that their own perspective is full of assumptions is more likely to maintain an open mind and be respectful of all people and not act as if their way was the only way or the best way to proceed. Cultural humility should always be present, even if a nurse feels they have worked and developed true cultural competency. This is necessary because even though the nurse may have extensive knowledge of a culture, he or she is not "living" that culture, which means there still will be differences between the nurse's perspectives from the actual members of the learned culture.

Impact of Diversity

The data presented here is to provide you with an overview of demographic data from the 2000 US Census and other government agencies (US Census Bureau, 2000). There is no doubt that the population of the United States is extremely diverse and becoming even more so with each passing year.

The total minority population of the United States is 100.7 million, which means one in three US residents is a minority (US Department of Commerce, 2007). During the period of July 2005–July 2006, the nation's Black population surpassed 40 million (US Department of Commerce, 2007).

Based on 2005 census data, the current population of the United States is 296.4 million. Of that number, 67% are considered "White" (non-Hispanic). Hispanics make up 14% of the population, African Americans 12%, Asians 4%, American Indian 0.4%, Native Hawaiian/Pacific Islander 0.1%, and 1% of our population was identified as belonging to two or more races (US Census Bureau, 2005). According to the most recent census data, our country continues toward even more diversity, as demonstrated by significant increases in the numbers and proportion of populations including Hispanics, Asians, and Pacific Islanders. Another key consideration in attempting to understand diversity is that in contemporary US society, many individuals, probably the majority, are or consider themselves to be bicultural. Membership in more than one culture is not the same as being biracial or multiracial (McGrath, 1998). A person may self-identify with more than one cultural group and that bicultural person sees both sides and can function in both worlds (McGrath, 1998).

There appears to be a correlation between race, economic status, and poor health (see Boxes 3-1 and 3-2). Twelve percent of nonelderly (age 65 or younger) Whites (non-Hispanics) are considered poor as they fall below the federal poverty level and 8% self-rated their health as fair or poor, 29% of nonelderly Hispanics are considered poor and 13% have fair or poor health, 33% of nonelderly African Americans are

Box 3-1

Nonelderly Population by Race/Ethnicity as of 2005					
White	African American	Hispanic	Asian	American Indian/Alaska Native	Two or More Races
166.6 million	32.6 million	40.8 million	11.8 million	1.5 million	4.2 million

---

Box 3-2

Poverty Status of the Nonelderly Population by Race/Ethnicity as of 2005

White	African American	Hispanic	Asian	American Indian/ Alaska Native	Two or More Races
74% Nonpoor (200% + FPL)	46% Nonpoor (200% + FPL)	42% Nonpoor (200% + FPL)	68% Nonpoor (200% + FPL)	43% Nonpoor (200% + FPL)	59% Nonpoor (200% + FPL)
14% Near poor (100–199% FPL)	21% Near poor (100–199% FPL)	29% Near poor (100–199% FPL)	16% Near poor (100–199% FPL)	23% Near poor (100–199% FPL)	20% Near poor (100–199% FPL)
12% Poor (Less than 100% FPL)	33% Poor (Less than 100% FPL)	29% Poor (Less than 100% FPL)	17% Poor (Less than 100% FPL)	34% Poor (Less than 100% FPL)	21% Poor (Less than 100% FPL)

FPL, federal poverty level.

---

considered poor and 15% have fair or poor health, 17% of nonelderly Asians are considered poor and 9% have fair or poor health, 34% of nonelderly American Indians are considered poor and 17% have fair or poor health, and 21% of the nonelderly members of two or more races are considered poor and 13% have fair or poor health (Urban Institute and Kaiser Commission, 2006). The federal poverty level was set by the government as income below $19,971 for a family of four.

Diversity also impacts health insurance coverage (Box 3-3). The racial group with the highest percentage of people lacking health insurance is the nonelderly Hispanic population at 34%. Whites, at 13%, have the lowest percentage of people lacking health insurance coverage (Urban Institute and Kaiser Commission, 2005).

Historically, our culture diversity has identified, separated, bound, and evolved us. The implication is that some cultural features are not

---

Box 3-3

Uninsured (Health Insurance) Percentage of the Nonelderly by Race/Ethnicity as of 2005

White	African American	Hispanic	Asian and Pacific Islander	American Indian/Alaska Native	Two or More Races
13%	21%	34%	19%	32%	14%

only different from others but are better than others. This is supported by the fact that all people have repeatedly chosen to abandon some feature of their own culture in order to replace it with something from another culture because the replacement feature is more effective. Some examples of this are the switch from Roman numerals (even in countries whose own cultures derived from Rome) to Arabic numerals and that produce that is indigenous to one area of the country is now being produced and exported from a different country (most rice is now grown in Africa but originated in Asia). One should view cultural diversity both internationally and historically as a dynamic competition in which what serves human kind survives and what does not disappears (Sowell, 1991). The will to survive is a common link as explorers moved throughout the globe to new worlds and lands. Just like the colonists in America learned survival skills from Native Americans, the first Europeans who entered Australia with its rough terrain learned from the Australian aborigines. The goal was survival and to meet that objective often requires change and adaptation. A given culture may not be superior in all settings and at all times, but certain cultural features of that specific culture may be superior for certain purposes and at certain times (Box 3-4).

Certain countries and civilizations have experienced different levels of cultural leadership over time (Sowell, 1991). There have been rises and falls of nations and empires throughout history: the Roman Empire, the Golden Age of Spain, the technology explosion in Japan, and the West of today. Certain cultural groups have been associated with certain skills or talents and occupations. Italians are known for wine production, Germans for beer making, and Jews in the apparel industry (Sowell, 1991). Geography has a role to play not only through the provision of or lack of natural resources but also because geography permits or limits opportunity for cultural interaction among different groups. The more isolated the geography, the more isolated the culture associated with that area. Access to water (either the sea at a port on the coastline or the river near or in a city) is another very

Box 3-4					
Percentage of People Without a Usual Source of Health Care: Adults 18–64, by Race/Ethnicity as of 2005					
White	African American	Hispanic	Asian	American Indian/Alaska Native	Two or More Races
15%	18%	31%	19%	21%	18%

important geographical determinant associated with sustaining life. Positive geographical features permit humans to interact with each other and with others, sharing their culture. Culture can exist in isolation as well. Culture dictates how we do all of the things that have to be done to live life where we are living it. Culture exists to serve the practical requirements of life: to structure society, to perpetuate life, to pass on hard earned knowledge and skills, and to spare the next generation the trial and error of learning how to live life.

How much culture a person chooses to retain is a personal decision. Every culture makes changes over time—how much of the old to retain and how much of the new to keep—and as such culture is dynamic.

Culturally Discordant Care

Although this growing diversity has been seen and continues to widen within the American population, the same cannot be said for our country's population of healthcare professionals. This lack of a parallel growth in the diversity among healthcare professionals impacts on healthcare delivery and suggests that many patients are receiving culturally discordant medical care. Culturally discordant care arises from unaddressed cultural differences between healthcare providers and their patients. Research has shown that significant disparities in health status, treatment, and medical outcomes between groups of patients who differ on the basis of gender, race, and/or ethnicity exist. Unconscious bias suggests that a provider's unconscious bias about a particular race, ethnicity, or culture and/or lack of effective cross-cultural communication skills may contribute to discordant medical care and health disparities. The most recent census data, which was analyzed in 2004, reveals that racial discordance in medical encounters is prevalent and often inevitable.

An example of this is that 12.2% of the US population is African American, yet only 2.2% of physicians and 10% of the nurse workforce is African American.

This suggests that all healthcare providers should know how to interact effectively with and provide care for patients whose ethnic and/or cultural background differs from their own to lessen the impact of culturally discordant care.

Health Disparities

It is also important to recognize that perception can impact our understanding of health disparities. Two studies conducted by the Kaiser Family Foundation are revelatory when physician and patient perceptions are compared to each other (Box 3-5). There was

---

Box 3-5

Physician Versus Public Perceptions of Disparities in Health Care

Question: Generally speaking, how often do you think our healthcare system treats people unfairly based on:

(Percent stating very/somewhat often)

What their race or ethnic background is?	29% physicians 47% patients
Whether they are male or female?	15% physicians 27% patients
How well they speak English?	43% physicians 58% patients

---

no significant difference found between physicians and the public in the perception of how often they thought our healthcare system treats people unfairly based on whether or not a patient had insurance (72% doctors and 70% patients).

Health disparities are defined as diseases, disorders, and conditions that disproportionately afflict individuals who are members of racial, ethnic minority, underserved, and other vulnerable groups (National Center on Minority Health and Health Disparities, 2002). Despite scientific medical advances, the poor and non-White ethnic minorities ranked lower in health status on numerous measures. The literature reveals that the reasons for the lower health status rankings are potentially many: genetic differences, gender differences, stereotyping, perceived discrimination, mistrust of the medical community, ineffective or poor communication, economic, clinical uncertainty by provider, biological treatment variations, and lack of access.

Impact of Diversity on Diagnosis and Treatment

At no time in the history of the United States has the health status of minority populations—African Americans, Native Americans, Hispanics, and some Asian subgroups—equaled or even approximated that of White Americans (Geiger, 2003). Despite the medical and scientific advances that occurred in the 20th century, the excess morbidity and decreased life expectancy for people of color have persisted. In 1995, the overall African American mortality rate was 60% higher than that of Whites—precisely what it had been in 1950. Despite steady improvement in the overall health of Americans, racial and ethnic minorities, with few exceptions, experience higher rates of morbidity and mortality than nonminorities. Table 3-2 lists

Table 3-2
Barriers to Cross-Cultural Communication That Can Impact Diagnosis and Treatment
1. Belief that cross-cultural communication entails learning the details of every existing cultural belief system.
2. Belief that such skills are impractical in that it is too time-consuming.
3. Belief that the Western biomedical model is the only valid model of health care.
4. Physician/nurse lack of experience.
Source: Hanson, M., Russel, L., Robb, A., & Tabak, D. (1996). *Cross-cultural interviewing: A guide for teaching and evaluation*. Toronto, Ontario: University of Toronto.

barriers to cross-cultural communication that can impact on the advance practice nurse or nurse's ability to properly diagnose and treat patients.

Barriers to Health Care

In order for people to receive adequate health care, a number of potential barriers need to be addressed: availability, accessibility, affordability, appropriateness, accountability, adaptability, acceptability, awareness, attitudes, approachability, alternative practices and additional services availability, fragmentation of care, and cultural insensitivity of healthcare providers. Quality care is not possible if the provider lacks sensitivity to the patient's culture (Cohen, 2003; Purnell & Paulanka, 2003; Geiger & Davidhizar, 2004; Saha, Komaromy, Koepsell, & Bindman, 1999). Effective patient care can be enhanced through awareness of one's own culture and how it may differ from other individuals' sociocultural experiences (Purnell & Paulanka, 2003). A healthcare provider who lacks awareness of cultural issues is culturally blind, and this type of provider requires the patient to accept the Western biomedical model of health, which may be in conflict with the patient's own views and beliefs. This type of narrow view, which is cultural blindness and/or cultural dogmatism, can lead to disaster as was evidenced in the book, *The Spirit Catches You and You Fall Down*, by Anne Fadiman (1997). The healthcare provider can overcome barriers and learn a lot by watching for varying interpretations of language, nonverbal interactions, and patient and provider responsibility.

Another barrier is the lack of understanding of the impact of cultural epidemiology.

Cultural epidemiology is often not emphasized in health professions training, even though the epidemiology of diseases and individual interpretation varies between populations. This means that a commitment to continuing education must be a focus of the nurse, and the nurse must seek out learning opportunities to learn more about various cultures. It is important to remember that with the vast number of ethnic and cultural groups in the United States, it is impossible for anyone to gain knowledge of all of the groups. A more reasonable approach may be to use the culture general approach. With the culture general approach, healthcare professionals develop the knowledge, skills, and approaches that may be effectively used with any group or individual who comes from a different cultural background (Taylor, 2005). This skill set would include acknowledgment of differences, advocacy for marginalized clients, and intolerance of inequity, bias, and stereotyping.

Ethnopharmacology

Ethnopharmacology is also an important consideration when attempting to provide culturally appropriate care. Ethnopharmacology (or ethnic pharmacology) is a field of study that investigates variant responses to drugs in ethnic and racial groups. This leads to an important consideration—in a world of mixed heritages, how does a nurse or physician even determine a patient's race? Promoting certain drugs for race-specific markets could lead to stereotyping and discrimination. The issue is further complicated because some feel that racial categories are a societal construct and not a scientific one. In an attempt to overcome these factors, new drug research is focusing on designing drugs to target certain genes, eliminating the need to weigh race or ethnicity.

Reasons for Health Disparities

The many reasons for health disparities are complex and require further investigation. What has been discovered indicates that socioeconomic differences, differences in health-related risk factors, environmental factors, discrimination, and barriers such as access, all play a role. Hispanics, Asian Americans, American Indians, Alaska Natives, and African Americans are all less likely than Whites to have health insurance, have more difficulty getting health care, and have fewer choices in where to receive that care. Hispanic and African American patients are more likely to receive care in hospital emergency rooms and are less likely than Whites to have a primary care provider.

Perhaps most disturbing is that when adjustments have been made to correct access issues, disparity still persists. Even when equivalent access to care exists, racial and ethnic minorities experience a lower quality of health services and are less likely to receive even routine medical procedures than White Americans. An example of this is that African Americans and Hispanics are less likely than Whites to receive appropriate cardiac medication (thrombolytic therapy, aspirin, and beta-blockers) or to undergo coronary artery bypass surgery.

In summary, racial and ethnic minorities are less likely than Whites to possess health insurance, are more likely to be beneficiaries of publicly funded health insurance, and even when insured, may face additional barriers to care because of other socioeconomic factors, such as high copayments, geographic factors such as the scarcity of healthcare providers in some minority communities, and insufficient transportation. Access-related factors are likely the most significant barriers to equitable care, and must be addressed in order to have any chance of eliminating healthcare disparities.

Global Healthcare Disparities

Public health experts have identified a significant deficit of resources to deal with the diseases that have a global impact. This deficit is referred to as the 90/10 gap. This means only 10% of the world's health research budget is spent on diseases that affect 90% of the world's population (Resnik, 2004). Global health disparities is such an apparent and pressing issue that the United Nations has set global mandates entitled the United Nations Millennium Development Goals (United Nations Development Programme, 2008). Nurses and other healthcare providers are being called on to care for patients from a widening and expanding range of cultural backgrounds. This explosion in diversity has resulted in an evolution in conceptualizing how nurses should function in global healthcare settings. The evolution has been from an initial awareness or sensitivity to cultural differences, to striving for competence or being able to interact effectively with people from a different culture than your own, to cultural humility. Cultural humility does not have an end point or the objective of mastery (which some experts' state is a lofty standard that few, if any, nurses will attain). Cultural humility places the emphasis on the evolution of the nurse as a continual active process of self-reflection and self-critique (which is an activity that any nurse can participate in) and is seen as a way of engaging in the world and developing a therapeutic relationship with those who are culturally different from ourselves.

As members of the global healthcare community, all nurses must engage in an ongoing dialogue with ourselves about the differences culture exerts on health outcomes, our own attitudes toward cultural differences, and our ability to objectively understand descriptions of cultural behaviors that are taken as explanatory. It is important that the descriptions we develop do not stereotype or constrain the different cultural groups that we come to work with and to care for.

Nurses and nursing programs in the United States are expanding their focus to other healthcare systems. Nursing schools are offering cultural immersion experiences in various parts of the world, and more and more nurses and nursing faculty are having global nursing experiences. There will be more opportunities for collaboration, and learning more about our fellow nurses utilizing cultural humility may permit us to find common ground and a true appreciation for the diversity within our global partners.

Global Diversity—The Role of Nursing

One would be mistaken to think that health disparities are a unique problem confined to the United States. Differential treatment of minorities is not a uniquely American phenomenon. Nursing practice is a critical place to build diverse relationships for the purpose of providing global optimal health for all. The building of diverse relationships is the key during times of nursing shortage globally. Nurses are challenged to view our patients from a variety of perspectives because of diverse global populations. Bridging the nurse/patient cultural gap can be a challenge. We must become aware of our differences to meet this challenge. One strategy to help with bridging the gap and to learn more about our differences is to follow the mnemonic of ASKED (Box 3-6) (Campinha-Bacote, 2003). Nurses are likely to feel helpless or powerless in effecting change when working with patients from another culture. Learning more about our differences may be helpful.

Disparities in health care continues to be a troubling issue for nursing and despite attention being given to the issue, it is still a worldwide

Box 3-6
ASKED Mnemonic
Awareness: Am I aware of my personal biases and prejudices toward cultural groups different than mine?
Skill: Do I have the skill to conduct a cultural assessment and perform a culturally based physical assessment in a sensitive manner?
Knowledge: Do I have knowledge of the patient's worldview and the field of biocultural ecology?
Encounters: How many face-to-face encounters have I had with patients from diverse cultural backgrounds?
Desire: What is my genuine desire to "want to be" culturally competent?
Source: Campinha-Bacote, J. (2003). Many faces: Addressing diversity in health care. *Online Journal of Issues in Nursing, 8,* 1. Retrieved September 8, 2009, from http://nursingworld.org/ MainMenuCategories/ANAMarketplace/ANAPeriodicals/OJIN.aspx

problem. Research and evidence-based nursing care are key to improving health care for all patients. Evidence-based nursing practice directed at how to effectively manage and treat diseases related to ethnic and racial minorities is imperative in overcoming current disparities in health care. In addition, more studies that listen to the voices of minority clients related to effective health interventions are needed to improve the quality of health care rendered to minority populations.

Cultural, ethnic, racial, language, and religious diversity exist in most nations in the world. One of the challenges to diverse democratic nation-states is to provide opportunities for different groups to maintain aspects of their community cultures while at the same time building a nation in which these groups are structurally included and to which they feel allegiance. A delicate balance of diversity and unity should be an essential goal of democratic nation-states and of teaching and learning in a democratic society. The challenge of balancing diversity and unity is intensifying as democratic nation-states such as the United States, Canada, Australia, the United Kingdom, and Japan become more diversified and as racial and ethnic groups within these nations try to attain cultural, political, and economic rights.

These nations share the democratic ideal of inclusion of diverse groups into the mainstream society, but they are also characterized by widespread inequality through racial, ethnic, and class stratification. The discrepancy between this democratic ideal and reality can result in protest. During the 1960s and 1970s in the United States, the civil rights movement resulted in major change. The US civil rights movement continues to spread throughout the world.

Because of technology, we are no longer just citizens of our country of origin but we are global citizens and as such we need the knowledge, skills, and attitudes to function in this cultural community and to maintain our diversity and unity. We are becoming a multicultural global community.

Culture of Poverty

Poverty is a global phenomenon. The cycle of poverty perpetuates itself from generation to generation. Often, the motivation for immigration is the search for a better life or as a way out of poverty—to break the cycle. A child born into poverty is more likely to have poor intellectual and physical development. Often, the child is housed in substandard housing in either a densely populated or remotely located rural area where water or other resources are scarce, resulting in poor nutrition and health. All of these poverty-related conditions result in high morbidity, substance abuse, and accidents and injury caused by violence.

United States

According to the US Census Bureau, despite the United States being the third most populous country on Earth (after China with 1,330,044,605 inhabitants and India with 1,147,995,898 people as of July 2008), it only comprises less than 5% of the total world's population (US Census Bureau, 2008). As of July 2008, the population of the United States was 304,228,257 (US Census Bureau, 2008). The size of a country's total population tells only a small part of its demographic story. A country's population growth rate and its age–sex composition indicate the challenges it faces in providing health care for its children and elderly, providing education to its youth, providing employment opportunities for its young adults, and supporting its elderly population. The population of the United States ranked fourth among all countries with 3% of the world's population younger-than-15 and ranked third among all countries in the number of elderly (ranking third among countries with 8% of the total). For the past 50 years, the United States (along with other more developed countries, moderately developed countries [MDCs], such as all of North America, Europe, Japan, Australia, and New Zealand) have differed from other less developed countries in fertility, mortality, and overall growth. The United States and all MDCs have typically had lower fertility, mortality, and population growth rates. This is now less true than in the past and in the area of population growth is particularly alarming. From 1990 to 2000, the US population increased by 13% (compared with only 2.5% for other MDCs combined).

Having these population numbers is essential for planning public policy to address many global issues. The distributions of the world's children and elderly older than age 80 indicates where the needs for children and elderly healthcare services are greatest in the world, and it is also used to predict where the needs for schooling and elderly support will be greatest in the coming years.

The country's age structure, its support ratios, and its national wealth indicate the extent to which it will be likely to address all of these age-related needs. Alarmingly, 60% of the world's children younger than 5 years of age live in just 10 countries, of which the United States is one. About 3% of the all children younger than 5 years of age and 13% of the world's oldest old (older than 80) live in the United States (US Census Bureau, 2000).

The US Census Bureau predicts that by 2025, the US population will be 23% larger when compared to the year 2000. More industrial nations as a group, including the United States, will be forced to support a growing elderly population with a smaller number of working adults. The good news is that despite this decrease in work support,

Figure 3-1

Top 10 Countries of the World by Population

Country	Population
1 China	1,330,044,605
2 India	1,147,995,898
3 United States	304,228,257
4 Indonesia	237,512,355
5 Brazil	196,342,587
6 Pakistan	172,800,051
7 Bangladesh	154,037,902
8 Nigeria	146,255,306
9 Russia	140,702,094
10 Japan	127,288,419

Source: US Census Bureau, 2008.

the impact is expected to be less here in the United States than elsewhere worldwide because fertility and immigration both tend to replenish our younger populations.

As of May 13, 2009, the population of the world is 6,779,501,177 and 306,416,608 in the United States. See Figure 3-1 for the top 10 countries of the world ranked by population as of 2008.

United Kingdom

As of December 15, 2008, the population of the United Kingdom was 60,944,000, and the life expectancy at birth was 79 years of age (US Census Bureau 2008). See Figure 3-2 for population pyramids for all countries described in this chapter from the year 2008 and estimated for the year 2025.

The transition of uniting the former countries into what today is the United Kingdom was a gradual process. Even after being recognized as one nation, there still remained hostility and cultural barriers. There had to be a new set of rules and guiding principles put into play in order to keep all satisfied. These guiding principles, such as the division of property, capitalism, and parliamentary democracy, along with technological advancements, are now present not only in the United Kingdom but also around the world. See Figure 3-3 for demographic information related to the United Kingdom.

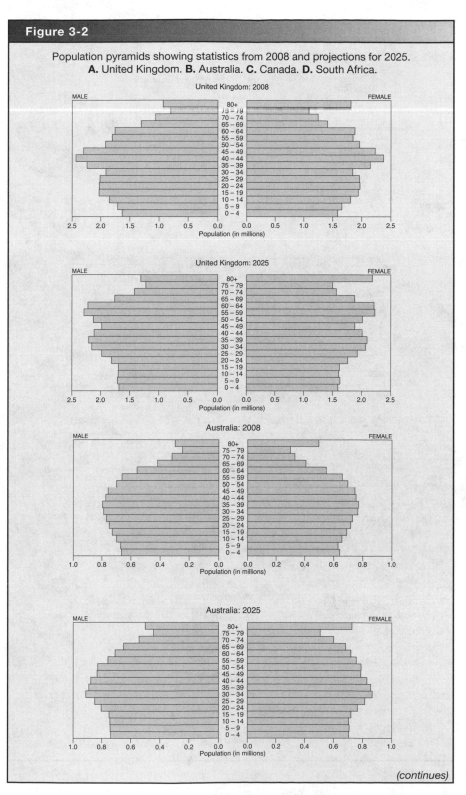

Figure 3-2

Population pyramids showing statistics from 2008 and projections for 2025.
A. United Kingdom. **B.** Australia. **C.** Canada. **D.** South Africa.

(continues)

Figure 3-2 *(continued)*

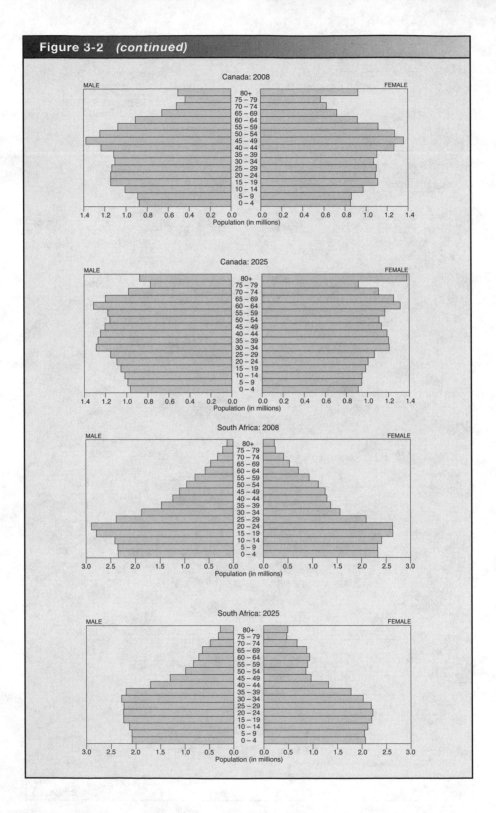

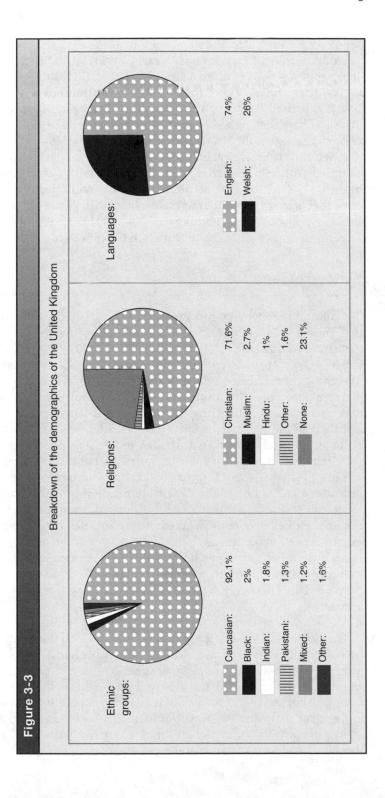

Figure 3-3

Breakdown of the demographics of the United Kingdom

Ethnic groups:

Caucasian:	92.1%
Black:	2%
Indian:	1.8%
Pakistani:	1.3%
Mixed:	1.2%
Other:	1.6%

Religions:

Christian:	71.6%
Muslim:	2.7%
Hindu:	1%
Other:	1.6%
None:	23.1%

Languages:

English:	74%
Welsh:	26%

Despite a high caloric diet and minimal exercise, the average life span in the United Kingdom is 79 years of age. Healthcare dollars are almost entirely derived from taxes. The National Health Service has been criticized for associated long waiting periods and obsolete equipment and praised for its high number of qualified physicians.

There have been published reports, since as early as 1981, which describe racism within the National Health Service in the United Kingdom. More recently, language other than English and social class have been associated with impaired continuity of care (Hemingway, Saunders, & Parsons, 1997). Another study found that non-White patients are referred for coronary revascularization less often than White patients with similar severity of disease (Hemingway et al., 2001). Obviously, diversity is having an impact on health outcomes in Great Britain.

Australia

The cultural competency movement is a global one and is making itself known in Australia. Australia is an extremely diverse nation. The population of Australia as of July 2008 was 21,007,000 (US Census Bureau, 2008). Australia's population comprises people with over 200 different ancestries. Over 200 languages are spoken and over 100 religions are observed. Almost one quarter of the population (22%) were born overseas and approximately 15% speak a language other than English at home (Australian Bureau of Statistics, 2001). In addition to this is the diversity within Australia's indigenous population who, at the last census, made up 2.4% of Australia's population (Australian Bureau of Statistics, 2001). Australia, like the United States, provides medical care according to the Western biomedical model. As has been discussed previously, for many client groups, this approach does not fit with their belief systems. When there is a mismatch between belief systems, health outcomes are likely to be poorer. The tendency of the health system (or more specifically medicine) to represent itself as a "culture of no culture" thus results in a culture-blind and ethnocentric approach. This effectively creates an exclusionary system which must be avoided.

Now, there is also a growing body of work being produced to respond to Australasian contexts, some of it addressing the relationship between cultural respect and working with Aboriginal peoples. The health care of Aboriginal people in Australia has been criticized repeatedly during the past 20 years. It is well documented that the health status of Aboriginal and Torres Strait Islander people is substantially poorer than that of nonindigenous Australians. Disadvantage across a range of socioeconomic factors impacts negatively on the health of Aboriginal and Torres Strait Islander people.

Both morbidity and mortality rates are higher, with indigenous people more likely to experience disability and reduced quality of life because of ill health. Life expectancy of indigenous Australians is estimated to be approximately 20 years lower than for other Australians (Australian Bureau of Statistics & Australian Institute of Health and Welfare, 2003). Stereotyping impacting the allocation of healthcare resources has also been described (Lowe, Kerridge, & Mitchell, 1995).

Canada

In Canada, the population in general, and thus the service area for health care, is becoming more diverse. As of July 2008, the total population of Canada was 33,213,000 (US Census Bureau, 2008). It has been estimated that one in eight Canadians is a member of a visible minority in a proportion that grew by 25% between 1996 and 2001, while overall population growth was just 4%. The population of First Nations peoples increased 22.2%, and there are now one million First Nations people in Canada. Thus, the diversity of the country has grown rapidly, and will continue to do so in the coming 50 years. Our neighbor to the North, Canada has also been experiencing a tremendous growth in immigration, specifically from internationally trained professionals. These "New Canadians" are changing the culture of Canada. Canada has recognized the need for its nurses to become culturally competent and the Registered Nurses' Association of Ontario has established nursing best practice guidelines on this important issue (Registered Nurses' Association of Ontario, 2007). The recommendation of this best practice guideline is that as Canada becomes more diverse, so must its healthcare system. Men and women from all cultures need to be recruited and welcomed into a profession that is committed to the care of others so they can learn from these diverse groups to create an environment that capitalizes on diversity and furthers the profession and the broader healthcare system (Registered Nurses' Association of Ontario, 2007).

Although Canada has a long-standing multicultural identity and a tradition of acceptance of diversity, reinforced, for example, by the Federal government's 1971 Multiculturalism Policy, government intentions have not been sufficient to achieve equity and integration. Racism and cultural oppression have been realities for many minority groups living in Canada, especially the First Nations peoples, resulting in poverty, poor health, loss of identity, and marginalization.

Numerous problems with the differential treatment of the Inuit people of Canada have also been described. These problems have resulted in a call for cultural competency in Canada to better meet the healthcare needs of the Inuits.

South Africa

South Africa is characterized as a multicultural society and has great diversity in geography, language, and culture. As of July 2008, the total population in South Africa was 48,783,000 (US Census Bureau, 2008). The family structure in many families tends to be extended rather than nuclear and may also be multigenerational. There tends to be a fatalistic approach to disability that can result in passivity when seeking out treatment or rehabilitation. Traditional healers may form an integral part of a family's approach to health and illness. Technology and Western medical practices may be viewed as an intrusion on accepted and respected traditional activities and rituals. The community view within South Africa is that the group takes precedence over the individual, and time is only a two-dimensional phenomenon. The concept of time is one of having a long past, a present, and no future.

During the time of apartheid in South Africa, profound inequality existed in the availability and content of medical and public health services, which resulted in serious consequences for the majority non-White population (Nightingale et al., 1990). Despite the fall of apartheid, there is evidence that discrimination in treatment persists (Geiger, 2003). This painful part of South Africa's history has resulted in a push toward cultural competency within the country. The Truth and Reconciliation Commission of South Africa was established by Former South African President Nelson Mandela; the commission's work has allowed the people of South Africa to openly discuss the pain and suffering caused by the intentional and enforced racial and cultural divisions within their country. The commission's activities have been credited with opening the doors to deeper cultural knowledge and positive change—key elements in the journey toward cultural competence.

Recommendations

To increase recognition among all healthcare providers that racial bias persists and can be overt or covert. These biases continue to impact treatment decisions of minority patients. Quality assurance programs should be expanded to track patterns of patient care by race and ethnicity. The elephant in the room must be acknowledged, and nursing students need to be made aware that this bias is out there and that they need to advocate for their patients when treatment decisions are not evidence-based. Curriculum should be expanded, not just as has been done with cultural competency concepts, but also including the importance of the nurse developing self-awareness and understanding the culture of medicine and how it may impact on the patient experience.

For example, nurse practitioners are taught to present a case according to the medical model. This approach has traditionally included the patient's race in the clinical presentation. It has been argued that labeling a patient by race is necessary to clarify biologic risk for particular diseases, critical for differential diagnosis formation, that it provided information about socioeconomic status by proxy, and that the practice should be continued (South-Paul, 2001). Others feel that the placement of the patient's race should be moved from its traditional position in the initial patient description and placed with the other psychosocial patient data (Anderson, Moscou, Fulchon, & Neuspiel, 2001). On the surface, the placement of the patient's race in the clinical presentation may appear trivial, but small changes may ultimately result in effective change within the culture of medicine (Geiger, 2003).

Summary

Diversity is a global phenomenon. As people who later become patients and as healthcare professionals immigrate into the United States, this global diversity will contribute to even greater diversity within the United States.

Related Web Sites

Key Facts: Race, Ethnicity and Medical Care. Available at: http://www.kff.org/minorityhealth/6069.cfm.

A joint initiative sponsored by Robert Wood Johnson and the Henry J. Kaiser Foundations to increase dialogue regarding health care disparities. Available at: www.kff.org/whythedifference.

Kaiser Health Disparities Report: A Weekly Look at Race, Ethnicity and Health. Available at: http://www.kaisernetwork.org/daily_reports/rep_hpolicy.cfm.

National Healthcare Disparities Report. Available at: http://www.ahrq.gov/qual/nhdr06/nhdr06.htm

Today's Topics in Health Disparities. Available at: http://www.kaisernetwork.org/todaystopics.

National Center on Minority Health and Health Disparities. Available at: http://ncmhd.nih.gov/.

HRSA Office of Minority Health. Available at: http://ask.hrsa.gov/Minority.cfm

Indian Health Service. Available at: http://www.ihs.gov.

References

Australian Bureau of Statistics (2001). National health survey. Summary of results, 2001. Canberra: ABS.

Australian Bureau of Statistics & Australian Institute of Health and Welfare. (2003). Retrieved September 8, 2009, from http://www.aihw.gov.au/publications/aus/ar02-03/ar02-03.pdf.

Anderson, M. R., Miscou, S., Fulchon, C., & Neuspiel, D. R. (2001). The role of race in the clinical presentation. Family Medicine, 33, 430–434.

Campinha-Bacote, J. (2003). Many faces: Addressing diversity in health care. Online Journal of Issues in Nursing, 8, 1. Retrieved September 8, 2009, from http://nursingworld.org/MainMenuCategories/ANAMarketplace/ANAPeriodicals/OJIN.aspx.

Cohen, J. J. (2003). Disparities in health care: An overview. Academic Emergency Medicine, 10, 11, 1155–1160.

Fadiman, A. (1998). The spirit catches you and you fall down. New York: Farrar, Straus, and Giroux.

Geiger, H. J. (2003). Racial and ethnic disparities in diagnosis and treatment: A review of the evidence and a consideration of causes. In B. D. Smedley, A. Y. Stith, & A. R. Nelson (Eds.), Unequal treatment: Confronting racial and ethnic disparities in health care (pp. 415–454). Washington, DC: The National Academies Press.

Giger, J. N., & Davidhizar, R. E. (2004). Transcultural nursing: Assessment and intervention (4th ed.). Philadelphia: Mosby.

Hanson, M., Russell, L., Robb, A., & Tabak, D. (1996). Cross-cultural interviewing: A guide for teaching and evaluation. Toronto, Ontario: University of Toronto.

Hemingway, H., Crook, A. M, Feder, G., Banerjee, S., Dawson, J. R., Magee, P., et al. (2001). Underuse of coronary revascularization procedures in patients considered appropriate candidates for revascularization. New England Journal of Medicine, 344, 645–654.

Hemingway, H., Saunders, D., & Parsons, I. (1997). Social class, spoken language, and pattern of care as determinants of continuity of care in maternity services in East London. Journal of Public Health Medicine, 19, 156–161.

The Institute of Medicine. (2003). Patient safety: Achieving a new standard of care. Washington, DC: The National Academies Press.

Kleinman, A. (1988). Rethinking psychiatry: From cultural category to personal experience. New York: Free Press.

Lowe, M., Kerridge, I. H. & Mitchell, K. R. (1995). "These sorts of people don't do very well": Race and allocation of health care resources. Journal of Medical Ethics, 21, 356–360.

Martin, J., & Fogel, S. (2006). Projecting the U.S. population to 2050: Four immigration scenarios. A report by the Federation for American Immigration Reform. Retrieved April 9, 2009, from http://www.fairus.org/site/DocServer/pop_projections.pdf?docID=901.

McGrath, B. B. (1998). Illness as a problem of meaning: Moving culture from the classroom to the clinic. Advances in Nursing Science, 21, 2, 17–29.

National Center on Minority Health and Health Disparities. (2002). Retrieved September 8, 2009, from http://www.health.gov/nhic/nhicscripts/entry.cfm?hrcode=hr3342.

Nightingale, E., Hannibal, K., Geiger, H. J., Hartmann, L., Lawrence, R., & Spurlock, J. (1990). Apartheid medicine: health and human rights in South Africa. *Journal of the American Medical Association, 264,* 2097–2102.

Purnell, L., & Paulanka, B. (Eds.). (2003). *Transcultural health care: A culturally competent approach* (2nd ed.). Philadelphia: F. A. Davis.

Registered Nurses' Association of Ontario. (2007). *Embracing cultural diversity in health care: Developing cultural competence.* Toronto, Canada: Registered Nurses' Association of Ontario.

Resnik, D. B. (2004). The distribution of biomedical research resources and international justice. *Developing World Bioethics, 4,* 42–67.

Rubio-Stipec, M., Hsiao-Rei Hicks, M., & Tsuang, M. T. (2000). Cultural factors influencing the selection, use and interpretation of psychiatric measures. In *Handbook of psychiatric measures* (pp. 33–41). Washington, DC: American Psychiatric Association.

Saha, S., Komaromy, M., Koepsell, T. D., & Bindman, A. B. (1999). Patient–physician racial concordance and the perceived quality and use of health care. *Archives of Internal Medicine, 159,* 9, 997–1004.

South-Paul, J. E. (2001). Racism in the examining room: Myths, realities and consequences. *Family Medicine, 33,* 473–475.

Sowell, T. (1991). A worldview of cultural diversity. *Cultural Consensus,* 37–44.

Stein, H. F. (1985). The culture of the patient as a red herring in clinical decision making: A case study. *Medical Anthropology Quarterly, 17,* 2–5.

Taylor, R. (2005). Addressing barriers to cultural competence. *Journal for Nurses in Staff Development, 21,* 4, 135–142.

United Nations Development Programme, 2008. Annual Report. Retrieved September 8, 2009, from http://www.undp.org/publications/annualreport2008/.

Urban Institute & Kaiser Commission on Medicaid and the Uninsured, analysis of March 2006 Current Population Survey. Retrieved September 8, 2009, from http://www.statehealthfacts.org/profileind.jsp?cat=9&sub=106&rgn=1.

US Department of Commerce, Bureau of the Census. (2000). 2000 Census data. Retrieved October 3, 2009, from http://www.census.gov/main/www/cen2000.html.

US Department of Commerce, Bureau of the Census. (2005). Race and Hispanic origin in 2005. Retrieved October 3, 2009, from http://www.census.gov/population/pop-profile/dynamic/RACEHO.pdf.

US Department of Commerce, Bureau of the Census. (2007). Retrieved October 3, 2009, from http://www.census.gov/Press-Release/www/releases/archives/population/010048.html.

US Department of Commerce, Bureau of the Census. (2008). USA quick facts. Retrieved October 3, 2009, from http://quickfacts.census.gov/qfd/states/00000.html.

Review Questions

Review Question 1:

Identify your own primary and secondary characteristics of culture.

Review Question 2:

How have these characteristics influenced you and your worldview?

Review Question 3:

Determine the racial and ethnic characteristics of the community where you practice or will practice nursing.

Review Question 4:

Define race and ethnicity. Differentiate the two terms.

Chapter **4**

Organization of Healthcare Delivery in the 21st Century

Chapter Objectives

Upon completion of this chapter, the nurse will be able to:

1. Describe standards of care, ethical, and legal influences related to healthcare delivery for the 21st century with an emphasis on the provision of safe, quality, culturally appropriate care by nurses and advance practice nurses.

2. Identify barriers to the provision of culturally appropriate patient-centered healthcare delivery.

3. Integrate cultural competency into primary care practice for nurse practitioners (NPs) and nursing practice for registered nurses (RNs) that accepts the rights of patients, shows respect to patients, and acknowledges personal biases that can impact nursing care.

4. Recognize cultural issues and interact with patients from other cultures in a culturally appropriate way that incorporates cultural preferences, health beliefs, and behaviors and traditional practices into the management of the nursing plan of care.

Key Terms

➤ Biopsychosocial Model

➤ Health Belief Model

➤ Interdisciplinary health care

➤ Patient-centered health care

➤ Unidisciplinary practice

➤ Western Biomedical Model

Introduction

This chapter will describe the organization of healthcare delivery in the 21st century such as the use of interdisciplinary or multidisciplinary teams for patient care. National standards related to quality, safety, and culturally appropriate care will be described. The shift in focus from the Western biomedical model (provider-focused model) to a health belief model (patient-focused model) will be included. Keeping the patient central to the planning process will help to ensure that cultural beliefs will be incorporated into the plan of care. Barriers impacting the patient and the system will also be described as well as offering some potential solutions. These barriers are communication issues, lack of access to preventive care, history of discrimination and abuse in some cultures, distrust of healthcare providers, nonadherence, and the refusal of some to enter the healthcare system for care or treatment at all. The impact of the provision of primary care by NPs will be described as well. The integration of cultural competency into primary care practice has been clarified in the National Organization of Nurse Practitioner Faculties (NONPF) document on cultural competency (Green-Hernandez, Quinn, Denman-Vitale, Falkenstern, & Judge-Ellis, 2004). It states that the NP demonstrates cultural competence when she or he shows respect for the inherent dignity of every human being, whatever their age, gender, religion, socioeconomic class, sexual orientation, and ethnic or cultural group; accepts the rights of individuals to choose their care provider, participate in care, and refuse care; acknowledges personal biases and prevents these from interfering with the delivery of quality care to persons of other cultures; recognizes cultural issues and interacts with clients from other cultures in culturally sensitive ways and incorporates cultural preferences, health beliefs, behaviors, and traditional practices into the management plan; develops client-appropriate educational materials that address the language and cultural beliefs of the client and accesses culturally appropriate resources to deliver care to clients from other cultures; and lastly, assists clients to access quality care within a dominant culture. Opportunities for the nurse to obtain cultural competency certification will finish up the content in this chapter.

National Standards: Culturally and Linguistically Appropriate Services

The Office of Minority Health of the US Department of Health and Human Services (USDHHS) (2001) issued its final report of national standards for culturally and linguistically appropriate services (CLAS). The 2001 report describes culturally competent care as care that is effective, compatible with the patient's culture, and communicated in a language that the patient fully understands (USDHHS, 2001). This USDHHS report was powerful in that it highlighted the need for culturally and linguistically appropriate healthcare services for diverse populations. CLAS consists of 14 national standards for providing CLAS in health care. These standards are based on a review of the law, regulation, and federal and state standards currently in place. Input was also provided by a national advisory committee made up of healthcare providers, researchers, and policymakers.

The CLAS standards are primarily directed at healthcare organizations but are helpful to the individual healthcare professional as well. The CLAS standards (Box 4-1) are organized by theme: culturally competent care (standards 1–3), language access services (standards 4–7), and organizational supports for cultural competence (standards 8–14). Each of the standards has varying stringency ranging from recommendations, to guidelines, to mandates. A mandate is required to be followed by all recipients of federal funds. The guidelines have been recommended by the Office of Minority Health to be adopted by accrediting agencies. The recommendations are suggested for voluntary adoption by healthcare organizations.

Standards of Care: Institute of Medicine

The recognition of the existence and persistence of healthcare disparities resulted in Congress in 1999 requesting that the Institute of Medicine (IOM) conduct a study. The study was to assess disparities in the kinds and quality of health care received by US racial and ethnic minorities and nonminorities. Congress requested that the IOM assess the extent of racial and ethnic differences in health care that are not attributable to known factors such as access to care, evaluate potential sources of disparities in health care (including bias, discrimination, and stereotyping), and perhaps most importantly, to provide recommendations regarding interventions to eliminate the disparities. The IOM committee defined health care as the continuum of services provided in traditional healthcare settings (public and private clinics, hospitals, community health centers, nursing homes, as well as home-based care). Disparities

Box 4-1

National Standards for Culturally and Linguistically Appropriate Services in Health Care

1. Healthcare organizations should ensure that patients receive from all staff members effective, understandable, and respectful care that is provided in a manner compatible with their cultural health beliefs and practices and preferred language.

2. Healthcare organizations should implement strategies to recruit, retain, and promote at all levels of the organization a diverse staff and leadership that are representative of the demographic characteristics of the service area.

3. Healthcare organizations should ensure that staff at all levels and across all disciplines receive ongoing education and training in culturally and linguistically appropriate service delivery.

4. Healthcare organizations must offer and provide language assistance services, including bilingual staff and interpreter services, at no cost to each patient with limited English proficiency at all points of contact, in a timely manner, during all hours of operation.

5. Healthcare organizations must provide to patients in their preferred language both verbal offers and written notices informing them of their right to receive language assistance services.

6. Healthcare organizations must assure the competence of language assistance provided to limited English-proficiency patients by interpreters and bilingual staff. Family and friends should not be used to provide interpretation services (except on request by the patient).

7. Healthcare organizations must make available easily understood patient-related materials and post signs in the languages of the commonly encountered groups and/or groups represented in the service area.

8. Healthcare organizations should develop, implement, and promote a written strategic plan that outlines clear goals, policies, operational plans, and management accountability/oversight mechanisms to provide culturally and linguistically appropriate services.

9. Healthcare organizations should conduct initial and ongoing organizational self-assessments of CLAS-related activities and are encouraged to integrate cultural and linguistic competence-related measures into their internal audits, performance improvement programs, patient satisfaction assessments, and outcomes-based evaluations.

10. Healthcare organizations should ensure that data on the individual patient's race, ethnicity, and spoken and written language are collected in health records, integrated into the organization's management information systems, and periodically updated.

11. Healthcare organizations should maintain a current demographic, cultural, and epidemiologic profile of the community as well as a needs assessment to accurately plan for and implement services that respond to the cultural and linguistic characteristics of the service area.

12. Healthcare organizations should develop participatory, collaborative partnerships with communities and utilize a variety of formal and informal mechanisms to facilitate community and patient involvement in designing and implementing CLAS-related activities.

13. Healthcare organizations should ensure that conflict and grievance resolution processes are culturally and linguistically sensitive and capable of identifying, preventing, and resolving cross-cultural conflicts or complaints by patients.

14. Healthcare organizations are encouraged to regularly make available to the public information about their progress and successful innovations in implementing the CLAS standards and to provide public notice in their communities about the availability of this information.

Source: US Department of Health and Human Services: Office of Minority Health. (2001). *National standards for culturally and linguistically appropriate services in health care. Final report*. Rockville, MD: Author. Retrieved April 14, 2009, from http://www.omhrc.gov/assets/pdf/checked/finalreport.pdf.

were defined by the IOM as racial or ethnic differences in the quality of health care that were not results of access-related factors or clinical needs, preferences, and appropriateness of intervention. Racial and ethnic groups were placed into the five categories for racial groups and two categories for ethnic groups established by the Federal Office of Management and Budget (2001) (Box 4-2).

Box 4-2

Revised Standards for the Classification of Federal Data on Race and Ethnicity

---

Categories for Race:

American Indian or Alaska Native: A person having origins in any of the original peoples of North or South America (including Central America) and maintains tribal affiliation or community attachment.

Asian: A person having origins in any of the original peoples of the Far East, Southeast Asia, or the Indian subcontinent including, for example, Cambodia, China, India, Japan, Korea, Malaysia, Pakistan, the Philippine Islands, Thailand, and Vietnam.

Black or African American: A person having origins in any of the Black racial groups of Africa. Terms such as "Haitian" or "Negro" can be used in addition to Black or African American.

Native Hawaiian or Other Pacific Islander: A person having origins in any of the original people of Hawaii, Guam, Samoa, or other Pacific Islands.

White: A person having origins in any of the original peoples of Europe, the Middle East, or North Africa.

Categories for Ethnicity:

Hispanic or Latino: A person of Cuban, Mexican, Puerto Rican, South or Central American, or other Spanish culture or origin, regardless of race. The term "Spanish origin" can be used in addition to "Hispanic or Latino."

Not Hispanic or Latino

Source: Federal Office of Management and Budget. (2001). Reports and bulletins. Retrieved June 9, 2009, from http://www.whitehouse.gov/omb.

The IOM study committee reviewed well over 100 studies that assessed the quality of health care for various racial and ethnic minority groups, while holding constant variations in insurance status, patient income, and other access-related factors. Many of these studies also controlled for other potential confounding factors, such as racial differences in the severity or stage of disease progression, the presence of comorbid illnesses, where care is received (e.g., public or private hospitals and health systems), and other patient demographic variables, such as age and gender. Some studies that employed more rigorous research designs followed patients prospectively, using clinical data abstracted from patients' charts, rather than administrative data used for insurance claims. The study reported the consistency of research findings indicated that minorities are less likely than Whites to receive needed services, including clinically necessary procedures. Minorities may experience a range of barriers to accessing care, even when they have health insurance comparable to Whites. These barriers include language, geography, and cultural factors. Financial, institutional, legal, regulatory, and policy factors also have a negative effect on a minority patient's ability to get quality health care. Health disparities were found to exist in a number of disease areas including cancer, cardiovascular disease, human immunodeficiency virus (HIV)/acquired immunodeficiency syndrome (AIDS), diabetes, and mental illness, and are found across a range of procedures, including routine treatments for common health problems. Alarmingly, the literature review conducted by the IOM (Smedley, Stith, & Nelson, 2003) found that racial and ethnic minorities experience a lower quality of healthcare services and are less likely to receive even routine medical procedures than are White Americans.

Even more alarming is the discovery that racial and ethnic minorities receive lower quality health care than Whites, even when they are insured to the same degree and when other healthcare access-related factors, such as the ability to pay for care, are the same. The IOM (Smedley et al., 2003) report concluded that prejudice and stereotyping on the part of healthcare providers may contribute to the differences in care. This conclusion was met with controversy within the healthcare community because the vast majority of healthcare professionals work hard under challenging circumstances to ensure that our patients receive the best possible health care. How could bias, prejudice, and stereotyping contribute to unequal treatment, particularly given that healthcare providers are sworn to beneficence and cannot, by law, discriminate against any patient on the basis of race, ethnicity, color, or national origin? Our professional organization, the American Nurses Association, states that all nurses are sworn to beneficence and cannot by law discriminate against any patient (American Nurses Association, 2004).

The IOM report (Smedley et al., 2003) found that many factors may contribute to the healthcare disparities observed in the reviewed studies. They found that some researchers suggest that there may be subtle differences in the way that members of different racial and ethnic groups respond to treatment, particularly with regard to some pharmaceutical interventions, suggesting that variations in some forms of treatment may be justified on the basis of patient race or ethnicity. In addition, patients vary in help-seeking behavior, and some racial and ethnic minorities may be more likely than Whites to avoid or delay seeking care. However, the majority of studies find disparities in clinical services that are equally effective for all racial and ethnic groups. Further, the studies that the IOM reviewed suggest that racial differences in patients' attitudes, such as their preferences for treatment, do not vary greatly and cannot fully explain racial and ethnic disparities in health care. This landmark report identified cultural competence training of health professionals as a potential strategy to improve the quality of care and to reduce health disparities between ethnic minorities and Whites (Smedley et al., 2003). The report advocates cross-cultural education from three conceptual approaches. The first focus is attitudes (cultural sensitivity/awareness), the second approach is knowledge (multicultural/categorical approach), and the third is skills (cross-cultural approach) (Smedley et al., 2003). Research does support this approach as training is effective in improving provider knowledge of cultural and behavioral aspects of health care and building effective communication strategies. The IOM (Smedley et al., 2003) report recommended that a broad sector approach, including healthcare providers, their patients, payors, health plan purchasers, and society at large, must work to ensure that all patients receive quality health care. This type of healthcare training shows promise as a strategy for improving healthcare professionals' knowledge, attitudes, skills, and patients' ratings of care.

The IOM (Smedley et al., 2003) study determined that despite scientific medical advances, the poor and non-White ethnic minorities ranked lower in health status on numerous measures. The IOM report (Smedley et al., 2003) states that a small number of studies find that African Americans are slightly more likely to reject medical recommendations for some treatments, but these differences in refusal rates are generally small (African Americans are only 3–6% more likely to reject recommended treatments, according to these studies). The IOM report (2003) recommends that more research is needed to fully understand the reason(s) for the refusal of treatment as this may lead to the development of different strategies to help patients make informed treatment decisions. The IOM report (Smedley et al., 2003) also highlighted the need to recruit more minorities to enter the health professions and for those already in practice to develop cultural competence. The report states that as the number of patients of diverse racial, ethnic, cultural, and linguistic backgrounds continues to increase in the United States, so will the need to produce culturally competent providers who incorporate the patients' worldview into patient management decisions. Cross-cultural training should have a significant role in improving quality of care for minorities and in attempting to eliminate racial and ethnic disparities.

Identified Barriers that Contribute to Healthcare Disparities

Classification by race and ethnicity is not an issue-free process. Definitions for race and ethnicity vary according to the source utilized, and they are often rife with criticism. Arguably, the most relevant criticism is that the use of the federal classifications does not permit a person to choose the label with which they self-identify. The five racial categories used are American Indian or Alaska Native, Asian, Black or African American, Native Hawaiian or other Pacific Islander, and White. The two ethnic categories are Hispanic or Latino and Not Hispanic or Latino.

It is difficult to attempt to determine the reasons why healthcare disparities exist in this country; it is a daunting process. To separate or attempt to quantify or qualify the relative contribution of any one factor or the interrelationship between factors increases the risk of not seeing the whole picture. For example, when trying to determine the reasons why segregation of housing persists, one must recognize that it is a byproduct of discrimination in the past and present, past, and contemporary racism, socioeconomic differences, and the legacy of less or poorer opportunities being available to minority groups in this country. Recognizing that the problems are a result of both historic and contemporary forces reinforces the importance of considering the impact of these forces that contribute to differences in access to quality health care when searching for solutions. Despite the inherent difficulty in the task, many connections and relationships were identified by the IOM study (Smedley et al., 2003).

Individual risk factors for poor health are pronounced among many racial and ethnic minorities. These risks are increased by the disproportionate representation of minorities in the lower socioeconomic levels. Socioeconomic status seems to be the most important predictor of health status. Socioeconomic position, in and of itself, is correlated with a health status independent of individual risk factors. This is a powerful discovery. As people move up the socioeconomic ladder, they tend to have better health.

Cultural factors also play an important part. Korenbrot and Moss (2000) found that among some immigrant Hispanic populations, birth outcomes were better than among those of their US-born peers. This may suggest that the risk of poor health status increases with each subsequent generation living in the United States. Negative environmental factors, such as air and water pollution, are more likely to exist in poorer communities. House and Williams (2000) conclude that these and other risk factors that are associated with health and poor health illustrate that racial and ethnic disparities in health status largely reflect differences in social, socioeconomic, and behavioral risk factors and environmental living conditions. If one accepts this conclusion to be true, then it becomes apparent that the solution to the problem of healthcare disparities cannot be solved by addressing the issue of healthcare delivery alone.

There were two other factors that may be associated with healthcare disparities, assuming that all populations have equal access to health care. The first sets of factors are those related to the operation of healthcare systems and the legal and regulatory climate in which they operate. These include factors such as cultural or linguistic barriers (e.g., the lack of interpreter services for patients with limited English proficiency), fragmentation of healthcare systems (as noted earlier, these include the possibility that minorities are disproportionately enrolled in lower-cost health plans that place greater per-patient limits on healthcare expenditures and available services), the types of incentives in place to contain costs (e.g., incentives to physicians to limit services), and where minorities tend to receive care (e.g., minorities are less likely to access care in a private physician's office, even when insured at the same level as Whites).

The second set of factors emerges from the clinical encounter. Three mechanisms might be operative in healthcare disparities from the provider's side of the exchange: bias (or prejudice) against minorities, greater clinical uncertainty when interacting with minority patients, and beliefs (or stereotypes) held by the provider about the behavior or health of minorities. Patients might also react to providers' behavior associated with these practices in a way that also contributes to disparities. The IOM report (Smedley et al., 2003) states that research on how patient race or ethnicity may influence physician decision making and the quality of care for minorities is still emerging, and as yet there is no direct evidence to illustrate how prejudice, stereotypes, or bias may influence care. In the absence of conclusive evidence, the study committee decided to draw upon a mix of theory and relevant research in an attempt to understand how these processes might operate in the clinical encounter.

Clinical Uncertainty

A concept that emerged was that of clinical uncertainty. Clinical uncertainty is the uncertainty a healthcare professional has, relative to the condition of the patient. Clinical uncertainty can contribute to disparities in treatment. The diagnosis that is formulated by the NP or physician must depend on inferences made about the severity of the illness. These inferences are made based on what is seen during the clinical encounter (this also includes the patient's race or ethnicity) often within a very short time frame. In the process of care, health professionals must come to judgments about patients' conditions and make decisions about treatment, often without complete and accurate information. In most cases, they must do so under severe time pressure and resource constraints. The responses of racial and ethnic minority patients to healthcare providers during the clinical encounter are also a potential source of disparities. Little research has been conducted as to how patients may influence the clinical encounter but in the IOM (Smedley et al., 2003) report, it was speculated that if patients convey mistrust, refuse treatment, or comply poorly with treatment, the provider may become less engaged in the treatment process, which can result in the patient being less likely to be provided with vigorous treatment and services. This type of patient response or reaction is understandable as a response to prior negative racial experiences whether they include real or perceived mistreatment by other providers in the past. Research indicates that minority patients perceive higher levels of racial discrimination in health care than nonminorities do. Patients' and providers' behaviors and attitudes may therefore influence each other concurrently.

Biases

Biases may exist subconsciously even among people who are strongly opposed to bigotry and discrimination and in people who strongly believe that they are not prejudiced. The rate of prejudice among White Americans is very high as estimates range from one half to three quarters of White Americans believe that relative to Whites, minorities—and particularly African Americans—are less intelligent, more prone to violence, and prefer to live off welfare (Smedley et al., 2003). With such a high prevalence rate, it would be unrealistic to assume that all healthcare professionals are without at least some of these prejudicial beliefs or the manifestation of these prejudicial beliefs in their own behaviors.

The IOM report (Smedley et al., 2003) states that there is significant evidence that well-intentioned Whites who are not overtly biased and who do not believe that they are prejudiced typically demonstrate unconscious implicit negative racial attitudes and stereotypes. Both implicit and explicit stereotypes significantly shape interpersonal interactions, influencing how information is recalled and guiding expectations and inferences in systematic ways. They can also produce self-fulfilling prophecies when the perceived stereotype influences the interaction in ways that conform to the stereotypical expectations.

Some of the identified areas requiring intervention from the IOM study (Smedley et al., 2003) are improving minority socioeconomic status, desegregating housing and making housing more equitable, improving educational opportunities, modifying individual behavioral risk factors, and improving access to and use of healthcare services. Healthcare delivery must strive to be egalitarian. Health care is a resource that should be tied to social justice. Society expects our healthcare providers adhere to the highest ethical standards to ensure fairness to all. Opposing this is the need for providers to be managers of the available healthcare resources. Poor decisions can result in the allocation of more resources for one or some than for others. An unequal distribution of healthcare resources can have serious consequences. First, some will receive inadequate care. Secondly, the trust of the public (already tenuous within some minority populations) would be further weakened. Lastly, a lack of access and/or lack of trust will negatively impact a patient's willingness to seek care and adhere to treatment recommendations.

Role of Education

Because of the identified factors/barriers that can impact on treatment decisions, it appears that education is the key tool to attempt to overcome healthcare disparities. Education needs to focus on all healthcare professionals as well as the patients. Healthcare providers should be made aware of racial and ethnic disparities in health care, and the fact that these disparities exist, often despite providers' best intentions. In addition, all current and future healthcare providers can benefit from cross-cultural education. Cross-cultural education programs have been developed to enhance health professionals' awareness of how cultural and social factors influence health care, while providing methods to obtain, negotiate, and manage this information clinically once it is obtained. Cross-cultural education can be divided into three conceptual approaches focusing on attitudes (cultural sensitivity/awareness approach), knowledge (multicultural/categorical approach), and skills (cross-cultural approach), and has been taught using a variety of interactive and experiential methodologies. Research to date demonstrates that training is effective in improving provider knowledge of cultural and behavioral aspects of health care and building effective communication strategies.

Impact on Public Health

The productivity of the workforce is inextricably linked to the health of the workforce. Therefore, if some members of the workforce receive substandard medical care, there will be both an individual and societal consequence. The individual impact on those workers is that they will become further disadvantaged and unable to advance both economically and professionally. The costs to society are loss of productivity and increased healthcare costs. This higher burden of disease and mortality among minorities has profound financial implications (higher costs for health care and rehabilitative care) and public health implications. All members of a community are affected by the health of other community members. This is the tenet of public health. All members of a community are affected by the poor health status of its least healthy members. An infectious disease outbreak can and will have devastating consequences to the entire community. Infectious diseases do not discriminate and do not recognize any racial or ethnic boundaries. This principle is so well recognized by public health advocates and the federal government that it guides policy for our country. For example, Healthy People 2010 (a federal healthcare initiative) has an overarching goal to eliminate health disparities. Imbedded in the Health People 2010 policy is the following statement: "the health of the individual is almost inseparable from the health of the larger community, and. . .the health of every community in every State and territory determines the overall health status of the Nation" (US Department of Health and Human Services, 2000, p. 15).

From an economic standpoint, failure to treat properly has repercussions. In the long run, it will cost more to treat the complications associated with a chronic disease process than the cost of doing the job right in the first place. For example, a patient with diabetes who is brought to control (hemoglobin A1C of less than 6) is less likely to develop serious complications of diabetes. A patient that is not well controlled is vulnerable to many serious and potentially life-threatening complications including dialysis, kidney transplantation, or amputation. This fact should be of importance to every taxpayer in the United States. Minority patients who are the beneficiaries of publicly funded health insurance are less likely to receive high-quality health care that will result in higher future healthcare costs not only for the beneficiary but also for the taxpayers. It is cheaper to do it right in the first place but it is also, according to distributive justice theory, the correct thing to do.

Discrimination and Equitable Quality Healthcare Delivery

Americans have widely held beliefs that abhor racial discrimination and believe that all Americans should (and do) enjoy equal opportunities in accessing health care (Morin, 2001). Most Americans are unaware that this ideal falls short in many areas of this country, most predominantly within our lower socioeconomic communities.

Evidence of unequal or substandard care for some segments of the population, particularly on the basis of group membership, should raise the concern that the provision of care may be inconsistently and subjectively administered. Inequities in care, therefore, expose a threat to quality care for all Americans (IOM, 2001).

Ethics

Normative ethics is the primary standard utilized for ethical decision making in nursing and medicine. Normative ethics include questions about what ethical principles and values should be adopted, what reasons count as ethical reasons, what actions should be performed in a certain situation, and why some principles or values should be chosen over other (Kuhse, 1997). Our values provide the framework for decision making. Our values give meaning to our lives and are derived from our family, societal norms, and may include a religious influence. Our morals are our personal standards for determining right from wrong. Behaviors that are in accordance with group norms, customs, and traditions are considered moral. Culture can play a role in group norms so moral behaviors can be individual and associated with certain cultural groups. This is different from ethics. Instead, ethics are societal standards of right or wrong and what ought to be and, as such, they guide conduct to ensure the protection of individual and/or the rights of

Box 4-3

Categories of Ethical Frameworks

Utilitarianism	Moral behavior is behavior that results in the greatest good; the individual has the responsibility to behavior that is for the good of the community.
Liberalism	Focuses on individual rights and freedom from coercion.
Contextualism	Ethics are bound to time and place and possess cultural relativism: "There is a moral, bounded or cultural relativism where ethical standards are dictated by the society and those in power, judged by the customs, rules and norms of the society, and grounded in the history of the community" (Rothschild, 2000, p. 31).
Deontology	Proposes that ethical standards are held absolutely and categorically.

Source: Leddy, S. K. (2006). *Integrative health promotion* (2nd ed.). Sudbury, MA: Jones and Bartlett; Rothschild (2000).

groups. Normative ethics have traditionally been considered impartial and possessing universal applicability.

There are several ethical frameworks under the normative umbrella. Each person must select the framework that is most acceptable to them. For some, one framework will be relied on exclusively, whereas others may change frameworks depending on the situation. The four main frameworks are utilitarianism, liberalism, contextualism, and deontology. See Box 4-3 for a description of each of these frameworks. The principles of biomedical ethics are autonomy (independence), nonmaleficence (avoidance of harm), beneficence (produce benefit), and justice (fairness). Many nurse scholars, such as Hall (1996), Nash (1999), and Schwarz (2000) have attempted to set a hierarchy for these principles, but according to Leddy (2006), none have provided justification for the rankings.

Informed consent arises from the ethical principle of autonomy. How much or little autonomy a patient wishes to possess is culturally mediated. In practice, obtaining consent is often done to meet an administrative requirement and as such does meet its true intent of ensuring that a patient understands and makes a rational, voluntary decision after adequate deliberation. The language on the consent form connotes compliance with the treatment plan and not collaboration—it does not permit or engage the patient and as such is not patient-centered. A way to become more culturally competent in one's nursing practice is to rethink the informed consent process that is being undertaken. Engage in a meaningful discussion with your patients about healing methods and the expected or desired outcome instead of just providing one-way communications that spells out the patients' alternatives and the associated risks and benefits, which truly permits informed decision making on the patient's and family's part.

Crossing the Quality Chasm

The purpose of the IOM report (2001) was to identify strategies that could substantially improve the quality of health care delivered to Americans with the focus on how to redesign the healthcare system to innovate and improve care. This redesign refers to a new perspective on the purpose and aims of the healthcare system, how patients and their clinicians should relate, and how care processes can be designed to optimize responsiveness to patient needs. The principles and guidance for redesign that are offered in this report represent fundamental changes in the way the system meets the needs of the people it serves. This redesign is not aimed only at the healthcare organizations and professionals that comprise the delivery system. Change is also required in the structures and processes of the environment in which those organizations and professionals function. Such change includes setting national priorities for improvement, creating better methods for disseminating and applying knowledge to practice, fostering the use of information technology in clinical care, creating payment policies that encourage innovation and reward improvement in performance, and enhancing educational programs to strengthen the healthcare workforce.

This report identified a quality gap in healthcare delivery as being either overuse, underuse, and misuse. The challenge is to bring the full potential benefit of effective health care to all Americans while avoiding unneeded and harmful interventions and eliminating preventable complications of care. This report was the result of an 8-year literature review of more than 70 publications which revealed abundant evidence that serious and extensive quality problems exist throughout American medicine, resulting in harm to many Americans. Four key aspects were identified: the growing complexity of science and technology, the increase in chronic conditions, a poorly organized healthcare delivery system, and constraints in fully embracing information technology revolution. Each of these four factors plays a role individually and each exacerbates the impact or effect of the other factors. The goal is quality health care, which the IOM (1990) defines as, "the degree to which healthcare services for individuals and populations increase the likelihood of desired outcomes and are consistent with current professional knowledge."

The commitment to quality health care for all is evidenced by the inclusion of the following goal as one of the six overarching goals of the IOM's Crossing the Quality Chasm Report (2001). The goal is to provide equitable health care that does not vary by patient race, ethnicity, gender, or age. The Crossing the Quality Chasm report and the desire to meet the goal of equitable health care was one of the motivating factors for Congress to request the IOM to determine if unequal or substandard health care exists.

As part of the data collection process for the IOM report (Smedley et al., 2003), themes were identified. The strongest and most consistent evidence was found in support of the existence of cardiovascular health disparities among minorities. This finding remained consistent even when potential confounding factors were controlled (e.g., race, ethnicity, access to care, disease severity, comorbidities, disease prevalence, tendency of Whites to overuse services, etc.), indicating that racial and ethnic disparities in cardiovascular care remain. Studies of racial disparities in cancer diagnosis and treatment are less clear and consistent than the cardiovascular studies. In any event, several studies indicate that racial and ethnic minorities are diagnosed at later stages of cancer progression and several studies demonstrated significant racial differences in the receipt of appropriate cancer treatment and analgesics.

The preponderance of studies reviewed by the IOM committee found generally lower rates of diagnostic and therapeutic procedures among African Americans with cerebrovascular disease.

African Americans are at greater risk for end-stage renal disease (ESRD) than White Americans. Although African Americans only make up 12% of the US population, they represent almost one third of those with ESRD. Despite these numbers, African American patients with ESRD are less likely than similar White patients to receive a kidney transplant (Epstein, Baldwin, & Bishop, 2000). It is important to keep in mind that in general, fewer African Americans than Whites desire or are appropriate for transplantation, and immunologic matching criteria result in fewer donor matches for African Americans than Whites. The bottom line is that several studies are consistent in finding that African American patients (and in some instances, other ethnic minority patients) are less likely to be judged as appropriate for transplantation, are less likely to appear on transplantation waiting lists, and are less likely to undergo transplantation procedures, even after patients' insurance status and other factors are considered.

HIV infection continues to spread more rapidly among African American and Hispanic populations than any other racial/ethnic group in the United States. African Americans with HIV infection are less likely to receive antiretroviral therapy, less likely to receive prophylaxis for pneumocystic pneumonia, and less likely to receive protease inhibitors than nonminorities with HIV. These disparities remain even after adjusting for age, gender, education, and insurance coverage.

African Americans, particularly those living in urban areas characterized by concentrated poverty, are at greater risk for morbidity and mortality caused by asthma. Management and control of the disease is affected by socioeconomic and cultural considerations. African Americans are more likely to receive treatment for asthma in the emergency department and are more likely to use inhaled bronchodilator medications than inhaled corticosteroids, suggesting the management of the disease in this population has been focused more on acute symptom control as opposed to suppression of chronic airway inflammation. African Americans, Hispanics, and Native Americans experience a 50–100% higher burden of illness and mortality caused by diabetes than White Americans, yet the disease appears to be more poorly managed among minority patients.

Given the role of cultural and linguistic factors in both patients' perception of pain and in physician's ability to accurately assess patients' pain, it is reasonable to suspect that healthcare disparities might be greater in pain treatment and other aspects of symptom management than in treatment of objectively verifiable disease.

Although large increases to internet access have occurred among most groups of Americans, regardless of income, education, race or ethnicity, location, age, or gender (US Department of Commerce, 2000), the IOM quality report (2001) identifies a "digital divide" in the use of technology existing in the disabled African American and Hispanic communities. Access to the Internet and other information technology permits the patient access to healthcare information unavailable before. The quality and completeness of this Internet information has a high degree of quality variability that may result in more problems than answers for patients.

Placing a focus on patient-centered care is a recommendation from the quality report (IOM, 2001). Culture plays a role here. As with communication styles, patients differ in their views about how active they wish to be in decision making. In some cases, patients demand a large role or wish a large role but are passive in making this known. In other cases, the patient may delegate decision making to another person—this could be a family member of the provider. The goal of patient centeredness is to customize care to the specific needs and circumstances of each individual patient. The care must be modified to respond to the person and their culture, not for the patient to modify to the care. Health care is not just any service industry as its fundamental nature is the delivery of care to people and their families in a time of illness. Because the outcome is uncertain, the stress and strain are considerable. The establishment of a trusting relationship between patient and nurse is essential and critical, and its absence contributes to a poor outcome. Change is a difficult concept for many. This appears to be especially true of healthcare professionals who traditionally are a conservative group who stress precedent and the avoidance of risk in practice (IOM, 2001). The result is that change is slow and difficult to achieve, especially when the perceived benefit is unclear or not valued.

Another important issue raised in this report is equity. The aim of equity is to ensure that all Americans receive the same benefit from our healthcare system. The goal of health care is to improve health status and to reduce health disparities by providing universal access—a promise that has not yet been kept. The report states unequivocally that with regard to equity in caregiving, all individuals rightly expect to

---

Box 4-4

Barriers to Healthcare Delivery: The 12 As

Availability—Is the service available at times when it will be needed?

Accessibility—Is transportation available? Are there geographic boundaries that are impenetrable?

Affordability—Does the patient have the financial resources to cover the cost?

Appropriateness—Are the offered services appropriate to the community?

Accountability—Do members of the healthcare team demonstrate accountability for their own education regarding the cultures being served?

Adaptability—Is the system designed for maximum flexibility or is it rigid?

Acceptability—Are the services culturally and linguistically acceptable to the patient population?

Awareness—Are potential patients and community members aware of all available services?

Attitudes—Are the attitudes of healthcare providers open to the inclusion of neutral or nonharmful traditional interventions?

Approachability—Do patients feel welcome when accessing care?

Alternative Practices—Are patient's alternative/complementary practices incorporated into the plan of care?

Additional Services—Is care delivery designed so that multiple services are available during the same hours?

Source: Lattanzi, J. B., & Purnell, L. D. (2006). *Developing cultural competence in physical therapy practice*. Philadelphia: F. A. Davis.

---

be treated fairly by social institutions, including healthcare organizations. The availability of care and quality of services should be based on individuals' particular needs and not on personal characteristics unrelated to the patient's condition or to the reason for seeking care. In particular, the quality of care should not differ because of such characteristics as gender, race, age, ethnicity, income, education, disability, sexual orientation, or location of residence.

Box 4-5

Pertinent Research Study

A retrospective study conducted by Enriquez et al. (2008) examined the impact of a bicultural/bilingual healthcare team on health-related outcomes among Hispanic/Latino adults who received care at an academic HIV specialty center (N = 43 subjects). The HIV center program manager brought together three Hispanic/Latino bilingual/bicultural care providers made up of a NP, case manager, and peer educator. All of the patient education and case management materials were revised and evaluated to ensure that they were culturally and linguistically appropriate. This was done by clinic staff and the Director of Interpreter Services for the institution, who was also bicultural/bilingual. Demographic and health data extracted from medical records were compared over two time periods: 1 year before and 1 year after the implementation of the care team. Results indicated that there were more clinic visits per patient and that a higher percentage of individuals had suppressed HIV viral loads to less than 50 copies/mL during the year after the team was implemented compared with the previous year. Results from this study suggest that provision of care by healthcare workers who are bilingual/bicultural, together with the use of linguistically and culturally appropriate materials may enhance health outcomes among Hispanic/Latino adults living with HIV infection. The team believed that the ability to interact with patients within the patient's cultural context improved communication, enhanced patient understanding of the treatment plan, and increased patient trust in the healthcare system.

Multidisciplinary and Interdisciplinary Teams

One approach advocated to provide for greater equity is the use of teams so that professionals from various disciplines contribute to patient care. Because some of the skills of NPs overlap with those of physicians, tension can often develop. Despite a difference in the training and education provided to all advance practice nurses who practice clinically (NP, nurse–midwife, certified RN assistant), there are subsets of skills that overlap with physicians. This complexity of rules across settings, and across state lines, makes it difficult for true multidisciplinary or interdisciplinary teams to be developed and fully implemented. Because licensure and scope of practice is determined at the state level, there is a great deal of variability in advance practice nursing roles. State licensure permits regulations are tailored to meet local needs, resources, and patient expectations. The resulting state-by-state variation is not always logical given the growth of the Internet and the formation of large, multistate provider groups that cut across geographic boundaries. The National Council of State Boards of Nursing has endorsed a mutual recognition model for interstate nursing practice that retains state licensure authority, but provides a mechanism for practice across state lines (similar to a driver's license that is granted by one state and recognized in other states). Still others have argued the relative merits of state-based versus national licensing systems. In any event, the care that is delivered must meet the individual needs of each patient to ensure quality health care for all Americans.

Clinical encounters are an interaction between the patient's culture and the culture of nursing/medicine. The patient culture and the medical culture both possess unique perspectives, knowledge, attitudes, skills, and behaviors. The patient and the nurse will each approach a clinical encounter from this viewpoint. The ability to find common ground is key to the ability to work effectively to collaboratively meet patient goals. To help find this common ground, it is important for the nurse to recognize that the patient will have an illness perspective (the subjective feeling of being unhealthy) while the nurse will plan care around the diagnosis of the patient (a medical label). The patient's beliefs provide the guidelines for how the patient will perceive, interpret, understand, and respond to the illness.

The practice of nursing with its emphasis on patient response to illness is compatible with a patient-centered approach. Medicine has a disease focus interpretation, which is not the same as the experience of illness related to individual perception. When a patient's beliefs about health and illness are closely aligned to the Western biomedical model, there is a high degree of likelihood of compatibility between patient and provider. On the other hand, when there is incompatibility between the patient's illness beliefs, there is the likelihood of resistance to biomedical treatment recommendations. The advance practice nurse, by virtue of education and philosophical focus, is in the best position to bridge such a gap if it is present. Taking the emphasis off of achieving medical goals and placing the emphasis on the concerns of the patient is the preferred approach. The nurse must attempt to understand the patient's health, illness, and health beliefs and not to impose his or her own personal cultural beliefs on them. Doing this is necessary to provide patient-centered care.

Need to Improve Diversity of Nursing and Healthcare Workforce

The National Advisory Council on Nursing Education and Policy (NACNEP) advises the Secretary of the US Department of Health and Human Services and the US Congress on policy issues related to programs authorized by Title VIII of the US Public Health Service Act and administered by the Health Resources and Services Administration, Bureau of Health Professions, Division of Nursing, including nurse workforce supply, education, and practice improvement. NACNEP in its sixth report entitled, "Meeting the Challenges of the New Millennium: Challenges Facing the Nurse Workforce in a Changing Health Care Environment," provided to the Secretary of Health and Human Services and to the Congress of the United States in 2008, stated that although more nurses are needed in the workforce, this is not the complete answer. Our increasingly diverse population requires increased cultural competence and sensitivity to receive the most effective care (NACNEP, 2008). Nurses play a critical role in making this a reality because nurses are the single largest component of the workforce in health care. Nurses not only provide the majority of direct care to patients, but also are major partners in healthcare management and policy. NACNEP predicts a nursing shortage that could expand to potentially insurmountable levels over the next 10 to 15 years because of an aging workforce and a faculty shortage that limits student enrollment, among other factors. Practicing nurses will also need to establish and further develop skills in critical thinking and to provide innovations in patient care delivery and increased cultural competence that corresponds to the patient population for which the nurse provides care (NACNEP, 2008).

The organization and delivery of health care in the United States is continually changing in order to meet new economic challenges and to adopt improvements and innovations in patient care. Delivery of healthcare services in the United States is becoming more demanding as the healthcare system is becoming more complex and the expectation for services is growing. At the same time, financial pressures are driving organizations to reduce costs, increase efficiency, and funders and consumers are demanding greater focus on the quality of health care and its impact on patients' outcomes. The healthcare system in the United States is becoming ever more complex at a time when an expanding, aging, and diverse population is demanding increasing amounts of healthcare services.

NACNEP (2008) has identified the capabilities, skills, and nursing resources required for today's modern nursing practice. The rapidly changing healthcare environment requires nurses with strong critical thinking and analytical skills as well as the ability to provide professional and compassionate care. These critical thinking and analytical skills are required to acquire and assimilate data in order to make appropriate patient care decisions. Nurses need interdisciplinary competencies supported by backgrounds in the sciences as well as the humanities. In order to ensure patient safety, provide quality care, and deliver patient care efficiently, nurses must be able to gather and synthesize new information and identify address needs as soon as they emerge. This is critical not only to nursing and the healthcare delivery system to provide for routine medical situations, but it is also complicated by the need for the healthcare workforce to be prepared to provide the necessary emergency response in the event of either natural or man-made disasters.

With the prospect of the nursing shortage worsening, nurse–patient staffing ratios also need to be considered when planning for nursing workforce design. There is a growing body of research that associates inadequate nurse staffing with adverse patient outcomes. A study by Aiken, Clarke, Sloane, Sochalski, and Silber (2002) found that each additional patient per nurse results in a 7% increase in the likelihood of dying within 30 days of hospital admission. Other studies have found associations between low nurse staffing levels and hospital-acquired pneumonia, urinary tract infection, sepsis, nosocomial infections, pressure ulcers, upper gastrointestinal bleeding, shock and cardiac arrest, medication errors, falls, and longer than expected length of stay (Needleman & Buerhaus, 2003). Evidence shows that having more nurses in the workforce is associated with better hospital outcomes (Needleman & Buerhaus, 2003).

Consideration must be given to the fact that inadequate or poor staffing not only increases the chance of a poor patient outcome, but its impact is felt by the nurse as well. Aiken et al. (2002) found RN job dissatisfaction levels were more elevated in hospitals with high patient-to-nurse ratios than in hospitals with lower patient-to-nurse ratios. Increased levels of nurse staffing means improved nurse-to-patient ratios. This leads to better patient safety (including more opportunities for patient monitoring and interaction) and reduces risks for unsafe conditions, thereby yielding better patient outcomes. Improved nurse-to-patient ratios also means more opportunities for patient monitoring and interaction, which includes attending to patients' psychosocial needs. Having more nurses available at a patient care site also improves the availability of cross coverage when one patient's care demands a greater proportion of an individual nurse's time.

According to the National Sample Survey of Registered Nurses (2004), the number of RNs in the United States grew by close to 200,000 between the years 2000 and 2004. The United States has one fifth of all of the world's nurses. Despite this growth, the demographic characteristics of RNs remain relatively unchanged (i.e., White females). The percentage of male RNs only increased very slightly from 5.4% in 2000 to 5.7% in 2004. Although there has been some increase in male student enrollment numbers, the representation of men in nursing education programs remains low. Men accounted for 8.8% of all baccalaureate graduates, 10.6% of master's graduates, and only 4.0% of doctoral program graduates in the year 2004. The numbers for minority student enrollments are also low. Racial and ethnic minorities accounted for 23.8% of undergraduate enrollees and 21.5% of graduate-level enrollees (Berlin, Wilsey, & Bednash, 2005). The average age of RNs increased by 6.5 years since 1980 to an average of 46.8 years in 2004, and 73.4% of all RNs were age 40 years or older.

Between 1977 and 1997, the number of RNs from minority backgrounds grew from 6.3% to 9.7% of the total population of RNs (Buerhaus & Auerbach, 1999). The 2004 National Sample Survey of Registered Nurses found 10.6% of RNs identified as non-White. Comparisons of racial/ethnic composition of the RN population across time are complicated because of changes in definitions of race/ethnicity initiated with the 2000 US census. Regardless of the difficulty of closely tracking changes over time, the US RN population in 2004 remained significantly less racially and ethnically diverse than the overall population of the United States: 88.4% of RNs identified as White and non-Hispanic, compared with 67.9% for the overall US population (Health Resources and Services Administration, 2004). Approximately 3.5% of RNs are foreign born and educated. The bottom line is that the nursing population in the United States does not reflect the population for whom we are asked to deliver care. The majority of RNs today are female, White, and aging.

Impact on Provision of Primary Care by Nurse Practitioners

During the past 5 years, the number of NPs has increased by nearly 4%, to 125,000, according to estimates from the American Academy of Nurse Practitioners (Rough, 2009). NPs need to continue the advocacy role of nursing and apply it to minority populations to help make a difference in the incidence of healthcare disparities over time. The movement to improve the quality of patient care and to minimize healthcare disparities places the focus on improving access to patient-centered and linguistically appropriate services (Nailon, 2007). NPs have traditionally gone to underserved areas to improve patient access throughout the years. Because NPs come from the nursing workforce, they are representative of the demographic characteristics of the global US nursing workforce in general. Based on the 2004 National Sample Survey of Registered Nurses, only about 11% of NPs are minorities. The fact that, again, the NP may not share the same cultural, racial, or ethnic background of the patients they care for underscores the need for NPs to be educated and to provide patient education to help decrease health disparities (Edmunds, 2008). NPs, just like other nurses, must acknowledge their beliefs and biases about specific groups of people because these biases and beliefs may be inadvertently communicated to the patient and his or her family through verbal and nonverbal communication or both. This can result in potentially offensive situations for both the patient and his or her family. NPs must find adaptive and creative ways to cross the cultural divide and to negotiate any language barriers so that all patients receive the quality health care they deserve and require.

The integration of cultural competency into primary care practice has been clarified in the NONPF document on cultural competency. It states that the NP demonstrates cultural competence when she or he shows respect for the inherent dignity of every human being, whatever their age, gender, religion, socioeconomic class, sexual orientation, and ethnic or cultural group; accepts the rights of individuals to choose their care provider, participate in care, and refuse care; acknowledges personal biases and prevents these from interfering with the delivery of quality care to persons of other cultures; recognizes cultural issues and interacts with clients from other cultures in culturally sensitive ways and incorporates cultural preferences, health beliefs, behaviors, and traditional practices into the management plan; develops client-appropriate educational materials that address the language and cultural beliefs of the client and accesses culturally appropriate resources to deliver care to clients from other cultures; and lastly, assists clients to access quality care within a dominant culture.

The American Association of Colleges of Nursing standards that are outlined in the Essentials of Masters Education for Advanced Practice Nurses states that NPs be exposed and complete diverse learning experiences in order to develop understanding of the impact of cultural diversity on human behavior (Van Zandt, Sloand, & Wilkins, 2008). Presently, NP educational guidelines do not specifically identify all of the unique skills that are required to provide advance practice nursing care to vulnerable groups.

An attempt to meet this challenge is the development and utilization of nurse-managed academic health centers which are community-based health practices that provide care to vulnerable populations that are managed by nurses. Because these staffs are often staffed by NPs, RNs, health educators, community health workers, social workers, dietitians/nutritional support, and collaborating or supervising physicians, among other healthcare professionals, it provides the opportunity for the student NPs to have a clinical placement to meet their educational requirements as well as the opportunity to can watch multidisciplinary and perhaps even interdisciplinary team in action.

Opportunities for Nurses to Attain Cultural Competency Certification

There are several opportunities already in existence for nurses to attain cultural competency certification. One such program is Cultural Competence Certification for Clinicians, which is offered by the Center for Professional Development at the School of Nursing at the University of Pennsylvania. Topics covered for the certification include appraisal of personal attitudes, values, and beliefs; impact of racial and ethnic disparities on quality of care; conceptual framework for discussions on ethnic diversity; and concerns of special populations. Other areas covered are assessments of diverse cultural health values and beliefs, strategies to facilitate cross-cultural communication, and working effectively with interpreters. The program also addresses issues surrounding ethnic pharmacology, dietary concerns, the use of complementary and alternative therapies, and religious issues with emphasis on healthcare decision making and treatment.

Another program focuses on the education of healthcare providers. This program is to educate healthcare leaders in promoting culturally appropriate care to all patients. It was developed by the American Hospital Association in collaboration with the National Healthcare Leadership Cultural Competence and is called the Leadership Fellowship. It is offered by the Health Resource Educational Trust.

Future Research

Future research should be designed to rely on standardized data collection. This IOM (Smedley et al., 2003) recommendation would result in improved identification of factors that are associated with healthcare disparities and avoid discriminatory practices. It is a difficult recommendation to implement, however, because of privacy concerns, cost, and resistance within the healthcare system. Research should also focus on the development of clinical practice guidelines that are culturally competent as well. In summary, a broad and comprehensive approach is required with full participation from all stakeholders, to keep the promise to all Americans of receiving high-quality health care.

Summary

Making the commitment to provide culturally competent nursing care within the changing healthcare environment takes time and dedication. The organization's mission statement, policies and procedures, and stated goals must also reflect this commitment as well. Areas of diversity that exist within the practice area must be identified, analyzed, and respected so that more can be learned about cultural beliefs and factors and the community's true healthcare needs. Lastly, the organization, often at the nurses urging, needs to provide training and education for all interdisciplinary and multidisciplinary team members on how to provide culturally appropriate care in the 21st century healthcare environment. The provision of culturally competent care will result in greater patient satisfaction, and if current research studies are correct, improved patient outcomes. This is an area that is ripe for further research opportunities as there are questions that still require answers and studies that need replication that are available for nurse researchers to tackle.

References

Aiken, L. H., Clarke, S. P., Sloane, D. M., Sochalski, J., & Silber, J. H. (2002). Hospital nurse staffing and patient mortality, nurse burnout, and job dissatisfaction. *Journal of the American Medical Association, 288,* 16, 1987–1993.

American Nurses Association. (2004). ANA position statements. Retrieved September 8, 2009, from http://www.nursingworld.org.

Berlin, L. E., Wilsey, S. J., & Bednash, G. D. (2005). *2004–2005 Enrollment and graduations in baccalaureate and graduate programs in nursing.* Washington, DC: American

Buerhaus, P., & Auerbach, D. (1999). Slow growth in the United States of the number of minorities in the RN workforce. *Image—the Journal of Nursing Scholarship, 31,* 2, 179–183.

Edmunds, M. W. (2008). Join us in resolving health disparities. *The Journal for Nurse Practitioners, 4,* 1, 7.

Enriquez, M., Farnan, R., Cheng, A., Almeida, A., Del Valle, D., Pulido-Parra, M., et al. (2008). Impact of a Bicultural/Bilingual Care Team on HIV-Related Outcomes. *Journal of the Association of Nurses in AIDS Care, 19,* 4, 295–301.

Epstein, N. B., Baldwin, L. M., & Bishop, D. S. (2000). Family assessment device. In K. Corcoran, & J. Fischer (Eds.), *Measures for clinical practice: A sourcebook.* New York: Jason Aronson, Inc.

Federal Office of Management and Budget. (2001). Reports and bulletins. Retrieved June 9, 2009, from http://www.whitehouse.gov/omb.

Green-Hernandez, C., Quinn, A. A., Denman-Vitale, S., Falkenstern, S. K., & Judge-Ellis, T. (2004). Making primary care culturally competent. *The Nurse Practitioner, 29,* 6, 49–55.

Hall, J. K. (1996). *Nursing ethics and law.* Philadelphia: W. B. Saunders.

Health Resources and Services Administration. (2004). The registered nurse population: Findings from the 2004 National Sample Survey of Registered Nurses. Retrieved October 3, 2009, from http://bhpr.hrsa.gov/healthworkforce/rnsurvey04/.

House, J. S., & Williams, D. (2000). Understanding and reducing socioeconomic and racial/ethnic disparities in health. In B. D. Smedley, & S. L. Syme (Eds.), *Promoting health: Intervention strategies from social and behavioral research* (pp. 81–124). Washington, DC: National Academy Press.

Institute of Medicine. (2001). *Crossing the quality chasm: A new health system for the 21st century.* Washington, DC: National Academies Press.

IInstitute of Medicine. (1990). *Medicare: A strategy for quality assurance: Executive summary IOM committee to design a strategy for quality review and assurance in Medicare.* Washington: National Academy Press.

Korenbrot, C. C., & Moss, N. E. (2000). Preconception, prenatal, perinatal, and post-natal influences on health. In B. D. Smedley, & S. L. Syme (Eds.), *Promoting health: Intervention strategies from social and behavioral research.* Washington DC: National Academy Press, 2000.

Kuhse, H. (1997). *Caring: Nurses, women and ethics.* Oxford, UK: Blackwell.

Lattanzi, J. B., & Purnell, L. D. (2006). *Developing cultural competence in physical therapy practice.* Philadelphia: F. A. Davis.

Leddy, S. K. (2006). *Integrative health promotion* (2nd ed.). Sudbury, MA: Jones & Bartlett.

Morin, R. (2001). Misperceptions cloud white's views of blacks. *The Washington Post,* July 11, 2001.

Nailon, R. E. (2007). The assessment and documentation of language and communication needs in healthcare systems: Current practices and future directions for coordinating safe, patient-centered care. Nursing Outlook, 55, 311–317.

Nash, R. A. (1999). The biomedical ethics of alternative, complementary, and integrative medicine. Alternative Therapies in Health and Medicine, 5, 92–95.

National Advisory Council on Nursing Education and Policy. (2008). Meeting the challenges of the new millennium: Challenges facing the nurse workforce in a changing health care environment. Retrieved May 23, 2009, from ftp://ftp.hrsa.gov/bhpr/nursing/sixth.pdf.

National Sample Survey of Registered Nurses. (2004). Retrieved October 3, 2009, from http://bhpr.hrsa.gov/healthworkforce/rnsurvey04/.

Needleman, J., & Buerhaus, P. (2003). Nurse staffing and patient safety: Current knowledge and implications for action. International Journal for Quality in Health Care, 15, 4, 275–277.

Office of Management and Budget. (1997). Recommendations from the Interagency Committee for the Review of the Racial and Ethnic Standards to the Office of Management and Budget concerning changes to the standards for the classification of federal data on race and ethnicity. Retrieved October 3, 2009, from http://www.whitehouse.gov/omb/fedreg_directive_15/.

Rothschild, M. L. (2000). Ethical considerations in support of the marketing of public health issues. American Journal of Health Behavior, 24, 26–35.

Rough, G. (2009). For many, a nurse practitioner is the doctor. The Arizona Republic, February 21, 2009.

Schwarz, J. K. (2000). Have we forgotten the patient? American Journal of Nursing, 100, 61–64.

Smedley, B. D., Stith, A. Y. & Nelson, A. R. (Eds.). (2003). Unequal treatment: Confronting racial and ethnic disparities in health care. Washington, DC: National Academies Press.

US Department of Commerce. (2000). How and when American goes online. CC Docket no. 99–301. Retrieved June 11, 2009, from http://www.ntia.doc.gov/ntiahome/dn/html/chapter4.htm.

US Department of Health and Human Services: Office of Minority Health. (2001). National standards for culturally and linguistically appropriate services in health care. Final report. Rockville, MD: Author. Retrieved April 14, 2009, from http://www.omhrc .gov/assets/pdf/checked/finalreport.pdf.

US Department of Health and Human Services. (2000). Healthy people 2010. Retrieved June 11, 2009, from http://www.healthypeople.gov/document/html/uih/uih_1.htm.

Van Zandt, S. E., Sloand, E., & Wilkins, A. (2008). Caring for vulnerable populations: Role of academic nurse—managed health centers in educating nurse practitioners. The Journal for Nurse Practitioners, 4, 2, 126–131.

Review Questions

Review Question 1:

Which potential areas of diversity exist in your practice community?

Review Question 2:

How might you learn more about your local community and its unique needs?

Review Question 3:

What reasons have you identified for you to make the commitment to strive toward cultural competence? What barriers are in your way? Can they be overcome?

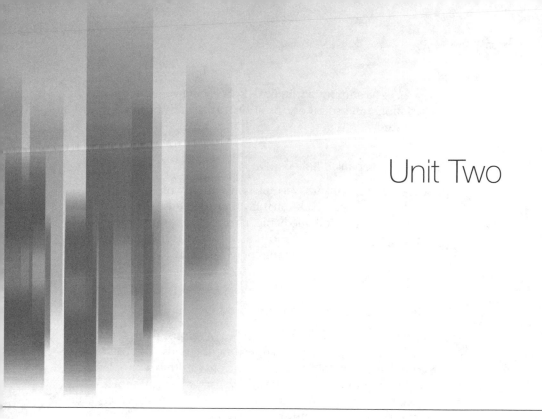

Unit Two

Impact of Culture on Health and Illness for Selected Cultural Groups

Overview

Unit Two consists of five chapters; each chapter describes a different ethnic group with an emphasis of the impact of health and illness on that group. The cultures selected for inclusion represent those most likely, based on numbers, to require nursing care from the nurse and advanced practice nurse currently practicing in the United States.

Unit Two is entitled, "Impact of Culture on Health and Illness for Selected Cultural Groups."

Chapter 5—Black Americans

Background/statistics, definition of health and illness, traditional healing methods, alternative and complementary folk medicine, current healthcare problems including mortality and morbidity, barriers (communication, time, space, environment, biologic variations, and social organization), faith and spirituality, case study

Chapter 6—Hispanics/Latinos

Background/statistics, various types of Hispanics, definition of health and illness, traditional healing methods, alternative and complementary folk medicine, current healthcare problems including mortality and morbidity, barriers (communication, time, space, environment, biologic variations, and social organization), faith and spirituality, case study

Chapter 7—Asians/Pacific Islanders

Background/statistics, various types of Asians, definition of health and illness, traditional healing methods, alternative and complementary folk medicine, current healthcare problems including mortality and morbidity, barriers (communication, time, space, environment, biologic variations, and social organization), faith and spirituality, case study

Chapter 8—Native Americans

Background/statistics, various types of Native Americans, definition of health and illness, traditional healing methods, alternative and complementary folk medicine, current healthcare problems including mortality and morbidity, barriers (communication, time, space, environment, biologic variations, and social organization), faith and spirituality, case study

Chapter 9—Whites (Non-Hispanic)

Background/statistics, various types of White Americans, definition of health and illness, traditional healing methods, alternative and complementary folk medicine, current health care problems including mortality and morbidity, barriers (communication, time, space, environment, biologic variations, and social organization), faith and spirituality, case study

Disclaimer

Every consideration will be given to be as accurate and comprehensive as possible. With that said, any attempt to provide cultural information has the potential to be viewed as discriminatory, an oversimplification, offensive, or at worst, all three. It is important that the reader recognizes that individual interpretation of the book's content by the reader will vary but the intent of the writer will not. The intent is to provide evidence-based information that is associated with the cultural groups being described in the book. The nurse must strive to learn about each individual patient and to find what if any of the included information the patient actually ascribes to. Every attempt was made to avoid stereotyping. Although the book strives to be a one-stop resource for the busy practicing nurse, the author does not in any way wish to imply that the culturally specific information that is included in the book is all inclusive or that it will be applicable to each and every patient under your care. Ultimately, experience is the best teacher so the nurse should attempt to broaden their practice—the best way to truly learn a culture is to work with patients and staff from that culture. Select the cultures that are most commonly seen in your practice to learn about first. Learning about cultural diversity will increase your understanding of the world in which we live; multicultural education is an important aspect of our personal and professional development.

Chapter 5

Black Americans

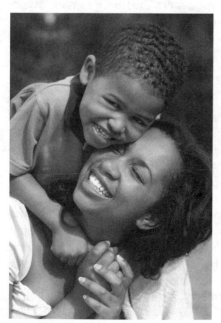

Source: © Studio 1One/ShutterStock, Inc.

Chapter Objectives

Upon completion of this chapter, the nurse will be able to:

1. Identify ways the Black American culture impacts healthcare beliefs and behavior.

2. Recognize biologic variations of the Black American patient.

3. Plan for the delivery of culturally aware nursing care for the Black American patient.

Introduction

Remember that all members of a cultural group are not the same. After reading this book, the assumption may be to generalize and stereotype members of various cultures as one. Striving to understand cultural trends should never overshadow the importance and uniqueness of the individual. Other factors can impact the situation as well, such as length of time in the United States, education, social status, whether people live in groups with other members of their cultural group or in isolation, or if they have assimilated into the mainstream culture.

It is neither possible nor necessary for every nurse to learn everything about every culture. What is important is for all nurses to recognize that there are major cultural differences not only in the beliefs and practices of the patients they care for, but also in their needs and expectations regarding care. Nurses should make an effort to learn more about the health beliefs of the particular cultural groups they are most likely to serve. This knowledge and awareness will boost nurses' competence even when they approach patients who belong to cultures with which they are unfamiliar. The key to cultural competence is an awareness and ability to identify differences in beliefs and practices about health maintenance and care and to evaluate their impact on patient satisfaction and adherence to care. Nurses need to view the practices of other cultures without judging them according to their own.

The nurse must always strive to understand the individual patient and to establish a therapeutic relationship. Recognizing that culture may impact on the patient's health beliefs and response to treatment is essential as a starting point to avoid a cultural mismatch or cultural gaffe, but the nurse must strive to learn as much as she or he can about the patient and be responsive to this information in planning nursing care. When nurses have developed these sensitivities, they will be better equipped to encourage the patients they care for to disclose any beliefs and practices that may have an impact on care and respond to them in an appropriate manner. The Giger and Davidhizar (2004) Transcultural Assessment Model is used as a framing guide for this textbook. Because not all Black Americans are from Africa, the term Black Americans will be used in place of African Americans. When caring for patients, the nurse should ask the patient how they wish to be identified as some prefer African American, some prefer Black, some prefer person of color, etc. Dark-skinned patients from the Caribbean may identify with the African culture but may prefer to be identified by their countries of origin such as Jamaican or Haitian. Newer immigrants from the continent of Africa may prefer to be called by their country of origin, such as Nigerian, and may feel disenfranchised from the African American community in the United States that has its roots in slavery.

Historical Background

The only racial group with ancestors who were forced immigrants to our country is African Americans. Most African Americans have their roots in Africa and the majority descend from people who were brought here, against their will, to be enslaved from the west coast of Africa. According to some sources, the first Black people to enter the United States arrived a year earlier than the Pilgrims in 1619, whereas other sources claim that Blacks arrived with Columbus in the 15th century (Bullough & Bullough, 1982). This means that the very first Blacks who came to the North American continent did not come as slaves. Between 1619 and 1860, more than 4 million people were transported to America as slaves. In 1619, the first African slaves arrived in Virginia. In 1808, Congress banned the importation of slaves from Africa. In 1820, the Missouri Compromise banned slavery north of the southern boundary of Missouri. Then a setback to the antislavery movement occurred when Congress passed the Kansas-Nebraska Act in 1854, establishing those two territories but repealing the Missouri Compromise. This inflamed tensions between proslavery and anti-slavery factions. In 1857, the Dred Scott case holds that Congress does not have the right to ban slavery in states and, further, that slaves are not citizens. In 1861, the Confederacy was founded when the South seceded from the Nation and the Civil War began. In 1863, President Abraham Lincoln signed the Emancipation Proclamation stating that all slaves "are and henceforward shall be free." In 1865, the Civil War ended, President Lincoln was assassinated, and the Thirteenth Amendment to the US Constitution abolished slavery throughout the United States. On June 19, 1865, slavery effectively ended when the last remaining slaves in Texas finally received word that the Civil War had ended 2 months earlier.

Despite the tremendous hardships endured by the slaves as well as the inhumane treatment, the Black culture survived and continued to grow. Despite overwhelming hardship and forced separations, Black people managed to maintain community awareness and family structure. The rich variety of traditional beliefs and practices that came with them from West Africa were maintained, continued, and passed down throughout the years. The religious traditions respected the spiritual power of ancestors. Many gods were initially worshipped, including gods who oversaw daily life (change of seasons, fertility, health, healing practices, etc.). Many aspects of current Christian religious practice are believed to have originated in these early practices. It has been estimated that between 10% and 30% of the slaves brought to America between 1711 and 1808 were Muslim, and some of these early religious customs have persisted until today.

Today, immigrants come voluntarily from African countries, the Dominican Republic, and other island countries such as Haiti, Jamaica, and the West Indian Islands.

New flows of immigrants from Africa and the Caribbean are a growing component of the US population. They are part of the racial and ethnic transformation of the United States in the 21st century. In 1800, about 20% of the 5 million people in the United States were Black compared to 13% of the nearly 300 million people in the country as of 2000. Although far outnumbered by non-Black Hispanic and Asian immigrants, the number of Black immigrants is growing at a remarkable rate. More than one fourth of the Black population in New York, Boston, and Miami is foreign-born. Immigration contributed at least one fifth of the growth in the US Black population between 2001 and 2006.

The foreign-born Black population increased nearly sevenfold between 1960 and 1980, and more than tripled between 1980 and 2005. The number of Haitians—the second-largest Caribbean group—nearly quadrupled between 1980 and 2005, and the number of Jamaicans—the largest Caribbean group—more than doubled. The increases were even more dramatic among African groups. The number of Ethiopians in 2005 was 13 times the 1960 number.

Overall, the number of foreign-born Blacks rose from 125,000 in 1980 to 2,815,000 in 2005, with a majority arriving just since 1990. About two thirds of Black foreign-born are from the Caribbean and Latin America, and one third from Africa. Only a small fraction of the new immigrants were born in Europe, Canada, or elsewhere. But the African share is growing. More African-born Blacks arrived between 2000 and 2005 than in the previous decade. Nearly two thirds of Caribbean-born Blacks live in the New York or Miami metropolitan areas. African-born Blacks are more dispersed throughout the United States. Among the top cities for African-born Blacks are New York, Washington, DC, Minneapolis, and Atlanta, but three fifths live in some other metropolitan areas, such as Philadelphia, Los Angeles, or Dallas. These immigrants have high educational attainment—38% of African-born and 20% of Caribbean or Latin American-born Blacks have a college degree. They tend to have low rates of unemployment and poverty compared with the general population, but they often are underpaid and underemployed given their educational achievements and experience. This new 21st-century Black immigration will have a tremendous impact on the American Black population as well as the whole population in general. According to the *New York Times* (Library Index), these immigrants from Africa have been "redefining what it means to be African American." Immigrants from Africa lack the perspective of American history that drove affirmative action and diversity programs. Many speak English, have been raised in large cities with capitalist economies, live in families headed by married couples, and are generally more highly educated than American-born Blacks. They also tend to have higher paying jobs.

Black or African American terminology is based on the definition used in the 2000 US Census. Black or African American refers to people having origins in any of the Black race groups of Africa. Most members of the present Black American community have their roots in Africa and the majority descended from people who were brought here as slaves from the west coast of Africa. Today, a number of Blacks have immigrated to the United States voluntarily from some African countries, the West Indian islands, the Dominican Republic, Haiti, and Jamaica. It is for the reason of inclusion that the term Black Americans or Blacks will be used in this textbook. There is no general agreement as to a preferred name for this racial group, so it is recommended to ask the patient how they prefer to be identified (Black, African American, colored, etc.).

There is a long history of blatant discrimination and racism that the Black population of the United States has had to endure. In the early 20th century, separate healthcare facilities were developed for African Americans. Churches were one of the most common sites used. Blacks who wished to become doctors were unable to attend White medical colleges. Black medical schools opened but they were not as well funded as the White counterparts. When Blacks were forced to have interactions with the White healthcare system, inequalities in care often resulted. This history coupled with the ethical violations that occurred at Tuskegee have contributed to a legacy of mistrust of the healthcare system that persists today. In the past, Blacks and other minorities were sent to either "all Black" hospitals, charity wards, or the basements of White hospitals for medical care (Myrdal, 1944). The scars from this segregation persist. Now the differential treatment that exists is much more subtle than in years past. Progress perhaps has been achieved but much more is required. The healthcare system has been slow to follow the governmental shift toward policy that supported discrimination toward one that supports the establishment of policies to dismantle healthcare discrimination and one of the consequences of this is healthcare disparities within the Black population.

Statistics

According to the most recent US Census data from July 2007, there were 40,744,132 African American residents in the United States. According to this most recently available population data, African Americans/Blacks made up 13.5% of the total population (up from 12.3% in the year 2000). It is predicted that by the year 2050, this group will make up 19% of the total population (US Census Bureau, 2008). The median age for both genders, as of July 2007, was 30.1 years old. This group has its origins in Black racial groups of Africa and the Caribbean islands (West Indies, Dominican Republic, Haiti, and Jamaica). Some Islanders resent and resist the label of African American because their roots are not from Africa. It is for this reason that it may be preferable to use the term "Black" instead when referring to this demographic group. The languages spoken can be English, French, Spanish, and African dialects. Although Blacks live in all parts of the United States, the majority live in the South. They are overall an economically deprived group, which impacts access to and quality of health care received: 12.7% of all Blacks of all ages are in fair or poor health and 12.3% of Black persons all ages have a limitation in usual activities caused by one or more chronic health conditions.

Figure 5-1

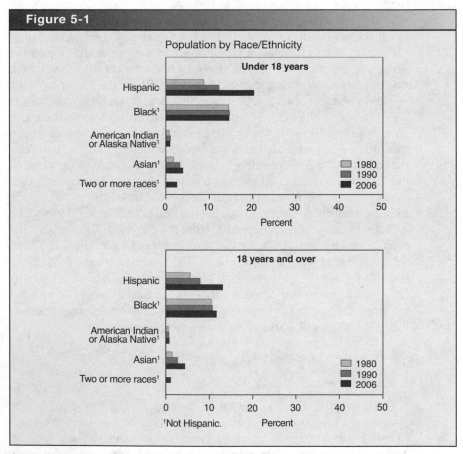

Source: National Center for Health Statistics Health. (2007). *Health, United States, 2007 with chartbook on trends in the health of Americans.* Hyattsville, MD: Author.

The state of health for African Americans is especially precarious. Chronic disease has an excessive impact on minority populations.

- The prevalence of diabetes among Blacks is about 70% higher than among White Americans.
- Infant mortality rates are twice as high for Blacks as for White Americans.
- The 5-year survival rate for cancer among Blacks diagnosed for 1986–1992 was about 44%, compared with 59% for White Americans.

The incidence of pregnancy is higher in this population, as are infant mortality rates. There has been some improvement in life expectancy in the Black population. Between 1990 and 2004, life expectancy at birth increased more for the Black than for the White population, thereby narrowing the gap in life expectancy between these two racial groups. In 1990, life expectancy at birth for the White population was 7.0 years longer than for the Black population. By 2004, the difference had narrowed to 5.2 years. The good news ends there, however. Overall mortality was 31% higher for Black Americans than for White Americans in 2004, compared with 37% higher in 1990. In 2004, age-adjusted death rates for the Black population exceeded those for the White population by 46% for stroke (cerebrovascular disease), 32% for heart disease, 23% for cancer (malignant neoplasm), and increased 787% for HIV disease. Large disparities in infant mortality rates among racial and ethnic groups continue to exist. In 2004, infant mortality rates were highest for infants of non-Hispanic Black mothers (13.6 deaths per 1000 live births). The homicide rate for Black males 15–24 years of age decreased sharply from the early to the late 1990s and has remained relatively stable since then. Homicide continues to be the leading cause of death for young Black males 15–24 years of age (Centers for Disease Control and Prevention [CDC], 2009).

Blacks and the US Healthcare System

African Americans understand and subscribe to the US Biomedical Model and, with little variation, hold mainstream cultural views about health and management of illness. It is important to keep in mind that caring for patients with English as their primary language does not eliminate the possibility of language impacting on the delivery of health care. Some African Americans believe they are treated unfairly and with disrespect in the healthcare system based on the way they speak English. This finding lends support to the belief that cultural differences between African Americans and their predominantly White physicians may exist despite language concordance (Johnson, Roter, Powe, & Cooper, 2004).

Blacks exhibit resilience and adaptive coping mechanisms when dealing with racism and poverty. They have a strong religious affiliation and the majority of households (greater than 51%) are headed by a woman. There is an extended network of caregivers from the family and the community. There is a high level of respect for elders, and small children are highly valued.

Definition of Health and Illness

The definition for health and illness has its roots in African beliefs. The major assumption is that all things, either living or dead, influence each other. It is felt that all people have control over their destiny and they can also have control over others either through behavior or knowledge. The possession of health means you are in harmony with nature, whereas illness is defined as disharmony with nature. Illness can result when a person is possessed by demons or evil spirits which causes illness or disharmony. The goal of treatment is to remove the demon or evil spirit through voodoo or traditional healers. Folk medicine is characterized by a belief in supernatural forces. From this perspective, health and illness are viewed as natural and unnatural. Some Blacks who were born and raised in the rural South may have grown up being treated by folk practitioners and may not have encountered a medical physician until adulthood. It is for this reason that it is essential for the nurse to question a patient about their geographic history. Careful questioning of African American women regarding menstruation is important. People steeped in African American folk tradition view menstrual blood as a pollutant. They believe that menstruation is the body's way of ridding itself of "bad blood." Some African Americans may consider medications that alter or reduce this flow to be harmful, fearing that this bad blood may back up and thicken, causing possible hemorrhage and death (Salimbene, 2000).

The traditional healers have extensive knowledge regarding the use of herbs and roots. Because the elderly have knowledge that resulted in their living a long and healthy life, they are held in high esteem in African society. Death is described as the passing from one realm to another. Funerals are often joyous events with a party following the burial. Today, many of the preventive treatments used by Blacks have their roots in Africa combined with approaches from Native Americans and tempered by the attitudes of the Whites with whom they interacted. Folk medicine still persists in the Black community for many reasons: lack of trust or respect in the system and its workers, fear, lack of money, lack of access especially in rural areas, and a history of bad experiences and humiliation encountered in the healthcare system.

Because of these reasons, seeking out healthcare services is often delayed. Blacks tend to seek prenatal care later, usually after the first trimester is completed. Haitian women are less likely than other groups to seek prenatal care.

Health is maintained by eating three meals a day, including a hot breakfast. Proper rest and a clean environment are also valued. Laxatives are also used to prevent constipation and to keep the system open, and cod liver oil is taken to prevent colds. Physicians are not consulted routinely and they are not generally viewed as important or necessary for disease prevention and health promotion.

The most common method today of treating illness in Blacks is prayer, which, for many, includes the laying on of hands.

Traditional Healing Methods

Providing health care to this group may be complicated by folk practices, including the belief that all animate and inanimate objects have good or evil spirits. Educational level or socioeconomic status does not appear to impact how some Blacks perceive folk practitioners. There are distinct types of folk practitioners. The healers may include family, a "granny," or a spiritualist. The granny or old lady acts as a local consultant. She is knowledgeable about home remedies made from spices, herbs, and roots that can be used to treat common illnesses. She may also give advice or make referrals to other folk practitioners with different expertise.

The spiritualist, another type of practitioner, is very prevalent. The spiritualist combines rituals, spiritual beliefs, and herbal medicines to affect a cure. The third type of practitioner is the voodoo priest or priestess. Voodoo is still practiced in some areas of the country. It is not just confined to the rural south, such as New Orleans, but can also be found in some urban areas as well. It is a belief in magic, both White magic, which is harmless, and Black magic, which is considered quite harmful. The nurse should be alert for terms such as "fix," "hex," or "spell." Many Black people continue to fear voodoo and become fearful when they fall ill.

Voodoo came to the United States around 1724 and was brought by slaves who had initially been sold in the West Indies. They were called "snake worshippers" and worshipped the god Vodu. Over time, the term changed to the more inclusive term voodoo (which also includes not only the god but the sect, the members, the priests and priestesses, the rites of passage, and all of the teachings). There are a large number of rituals associated with voodoo. The ceremonies are held with large groups, usually at night in the open air and include blood drinking (animal blood, such as from a young goat or cat, or from children) and animal sacrifice.

In some urban settings, the voodoo practitioner can be a man, but in some rural areas of the United States, the practitioner must be a woman who has inherited the title by birthright or by a perceived special gift. In New Orleans, the priestess must possess certain physical characteristics as well: She must be African American and, more specifically, she must be of mixed ancestry either one-eighth Black ancestry (an octoroon) or one-fourth Black ancestry (a quadroon) for her powers to be superior. In contrast to this type of voodoo priestess, the type of voodoo priest or priestess found in some larger urban areas such as Chicago, Queens or Jamaica, New York, or Los Angeles can be male or female and does not have to have inherited the right to practice by special powers or birth. The voodoo ceremonies that exist today have evolved from in primitive African rites and the addition of Christian rituals.

Folk practices may include the use of pica (ingestion of nonfood items such as starch and clay) and the wearing of garlic, amulets, and copper or silver bracelets. The practice of witchcraft is also widespread throughout the world. The practice of witchcraft is not limited to any one particular cultural group. Persons who believe in witchcraft feel that it can be used to cure illness or disease—but also to cause it. The fundamental belief of witchcraft is that some people possess the ability to use the forces of good and evil utilizing the principles of sympathetic magic. The principle of sympathetic magic is an important concept to all folk medicine practice, and its basic premise is that everything in the universe is connected. Any action taken against any part of the body or person causes an action against the whole of the person. A recurring theme is that dead animals that have been pulverized and ingested in one's food or drink can cause illness. Therefore, it is not uncommon for those who believe in witchcraft to refuse food or drink by someone they believe may have put a hex on them. The nurse should be aware that many patients who believe they have been hexed present at health fairs or healthcare settings with symptoms that refer to reptiles, snakes, lizards, toads, and spiders. Convincing these patients that a physician can be very difficult if not impossible, as they do not believe the hex can be fixed by western medicine.

Folk medicine in the Black community is viewed as effective—tried and tested. The terminology that may be used to describe folk medicine practitioners in the Black community are unique from titles used by other cultural groups. Some of the titles used by Blacks include "conjure doctor," "underworld man," "father divine," the "root doctor," or "root worker" (Jacques, 1976). One of the reasons the use of folk medicine practices has persisted is because of the fundamental practice of equality, fairness, and honesty. This tradition of equality of care contributes to the faith of the people in its effectiveness. Another reason folk medicine has persisted is access. In rural areas where access to health care is difficult, folk medicine may be the difference between living and dying.

Current Health Problems

Despite steady improvement in the overall health of Americans, racial and ethnic minorities, with few exceptions, linger behind. This is especially true of African Americans as numerous research studies point out African Americans experience the highest rates of mortality from heart disease, cancer, cerebrovascular disease, and HIV/AIDS than any other US racial or ethnic group.

The prevalence of hypertension in African Americans is among the highest in the world. Compared with Whites, hypertension develops earlier in life and average blood pressures are much higher in African Americans. African Americans have higher rates of stage 3 hypertension than Whites, causing a greater burden of hypertension complications. This earlier onset, higher prevalence, and greater rate of stage 3 hypertension in African Americans is accompanied by an 80% higher stroke mortality rate, a 50% higher heart disease mortality rate, and a 320% greater rate of hypertension-related end-stage renal disease (ESRD) than seen in the general population.

Available evidence indicates that, compared with Whites, African Americans receiving adequate treatment will achieve similar overall declines in blood pressure and may experience a lower incidence of cardiovascular disease. However, African Americans often do not receive treatment until blood pressure has been elevated a long time and target organ damage is present. This may also account for the higher incidence of hypertension-related morbidity and mortality in the African American population, including ESRD. Because of the high prevalence of cardiovascular risk factors in African Americans, such as obesity, cigarette smoking, and type 2 diabetes, as well as increased responsiveness to reduced salt intake, lifestyle modifications are particularly important.

In African Americans, as well as in Whites, diuretics have been proven in controlled trials to reduce hypertensive morbidity and mortality; thus, diuretics should be the agent of first choice in the absence of conditions that prohibit their use. Calcium antagonists and alpha-beta blockers are also effective in lowering blood pressure. Monotherapy with beta-blockers or angiotensin-converting enzyme (ACE) inhibitors is less effective, but the addition of diuretics markedly improves response. However, these agents are indicated regardless of ethnicity when patients have other specific indications (e.g., beta-blockers for angina or postmyocardial infarction, ACE inhibitors for diabetic nephropathy, or left ventricular systolic dysfunction). Large, long-term clinical trials of antihypertensive treatment have included both men and women and have not demonstrated clinically significant sex differences in blood pressure response and outcomes. Recent trials of older persons support a similar approach to hypertension

Box 5-1

Pertinent Research Studies

Study 1

Jacobs, Rolle, Ferrans, Whitaker, & Warnecke (2006) attempted to determine what trust and distrust in physicians means to African Americans. They found in their study that the establishment of trust is determined by a perception of interpersonal and technical competence. Trust appears to facilitate care-seeking behavior and promotes patient honesty and adherence. Conversely, distrust inhibits care-seeking behavior; it can result in the patient changing physician and also result in nonadherence. Perhaps even more alarming was the finding in this study that the subjects had an expectation that discrimination would occur during interactions with physicians. Many of the study subjects reported experiences with racial and financial discrimination by physicians in the past; in fact, it was reported as having occurred in all of the focus groups. This finding corresponds with the Institute of Medicine (IOM) report (Smedley, Stith, & Nelson, 2003) report that discrimination (and perceived discrimination) by physicians and healthcare organizations is a cause of health disparities. The IOM report (Smedley et al., 2003) was congressionally mandated. Its publication contributed greatly to the cultural competency movement. The report concluded that minority patients receive a lower quality of health care than Whites—even after taking into account differences in health insurance and other economic and health factors. It was authored by a blue-ribbon panel assembled by the nation's foremost health and science advisory body (the IOM). The report went on to say that such inequalities in health care carry a significant human and economic toll and therefore are "unacceptable" (Smedley et al., 2003), concluding that minority patients receive a lower quality of health care than Whites. The report was critically important because it highlights that unequal opportunity exists to accessing and/or receiving quality health care, which runs contrary to our national value that everyone should be treated equally. Smedley and Jenkins (2007) stated that while inequality continues to persist today in many ethnic groups, it is especially true in the African American population. Insured African American patients are less likely than insured Whites to receive many potentially life-saving or life-extending procedures—particularly high-tech care such as cardiac catheterization, bypass graft surgery, or kidney transplantation. Black cancer patients fail to get the same combinations of surgical and chemotherapy treatments that White patients with the same disease presentation receive. Even routine care suffers. Black (as well as Latino) patients are less likely than Whites to receive aspirin upon discharge following a heart attack, to receive appropriate care for pneumonia and to have pain—such as the kind resulting from broken bones—appropriately treated (Smedley & Jenkins, 2007).

Study 2

In a research study conducted in 2005, the first national study of its kind, a University of California, Irvine, sociologist found that Black immigrants who arrive in America from Black majority regions of the world are healthier than those from White majority regions; still, regardless of how healthy Black immigrants are when they come to the United States, the longer they stay, the more their health erodes. The findings suggest racial discrimination is a major cause of poor health for American Blacks—native and foreign born alike (Read & Emerson, 2005).

University of California, Irvine, Professor Jen'nan Ghazal Read and Rice University's Professor Michael O. Emerson examined the health of more than 2900 Black immigrants coming from the top regions of emigration: the West Indies, Africa, South America, and Europe. Compared to US-born Blacks, those born in Europe—a majority-White region that most closely resembles the US racial structure—are the least healthy, faring no better than American-born Blacks. Blacks born in Africa and South America, where Whites are the minority, are much healthier than US-born Blacks. Those born in the West Indies, a racially mixed region, are healthier than US-born Blacks, but less healthy than those from Black majority regions. According to Read, racial minorities are exposed to more stressful life events caused by discrimination. Stress, a key risk factor for many ailments, accumulates over the life course to harm health. "These findings do not bode well for the persistent Black/White health gap in America," said Read, "Any health advantage that Black immigrants have when they arrive is lost as they, and then their children, blend into America's racial landscape and suffer the consequences of being Black in the United States." Read explains that although this study does not provide the definitive explanation for the Black/White health gap in America, it encourages researchers and policy makers to take a much harder look at how racial discrimination harms health (Read & Emerson, 2005).

The researchers looked at three measures to assess peoples' health: self-rated health, disability, and hypertension. Their primary data came from the 2000–2002 National Health Interview Surveys, which were conducted by the National Center for Health Statistics and Centers for Disease Control and Prevention, and included a question on region of birth for the first time in 2000. Additional data for the study came from the US Census Bureau, the Office of Immigration Statistics, and the *CIA's World Factbook*. The study was published in the September 2005 issue of *Social Forces* (Read & Emerson, 2005).

management in men and women. Because of their greater prevalence of stage 3 hypertension, many African American patients require multidrug therapy. Every effort should be made to achieve a goal blood pressure of below 130/80 mm Hg; tight control is especially important in hypertensive patients with renal insufficiency.

Despite the high prevalence of heart disease in the African American population, this group is less likely to receive the appropriate medication therapy (thrombolytics, aspirin, and beta-blockers) or receive a coronary artery bypass surgery than White patients (Ayanian, Udvarhelyi, Gatsonis, Pashos, & Epstein, 1993; Canto et al., 2000; Hannan Jr., Kilburn, O'Donnell, Lukacik, & Shields, 1991; Johnson, Lee, Cook, Rouan, & Goldman, 1993). As just one example of healthcare disparities between African Americans and Whites, recent studies indicate that differences persist between these two racial groups in terms of coronary reperfusion therapy and coronary angiography (Canto et al., 2000; Cromwell, McCall, Burton, & Urato, 2005). White patients were more likely than African American patients to undergo the potentially lifesaving procedures such as coronary revascularization or reperfusion (Canto et al., 2000; Cromwell et al., 2005). African Americans with ESRD are less likely to receive peritoneal dialysis and to receive a kidney transplant (Kasiske, London, & Ellison, 1998; Barker-Cummings, McClellan, Soucie, & Krisher, 1995; Gaylin et al., 1993). African Americans (along with Hispanics) are less likely to receive analgesia than Whites for a bone fracture (Todd, Deaton, D'Adamo, & Goe, 2000; Todd, Samaroo, & Hoffman, 1993). This is especially distressing in light of the studies that show that the African American pain experience is unique. One study found after subjecting 108 women of different ethnicities to the same pain stimulus by immersing an extremity in cold water, that White non-Hispanics showed greater pain tolerance than African Americans (Reid, 1992). A study of African American Medicare patients revealed that patients with congestive heart failure or pneumonia received care that was inferior to that of White patients and that this receipt of substandard care was associated with increased mortality for the African American patients (Ayanian, Weissman, Chasan-Taber, & Epstein, 1999; Peterson et al., 1997).

As has been demonstrated, many African Americans tend to be suspicious of healthcare professionals, which means they may see a physician or nurse only when absolutely necessary. Also, many African Americans take medications differently from how they were prescribed. This is especially a problem when medications are used to treat pain and hypertension (Campinha-Bacote, 1999). Many African American patients take the antihypertensive medicine on an "as needed" basis (Campinha-Bacote, 1999). Pain is often perceived by African Americans as a sign of illness or diseases so many only take regularly prescribed medication for hypertension when they experience head or neck pain (Campinha-Bacote, 1999). Campinha-Bacote (1999) theorizes that taking medication only sporadically or as perceived when needed by the patient may be a major contributor to the high mortality and morbidity found among African Americans with hypertension. Another contributing factor may be that Blacks have high rates of hypertension, and they may have more disease risk than other populations.

In general, it is difficult to get African Americans to participate in screening programs (Bailey, 1987; Caplan, Wells, & Haynes, 1992; Naumburg, Franks, Bell, Gold, & Engerman, 1993). It is also important to point out that the determination of the applicability of screening criteria to diverse patient populations is vital to healthcare professionals in order to provide culturally competent care to their patients (Prussian, Barksdale-Brown, & Dieckmann, 2007). The purpose of screening tools is to assist in determining the risk of or the presence of a suspected disease. Providers have limited time to spend with patients, which requires reliance on rapid, accurate, and acceptable screening tests to ensure the delivery of culturally competent health care. We have a responsibility to ensure that acceptable screening tools are available and appropriate for use with various ethnic groups who live within the United States.

Despite the major medical advances of the 20th century, African Americans are still lagging behind. This is especially evident at the beginning and end of life. African American infant mortality rates are 2.5 times higher than the rates for Whites (Collins, Hall, & Neuhaus, 1999). The life expectancy of African American males is much less than that of White males. African American men in 1960 had an average life expectancy of 61 years compared to 67 years for White men. In 1996, the gap widened to 8 years. White males now have an average life expectancy of 74 years compared to only 66 years for the African American male.

Disparities

Psychiatric Care

African Americans are more likely than Whites to be diagnosed as psychotic but are less likely to be given antipsychotic medications. They are also more likely to be hospitalized involuntarily, to be regarded as potentially violent, and to be placed in restraints or isolation—differences that are found at every age level and in both outpatient and inpatient services (Benson, 1983; DelBello, Lopez-Larson, Soutullo, & Strakowski, 2001; Kales, Blow, Bingham, Copeland, & Mellow, 2000; Mukherjee, Shukla, Woodle, Rosen, & Olarte, 1983; Rosenfield, 1984; Sleath, Svardstat, and Roter, 1998; Whaley, 1998).

Asthma

A study of Black and White Medicaid-insured children in Detroit found that African American children were much more likely than their White counterparts to receive inadequate therapy, obsolete fixed-combination medications rather than the recommended single-entity prescriptions, and were less likely to receive steroid or an adrenergic inhaler (Bosco, Gerstman & Tomita, 1993; Joseph, Havstad, Ownby, Johnson, & Tilley, 1998) despite higher rates of healthcare visits and higher rates of hospitalization.

Diabetes

Diabetes strikes 1 out of 14 Blacks. Once diagnosed, African Americans are less likely than Whites to undergo hemoglobulin A1C testing, have lipids tested, have an ophthalmology visit, have a physician visit, and have vaccinations. African Americans with diabetes are also more likely to visit an emergency room or have a hospitalization than other groups.

Twenty-six percent of African American women and 16% of African American men qualify to have metabolic syndrome. The African American population is at a very high cardiovascular risk. Blacks have the highest rate of strokes among different populations in the United States. They have very high rates of hypertension, which certainly increases the risk for cardiovascular disease. Sixty-five percent of African American women are overweight (compared to the general population which has a rate of 50–60%). Fifty-seven percent of African American men are overweight. Overall, lipid levels are good (triglycerides and high-density lipoprotein), yet stroke level is so very high for these reasons as well as the prevalence of hypertension in this population.

Preventive Care

Medicare-insured African Americans were less likely than Whites to receive preventive services (Gornick et al., 1996).

Mistrust of the Healthcare System

There are many studies, some very recent, which reveal that Blacks generally mistrust the healthcare system (Boulware, Cooper, Ratner, LaVeist, & Powe, 2003; Voils et al., 2005), receive lower quality of care (Saha, Arbelaez, & Cooper, 2003; Smedley et al., 2003), and use fewer medical services in general than Whites (Mayberry, Mili, & Ofili, 2000; Wallace, Levy-Storms, Kington, & Andersen, 1998).

Barriers to Care

African Americans are less likely to have access to and to use healthcare services including preventive care. Studies show colorectal cancer screening disparities between Whites and African Americans, especially for sigmoidoscopy. African Americans have exhibited higher rates of late-stage colorectal cancer diagnosis and less overall decline in colorectal deaths than Whites over the past decade. One study found that psychosocial, cultural, and socioeconomic variables explained the difference between late-stage presentation of breast cancer between African American and White women (Lannin et al., 1998). There is significant fear of the healthcare system in general and fatalism associated with cancer.

African Americans are less likely than Whites to receive arthritis-related joint replacement, even when controlling for other demographic factors and access to care. African Americans are also more likely to be dissatisfied with the interpersonal aspects of the medical encounter than Whites (Barr, 2004).

Needed healthcare services may not be affordable for those in lower socioeconomic groups, or if they are available, they may not be culturally relevant. There are several identified barriers to health care that African Americans perceive. One major barrier, according to Underwood (1999), is that the history of discrimination and abuse against African Americans causes some to believe that their lives are not valued by most healthcare professionals, who may provide differential care according to race. Another perception of some African Americans is that some providers take risks with their lives when rendering care (Underwood, 1999). There is a general distrust of healthcare professionals, practitioners, and the healthcare system within the African American community in general. Saha, Komaromy, Koepsell, and Bindman (1999) found in their study that African American respondents who had African American physicians were more likely than those with non–African American physicians to rate their physicians as excellent (adjusted odds ratio 2.40; 95% confidence interval) and reported receiving preventive care (adjusted odds ratio 1.74; 95% confidence interval) and all required medical care (adjusted odds ratio 2.94; 95% confidence interval). This study emphasizes the importance of providing racially concordant care whenever possible to African Americans, and in the alternative, at a minimum, the provision of culturally competent care.

Physicians are somewhat less likely to have positive perceptions of Black than White patients on a number of dimensions. Blacks are often perceived as having a higher risk of substance abuse, more likely to be noncompliant than Whites, less likely to desire an active lifestyle compared to Whites, and less likely to participate in cardiac rehabilitation if it is prescribed (Van Ryn & Burke, 2000). In addition, Black patients are rated as less intelligent and educated than Whites (even when controlling for socioeconomic status and other standard covariates), and it is felt that they will have less social support (Van Ryn & Burke, 2000). Van Ryn and Burke concluded that this study found that physicians are applying general race characteristics to their impressions of individual patients and failing to incorporate disconfirming individual information.

Other studies have focused on distrust of the motives of the medical profession in withdrawal of life-sustaining technology, pursuit of organ donation, research, and health care overall (Gamble, 1997; Mechanic & Meyer, 2000; Thom & Campbell, 1997). A finding of importance in the Jacobs et al. (2006) study that has major implication for the cultural competence movement is that sharing the same race as the patient is not what was deemed as important: What was deemed important by the majority of respondents was the ability of the provider to communicate across language and cultural barriers.

Many African Americans are still dealing with the impact of slavery. The legacy of slavery is a serious mistrust of the medical establishment by the African American population. According to Smith (1999), the African American community's response to the AIDS epidemic has been in response to and has reflected the profound mistrust of the medical establishment which many African Americans feel. Among African Americans, the belief that the epidemic originated in a genocidal plot is widespread (Smith, 1999). It is thought that organized medicine has been significantly involved in this plot. If we look at African Americans' historical relationship to the medical establishment from the era of slavery to the recent past, the suspicious attitudes that make such beliefs possible may be seen as an intelligible response to a new disease that disproportionately affects African American. Successful medical and public health responses have depended and will continue to depend on overcoming the historical legacy of suspicion of the medical establishment and gaining the trust of the African American community. This view was stated even earlier by Charatz-Litt (1992), with an indictment of medical care to African Americans. According to Charatz-Litt, at no time in history has the health of Black Americans equaled that of White Americans. This is particularly evident in the South, where Blacks have been subjected to governmental policies promoting discrimination and segregation (Charatz-Litt, 1992). The rationale presented in the Charatz-Litt article to explain this unequal health status is that the health of Blacks in the United States has been greatly affected by the attitudes and perceptions of White physicians. This belief is supported in later studies conducted by Malat, Van Ryn, and Purcell (2006) and Van Ryn and Burke (2000).

Pertinent to the African American population is that African American men have prostate cancer at nearly twice the rates of White Americans and African Americans have the highest rates of hypertension of all ethnic groups (Office of Minority Health, 2005). According to data from the year 2003, the life expectancy for African American men was 69.2 years compared to 75.4 years for White males.

Impact of Communication

Differences in dialect are based on geography and social stratification (ethnic orientation, economic level, class status). Black English refers to the dialect that is spoken by many African Americans. It is significantly different from standard English in pronunciation, grammar, and syntax. The use of Black English by most African Americans is systematic and predictable, making it possible for others to understand it. This ability for understanding is key. It was estimated that approximately 80% of African Americans use Black English at least some of the time (Dillard, 1972). The use of Black English is not consistent among all African Americans, nor is it consistently used all of the time. It is felt that this variability is related to educational level and socioeconomic status. It has been described that the use of Black English is a way for African Americans to maintain their cultural and ethnic identity. It is not uncommon for some African Americans to speak standard English while interacting with general society and to use Black English when interacting with peers. A lack of comfort with standard English can serve as a barrier to the delivery of health care as the caregiver may perceive a quiet African American as hostile or submissive when in reality, they may be uncomfortable because of language. It is also important for the caregiver not to impart any judgment regarding the speaker as being substandard or ungrammatical because it is possible for Black English to be readily understood. Some characteristic traits of Black English are to pronounce certain syllables differently. For example "th" can be pronounced as "d," so "the" becomes "de," "these" becomes "dees," and "them" becomes "dem" (Dillard, 1972; Wolfram & Clark, 1971). There can also be the tendency to drop the final "r" or "g" from words. Slang may be a part of the language, and these slang words may not convey the same meaning and may be different from the slang words used in other dialects. For example, the word "bad" in Black English can mean good—the opposite of its definition in standard English. For this reason, it is essential that the nurse seek clarification if the African American patient states a medical experience was "bad." It is always essential to seek clarity of definition when slang words are used. It is also important to consider nonverbal communication. While the speech of some African Americans is very colorful and dynamic, they also tend to use a wide range of body movements (facial gestures, hand/arm

---

Box 5-2

Commonly Used Medical Terms With Equivalent Black English Subsitution Words

Medical Conditions	Equivalent Black English Term
Diabetes	Sugar
Pain	Miseries
Syphilis	Bad blood, pox
Anemia	Low blood, tired blood
Vomiting	Throw up
Medical Functions	**Equivalent Black English Term**
Constipation	Locked bowels
Diarrhea	Running off, grip
Menstruation	Red flag, the curse
Urinate	Urine/pass water, pee pee, tinkle

Source: Stokes, L. G. (1977). Delivering health services in a Black community. In A. M. Reinhardt, & M. B. Quinn (Eds.), *Current practice in family centered community nursing.* St. Louis: Mosby.

---

movements, hand signals and unique handshakes, expressive dance). The nurse must recognize when working with the African American population that frequent head nodding, good eye contact, or frequent smiling do not necessarily indicate that the patient is paying attention or is fully accepting of the message being sent. With that said, the nurse still needs to focus on all communication (verbal and nonverbal) in an attempt to fully grasp the context of the message. This is especially important when the language of the patient and the caregiver are technically the same (in this case English) to ensure that the perception of what message is being received matches the intent of the message being sent.

Giger and Davidhizar (2004) states it is essential that the nurse fully comprehends what is happening to the patient psychologically and physiologically, and to help with this process, they advocate substituting terms commonly understood by African Americans for complicated medical terminology. It is felt that this substitution will improve care delivery and patient satisfaction. Box 5-2 shows some examples from Stokes (1977) of commonly used medical terms with equivalent Black English words that can be substituted.

Impact of Time and Space

The time orientation of the Black American is dependent on how they have assimilated into the mainstream. The mainstream dominant culture is time conscious and future-oriented. This means being effective and on time is valued and punctuality is strived for. Other Blacks have a present time orientation. It is felt that this is a legacy from slavery. Planning for the future is viewed as hopeless since the future will be unchanged from the person's present and past. Blacks who are present time oriented are unlikely to value time. This can result in being tardy for or missing medical appointments. Some Blacks believe that lateness of 30 minutes up to 60 minutes is acceptable. An effective strategy to try for the patient who has a pattern of arriving late is to tell them their appointment time is 60 minutes earlier than the actual appointment time.

Other Blacks are future-oriented because of a strong religious belief. Future-oriented people are so future-focused that they plan for their funerals, even purchasing burial plots, long before illness even sets in. Nurses should consider that Black Americans view time as elastic and flexible. The nurse should help the patient identify activities where time can be flexible (such as grooming or exercising) as opposed to activities where time is inflexible such as medication administration. When dealing with the present-oriented patient, remember that they may be more likely to be flexible with keeping appointments and will feel that there immediate concerns are more important than any possible future ones.

African Americans tend to prefer closeness in personal space. Personal space refers to the amount of actual physical closeness a person is comfortable with during interactions with others. Whites prefer a personal space distance of 18–36 inches, whereas African Americans are comfortable with a much shorter personal distance span of only 5–10 inches (Hegner, Acello, & Caldwell, 2004). The nurse should consider this personal space difference when planning for and delivering nursing care. A violation in the personal space provided by the nurse may lead to patient discomfort during nursing interactions, especially if this need for closeness is violated or not respected.

Impact of Environment

It is important for the nurse to recognize whether a health practice is helpful (efficacious), neutral, or harmful (dysfunctional). Practices that are helpful should be actively encouraged by the nurse because a treatment plan that includes the patient's own health beliefs is more likely to be followed and successful. If the practice is deemed neutral, it should still be considered for incorporation in the plan of care because there may be psychologic benefits to its inclusion for the patient. Difficulty is encountered when the patient wishes to have dysfunctional health practices included in the plan of care.

The nurse must also determine whether the patient perceives their illness as natural or unnatural. Natural illnesses occur because the patient is affected by natural forces without adequate protection.

Patient education by the nurse may help the patient avoid these types of illnesses (e.g., cold or flu) in the future. Some African American patients believe in unnatural illnesses which are the result of evil influences (such as voodoo and witchcraft). In this case, it is often very difficult for the nurse to get the patient to accept that the treatment plan can be effective. Although the nurse may not believe in these cultural beliefs, it is essential that the nurse recognize that the patient does and that these beliefs must be identified and incorporated, whenever possible, into the plan of care for treatment to be effective.

Lastly, the nurse should recognize the importance of the church to African Americans and their recovery from illness. The African American minister can be a bridge between the client and the healthcare team because the African American minister fully understands the culture and beliefs of the patient.

Impact of Biologic Variations

Most healthcare providers, unless very recently educated, were taught the biopsychosocial characteristics of the dominant White culture in the United States. This resulted in members of the nondominant culture, such as African Americans, receiving care that was less than optimal. An essential component of providing culturally competent care is the recognition of differences and then incorporation of these differences from the dominant White culture into our plans of care. Understanding biologic variations is essential. This understanding needs to be more than just skin deep, which means recognizing that racial differences involve more than just skin color and the texture of hair. African Americans have unique and distinctive genotypes and phenotypes that characterize them as a racial group and as different from other racial groups. In addition, there are ethnic and cultural differences that differ from other ethnic and cultural groups. Understanding biologic variations is essential to avoid racial and ethnic disparities in health care. Important biologic variations include body size, birth weight, and body proportion. African American children younger than the age of 2 tend to weigh less and be shorter than White children. African American children tend to have less subcutaneous fat than White children but are taller and heavier by 2 years of age. The average weight for an African American woman is consistently higher than that for her White counterpart. There has been found a direct relationship between skin pigmentation and hypertension, which supports the need for hypertension screening in the African American population. There is also a higher incidence of lactose intolerance in this population that should be considered when providing nutritional education. Since 35% of the African American population has glucose-6-phosphate dehydrogenase (G6PD) deficiency (a hematologic problem), it is essential that nurses advocate for screening for this deficiency through the use of the fluorescent spot test.

The seven major chronic illnesses that impact African Americans are HIV/AIDS, asthma, coronary heart disease (CHD), diabetes, hypertension, sickle cell anemia, and cerebral vascular accident/stroke.

Human Immunodeficiency Infection/Acquired Immunodeficiency Sydrome

According to the US Centers for Disease Control and Prevention (CDC), the prevalence of AIDS is six times higher in African Americans and three times higher among Hispanics than among Whites (CDC, 2009).

Asthma

Asthma affects more than 5% of the US population. African Americans are three to four times more likely than Whites to be hospitalized for asthma, and are four to six times more likely to die from asthma than Whites (Asthma and Allergy Foundation of America, 2005).

Coronary Heart Disease

Research on CHD has contributed to the decline in cardiovascular disease morbidity and mortality that has occurred during the past three decades in the United States. However, life expectancy and rates of illness and death from CHD have not improved as much for Blacks as for Whites. Blacks have not experienced the full benefit of research advancements for a variety of reasons, including insufficient scientific data, lack of research focused on minority populations, and limited access to healthcare resources and technology. Consistent and universally accepted racial and ethnic categories have not been established, and definitions may vary according to the social and scientific context. The limited database currently available leaves a number of paradoxes unresolved. Controversy remains, in particular, regarding both chest pain and sudden death. Available data indicate that the probability of dying from CHD is greater in Black Americans than in White Americans and that there is a higher prevalence of smoking, hypertension, diabetes, obesity, and left ventricular hypertrophy (LVH) in Blacks. Blacks are also less likely to receive coronary angiography or coronary revascularization.

Although major advances in therapy for CHD have occurred in recent years, few data are available on the clinical value, effectiveness, and efficacy of newer therapeutic modalities in Blacks. Innovative therapeutic approaches to CHD have been based on data obtained primarily in White male populations. Blacks, especially women, are at greater CHD risk. Therapeutic algorithms focused primarily on the relief of chest pain have been refined in majority populations, but other algorithms may be more efficacious in populations with higher prevalence of hypertension, diabetes, and differing clinical presentations. Although information regarding the interactions of LVH, hypertension, and CHD has increased, there are few data in Blacks.

Diabetes

Approximately 2.7 million or 11.4% of all African Americans aged 20 years or older have diabetes (National Diabetes Statistics, 2007). However, one third of them do not know it. The following additional statistics illustrate the magnitude of diabetes among African Americans.

- For every African American diagnosed with diabetes, there is at least one undiagnosed case.
- For every White American who gets diabetes, 1.6 African Americans get diabetes.
- One in four Black women, 55 years of age or older, has diabetes. (Among African Americans, women are more likely than men to have diabetes.)
- Twenty-five percent of Blacks between the ages of 65 and 74 have diabetes.
- African Americans with diabetes are more likely to develop diabetes complications and experience greater disability from the complications than White Americans with diabetes.

There are genetic risk factors impacting African Americans. Research suggests that African Americans and recent African immigrants to America have inherited a "thrifty gene" from their African ancestors. Years ago, this gene enabled Africans, during "feast and famine" cycles, to use food energy more efficiently when food was scarce. Today, with fewer feast and famine cycles, the thrifty gene that developed for survival may instead make weight control more difficult. This genetic predisposition, along with impaired glucose tolerance (IGT), often occurs together with the genetic tendency toward high blood pressure.

African American ancestry is also an important predictor of the development of diabetes. To understand how rates of diabetes vary among African Americans, it is important to look at the historical origins of Black populations in America. Genetic predisposition to diabetes is based, in part, on a person's lineage. The African American population formed from a genetic admixture across African ethnic groups and with other racial groups, primarily European and North American White.

Another concern is the incidence of IGT. People with IGT have higher-than-normal blood glucose levels but not high enough to be diagnosed as diabetes. Some argue that IGT is actually an early stage of diabetes. African American men and women differ in their development of IGT. As Black men grow older, they develop IGT at about the same rates as White American men and women. African American women, who have higher rates of diabetes risk factors, convert more rapidly from IGT to overt diabetes than Black men and White women and men.

Some recent evidence shows that the degree to which obesity is a risk factor for diabetes may depend on the location of the excess weight. The presence of truncal, or upper body, obesity is a greater risk factor for type 2 diabetes, compared to excess weight carried below the waist. Blacks have a greater tendency to develop upper-body obesity, which increases their risk of type 2 diabetes. Although Blacks have higher rates of obesity, researchers do not believe that obesity alone accounts for their higher prevalence of diabetes. Even when compared to White Americans with the same levels of obesity, age, and socio-economic status, African Americans still have higher rates of diabetes. Other factors, yet to be understood, appear to be at work.

Compared to White Americans, African Americans experience higher rates of three diabetes complications: blindness, kidney failure, and amputations. They also experience greater disability from these complications. Some factors that influence the frequency of these complications, such as delay in diagnosis and treatment of diabetes, denial of diabetes, abnormal blood lipids, high blood pressure, and cigarette smoking, can be influenced by proper diabetes management.

Kidney Failure

African Americans experience kidney failure, also called ESRD, from 2.5 to 5.5 times more often than White Americans. Interestingly though, hypertension, not diabetes, is the leading cause of kidney failure in Black Americans. Hypertension accounts for almost 38% of ESRD cases in African Americans, whereas diabetes causes 32.5%. In spite of their high rates of the disease, African Americans have better survival rates from kidney failure than White Americans (Cooper, Brinkman, Petersen, & Guyton, 2003).

Visual Impairment

The frequency of severe visual impairment is 40% higher in African Americans with diabetes than in White Americans. Blindness caused by diabetic retinopathy is twice as common in Blacks as in Whites. Compared to White women, Black women are three times more likely to become blind from diabetes. African American men have a 30% higher rate of blindness from diabetes than White American men. Diabetic retinopathy may occur more frequently in Black Americans than Whites because of their higher rate of hypertension (Roy & Affouf, 2006).

Amputations

African Americans undergo more diabetes-related lower-extremity amputations than White or Hispanic Americans.

Hypertension

African Americans are at higher risk for this serious disease than any other race or ethnic group. High blood pressure tends to be more common, happens at an earlier age, and is more severe for many African Americans.

Sickle Cell Anemia

The sickle cell disorders are found in people of African, Mediterranean, Indian, and Middle Eastern heritage. In the United States, these disorders are most commonly observed in African Americans and Hispanics from the Caribbean, Central America, and parts of South America. An additional and less recognized problem is that sickle cell patients live under considerable psychosocial stress. Not only do they experience stresses common to other painful chronic illnesses, but they must also cope with the unpredictable nature of their illness. The recurrent and unpredictable nature of the disease can adversely affect both school and work attendance and has the potential of reducing the patient's sense of self-esteem.

Cerebral Vascular Accident/Stroke

Age-adjusted stroke deaths are higher in African Americans and men. High blood pressure has long been established as the major risk factor for stroke. More recently, cigarette smoking and obesity also have been found to be significant risk factors for stroke.

The bottom line is that the nurse who denies or who does not believe that race is a factor denies a significant part of the patient's being. All aspects of care must be adapted to the patient's culture, socioeconomic status, and educational background.

Impact on Social Organization

The majority of Black homes have a female-headed family structure. Most Blacks are demonstrative and comfortable with physical contact and emotional sharing. The legacy of slavery is that African Americans are the only cultural group in the United States who have not been fully assimilated into mainstream society. Historically, as a result of slavery, African Americans were kept isolated or segregated from other cultural groups. Even today, African Americans maintain separate and, in most cases, a lower socioeconomic lifestyle compared to mainstream society. Slavery also resulted in negatively impacting the role of the man in the family. Because the African American male was someone else's property, it kept him from being the head of the household or the protector of the family from his White slave owner. This resulted in the female becoming the dominant force in the family, which to this day is still true in the majority of households in the United States. It is important for the nurse to recognize that the African American family is matrifocal, which means the woman is responsible for the health of the family. The woman is responsible for sharing information and to assist the patient with all decision making, including treatment decisions. The recognition of the importance of the female role to the family should not permit the nurse to ignore or minimize the role of the Black man in the decision-making process.

Impact on Faith and Spirituality

Black people have a strong religious foundation and commitment. The most popular religions are Southern Baptist, fundamentalist, and Muslim. Many African Americans believe in the power of some people to heal and help others. Many have a belief in the healing powers of religion. A reliance on healers reflects the deep religious faith within this group.

An understanding of religion is also important because of its impact on nutrition and the patient's diet. Islamic dietary restrictions consist of eating a strictly Halal diet (no pork or pork products or soul foods such as Black eyed peas, kidney beans, ham hocks, bacon, or pork chops) and the philosophy that a "person is what he eats." These foods are considered to be filthy. It is felt that food affects the way a person thinks and acts. Alcohol should be avoided because it dulls the senses and it is felt that it causes illness. Muslims fast for a 30-day period during the year (fast of Ramadan) which means no consumption of meat from land animals and only one meal per day in the evening. Nothing is taken by mouth from 5:00 A.M. until sundown. Ill Muslims, small children, and pregnant women are exempt from this rule. Muslims believe in self-help and assisting in uplifting each other, and the lifestyle is not so rigid that people are not permitted to have a good time. To Muslims, life is precious. They will accept blood transfusions but no treatments that have a pork base (e.g., pork-based insulin) because of the belief that it is unclean and the avoidance of pork and pork products in a Halal diet. It is important to realize that many Muslims differ in their practice and philosophy of Islam. Some Muslims dress in distinctive clothing (e.g., long skirts and head coverings for women). Other sects are less strict regarding dress. Some do not follow the Halal diet and are allowed to smoke and drink alcoholic beverages in moderation. In some sects, it is acceptable for men to practice polygamy and for men to have many sexual partners. It is important for the nurse to determine which sect the Muslim African American patient belongs to in order to provide culturally competent care.

Summary

When caring for Black patients, the nurse must not only recognize the impact that culture has on the Black patient's experience, but also incorporate this knowledge of culture into the plan of nursing care. Adjustments in care may be necessary when the culture of the patient does not match the culture of the nurse. Even when the cultures match, there still is the potential for cross-cultural clashes because the nurse has been assimilated into the philosophy of Western medicine. Failing to recognize the impact of culture makes it impossible for the nurse to fully know the patient because race and culture contribute so much to the patient's entire being.

Black people, as a group, have disproportionate morbidity and mortality rates compared to the White majority group. Research to date, including the IOM report (Smedley et al., 2003), concludes that this is caused by discriminatory practices as well as inequalities in educational preparation, social status, and economics. This is considered to be of much more significance than racial or genetic/biologic factors. According to census data, Blacks are more likely to live in poverty and have less education than other racial and ethnic groups, and these two factors underlie many of the health disparities in this country. A public health focus that only considers the factors of socioeconomic status, access to care, and poverty would not be adequate. Even when these variables are controlled, health disparities remain constant along racial lines, and this was especially true among Blacks (Braithwaite & Taylor, 2001). Healthcare providers must be aware that unequal treatment and cultural incompetence is prevalent and that changing health outcomes requires all team members to recognize and acknowledge the patient's racial, cultural, and ethnic background because it is in these areas that the patient experience becomes unique. Nurses must consider and plan for any required changes in care to ensure that nursing care has been individualized. This requires the care to be adapted to consider the patient's cultural experiences, educational level, and socioeconomic background. As patient advocates, it falls to the nurse to ensure that a cultural assessment is performed, documented, and communicated clearly among all healthcare team members in order to narrow the gap in healthcare disparities in the United States.

Case Study 5-1

The "Hexed" Patient

C. I., a 56-year-old migrant Black construction and farm worker, had considerable difficulty explaining and describing his symptoms of back pain, right upper quadrant pain, and jaw pain. When nothing was found to explain his symptoms by radiograph or laboratory studies, he began to feel that they were secondary to a hex. He felt that a man was working "roots" on him and he wanted to see a root doctor. Suddenly, he developed a paraplegia and a granulomatous lesion was found in his vertebral column with cord compression. He has not had a return of function since surgery but still tends to think that the hex might have caused his problems.

Rationale: The perception of the nurse versus the patient in this situation will be very different. The potential for a cultural gaffe is great. While the patient believes he has been hexed, the nurse may believe the patient is delusional. Hex and voodoo are cultural beliefs found in some Blacks that an illness is caused by hexing or an evil influence brought about by another person. These traditional beliefs have persisted and are more prevalent in different parts of the United States and the world. These beliefs can be found in some developed areas that the nurse should keep in mind. A distinction is made between natural conditions that are perceived as God's will or unnatural conditions that are a result of disharmony or conflict with God's will or the result of evil influence. Symptoms can be quite varied but frequently include those associated with a generalized anxiety disorder: nausea, vomiting, dizziness, weakness, diarrhea, and fears ranging from being poisoned to being killed (Voodoo death). A culture-bound treatment for this is rootwork, which is the use of dried roots from plants in charms and spells and is quite common in the South among the African American population.

Case Study 5-2

Female Genital Mutilation

Female genital mutilation (FGM) was not known about widely in the United States until the case of Fauziya Kassindja, a then 17-year-old from Togo, who was requesting political asylum in the United States in 1994. She had run away on the eve of her arranged wedding to avoid FGM. At that time, our government thought she was attempting to immigrate to our country and held her for 1.5 years in prison, often in solitary confinement. Despite human rights advocates speaking out on her behalf, the court did not deem her case to be credible. It was only when the story gained widespread notice in the media that she was freed and the spotlight began to shine on the issue of FGM. It has taken many years for the public to become aware of this practice and still more awareness needs to occur as it is still practiced in many countries. The practice began 2000 years ago either in Egypt or the "Horn of Africa" (what is now Eritrea, Djibouti, Ethiopia, and Somalia). The World Health Organization estimates that it will take a minimum of 10 years to reduce the prevalence of FGM and three generations to eradicate it because it is such a firmly entrenched ritual that is valued by those cultures. Because it is a practice that will likely continue for some time, nurses need to be aware of it and how best to proceed with caring for these women and their families.

Rationale: An increasing number of the countries with a long tradition of performing circumcision rites, widely referred to as FGM, are beginning to re-examine and legislate against this practice. However, the custom of circumcising young girls may take several generations to change. The World Health Organization, which promotes the elimination of FGM, has estimated that between 100 and 140 million women have undergone FGM and that 2 million more undergo some form of FGM every year. The US Centers for Disease Control and Prevention has estimated that 168,000 women (48,000 under the age of 18) who have had FGM are living in the United States today (World Health Organization, 2000).

FGM is typically performed when a girl is between 4 and 8 years old. It is practiced in about 28 African countries, Asia, the Middle East, and increasingly in Europe, Australia, Canada, and the United States. The World Health Organization (2000) has identified four types of FGM. Type I, which is the only type that can accurately be referred to as female circumcision, is a clitoridectomy. The prepuce and all or parts of the clitoris are removed. This does not usually result in long-term complications. Type II involves an excision by which the clitoris and inner labia are removed. Women who have undergone this procedure may suffer from pain during intercourse and experience other long-term problems. Type III is infibulation or an extreme form of circumcision. The clitoris is removed, at least two thirds of the labia majora are cut off, as well as the entire labia minora. Incisions are made in the majora to create raw surfaces, which are then stitched or held together (sometimes by tying the woman's legs together), until a hood of skin grows to cover the urethra and vagina. A small hole, about the diameter of a matchstick, is made to allow menstrual blood and urine to escape. Type IV is pricking, piercing, or incising the clitoris and/or labia or cauterization by burning of the clitoris and surrounding tissue. Adverse effects include formation of cysts, abscesses, and scar tissue; sexual dysfunction; dysmenorrhea and chronic pelvic infections; damage to the urethra; incontinence; chronic pelvic and back pain; chronic urinary tract infections; and difficulties with childbirth (World Health Organization, 2000).

FGM refers to a range of practices involving the cutting, removal, and sometimes sewing up of the female genitalia for cultural or other nontherapeutic reasons. Women who have undergone FGM have been taught to believe that this rite of passage is normal. Reasons for having FGM include identification with cultural heritage and the initiation of girls into womanhood. The possible consequences of FGM are numerous including psychologic trauma, difficulty with childbirth, gynecological problems, infection, and even death.

Nursing implications: Nurses working with women are likely to encounter women who have had FGM in their clinical practice. It is important not to assume that all these women want this condition reversed. In their culture, reversal of circumcision would make them unsuitable for marriage, libel for divorce, and virtually an outcast in their communities. Make sure that your assessment questions are culturally appropriate, asking how the circumcision is impacting their life, urination, and menstruation. If the patient seems open to the possibility of surgical correction, it is recommended to refer the patient to healthcare providers and counselors that share her same cultural background.

References

Asthma and Allergy Foundation of America. (2005). Disparities in asthma care. Retrieved June 12, 2009, from https://www.aafa.org/pdfs/Disparities.PDF

Ayanian, J. Z., Udvarhelyi, I. S., Gatsonis, C. A., Pashos, C. L., & Epstein, A. M. (1993). Racial differences in the use of revascularization procedures after coronary angiography. *Journal of the American Medical Association, 269,* 20, 2642–2646.

Ayanian, J. Z., Weissman, J. S., Chasan-Taber, S., & Epstein, A. M. (1999). Quality care by race and gender for congestive heart failure and pneumonia. *Medical Care, 37,* 1260–1269.

Bailey, G. (1987). Divergence. *American Speech, 56,* 75–80.

Barker-Cummings, C., McClellan, W., Soucie, J. M., & Krisher, J. (1995). Ethnic differences in the use of peritoneal dialysis as initial treatment for end stage renal disease. *Journal of American Medical Association, 274,* 23, 1858–1862.

Barr, D. A. (2004). Race/ethnicity and patient satisfaction: Using the appropriate method to test perceived differences in care. *Journal of General Internal Medicine, 19,* 937–943.

Benson, P. R. (1983). Factors associated with antipsychotic drugs prescribing by southern psychiatrists. *Medical Care, 21,* 639–654.

Bosco, L. A., Gerstman, B. B., & Tomita, D. K. (1993). Variations in the use of medication for the treatment of childhood asthma in the michigan medicaid population, 1980–1986. *Chest, 104,* 1727–1732.

Boulware, L. E., Cooper, L. A., Ratner, L. E., LaVeist, T. A., & Powe, N. R. (2003). Race and trust in the health care system. *Public Health Reports, 118,* 358–365.

Braithwaite, R., & Taylor, S. (2001). *Health issues in the Black community* (2nd ed.). San Francisco: Jossey-Bass.

Bullough, V. L., & Bullough, B. (1982). *Health care for the other Americans.* East Norwalk, CT: Appleton-Century-Crofts.

Campinha-Bacote, J. (1999). A model and instrument for addressing cultural competence in health care. *Journal of Nursing Education, 38,* 203–207.

Canto, J. G., Allison, J. J., Kiefe, C. I., Fincher, C., Farmer, R., Sekar, R., et al. (2000). Relation of race and sex to the use of reperfusion therapy in Medicare beneficiaries with acute miocardial infarction. *New England Journal of Medicine, 342,* 1094–1100.

Caplan, L. S., Wells, B. L., & Haynes, S. (1992). Breast cancer screening among older racial/ethnic minorities and Whites: Barriers to early detection. *Journal of Gerontology, 47,* 101–110.

Centers for Disease Control and Prevention. Retrieved June 11, 2009, from http://www.cdc.gov/mmwr/preview/mmwrhtml/00001849.htmv.

Charatz-Litt, C. (1992). A chronicle of racism: The effects of the White medical community on Black health. *Journal National Medical Association, 84,* 8, 717–725.

Collins, K. S., Hall, A., & Neuhaus, C. (1999). *U.S. minority health: A chartbook.* New York: The Commonwealth Fund.

Cooper, W. A., Brinkman, W., Petersen, R. J., & Guyton, R. A. (2003). Impact of renal disease in cardiovascular surgery: Emphasis on the African American patient. *Annals of Thoracic Surgery, 76,* S1370–S1376.

Cromwell, J., McCall, N. T., Burton, J., & Urato, C. (2005). Race/ethnic disparities in utilization of lifesaving technologies by Medicare ischemic heart disease beneficiaries. *Medical Care, 43,* 330–337.

DelBello, M. P., Lopez-Larson, M. P., Soutullo, C. A., & Strakowski, S. M. (2001). Effects of race on psychiatric diagnosis of hospitalized adolescents: A retrospective chart review. *Journal of Child and Adolescent Psychopharmacology*, 11, 95–103.

Dillard, J. L. (1972). *Black English: Its history and usage in the United States.* New York: Vintage Books.

Gamble, V. N. (1997). Under the shadow of Tuskegee: African Americans and health care. *American Journal of Public Health*, 87, 1773–1778.

Gaylin, D. S., Held, P. J., Port, F. K., Hunsicker, L. G., Wolfe, R. A., Kahan, B. D., et al. (1993). The impact of comorbid and sociodemographic factors on access to renal transplantation. *Journal of the American Medical Association*, 269, 5, 603–608.

Giger, J. N., & Davidhizar, R. E. (2004). *Transcultural nursing: Assessment and intervention.* (4th ed.). St. Louis, MO: Mosby.

Gornick, M. E., Eggers, P. W., Reilly, T. W., Mentnech, R. M., Fitterman, L. K., Kucken L. E., et al. (1996). Effects of race and income on mortality and use of services among medicare beneficiaries. *New England Journal of Medicine*, 335, 791–799.

Hannan, E. L., Kilburn, H., Jr., O'Donnell, J. F., Lukacik, G., & Shields, E. P. (1991). Interracial access to selected cardiac procedures for patients hospitalized with coronary artery disease in New York state. *Medical Care*, 29, 5, 430–441.

Hegner, B. R., Acello, B., & Caldwell, E. (2004). *Nursing assistant: A nursing process approach* (p. 190). Clifton Park, NY: Thomson Learning.

Jacobs, E. A., Rolle, I., Ferrans, C. E., Whitaker, E. E. & Warnecke, R. B. (2006). Understanding African Americans' views of the trustworthiness of physicians. *Journal of General Internal Medicine*, 21, 6, 642–647.

Jacques, G. (1976). Cultural health traditions: A Black perspective. In M. F. Branch, & P. P. Paxton (Eds.), *Providing safe nursing care for ethnic people of color.* East Norwalk, CT: Appleton-Century-Crofts.

Johnson, P. A., Lee, T. H., Cook, E. F., Rouan, G. W., & Goldman, L. (1993). Effect of race on the presentation and management of patients with acute chest pain. *Annals of Internal Medicine*, 118, 593–601.

Johnson, R. L., Roter, D., Powe, N. R., & Cooper, L. A. (2004). Patient race/ethnicity and quality of patient-physician communication during medical visits. *American Journal of Public Health*, 94, 12, 2084–2090.

Joseph, C. L., Havstad, S. L., Ownby, D. R., Johnson, C. C., & Tilley, B. C. (1998). Racial differences in emergency department use persist despite allergist visits and prescriptions filled for anti-inflammatory medications. *Journal of Allergy and Clinical Immunology*, 101, 484–490.

Kales, H. C., Blow, P. C., Bingham, C. R., Copeland, L. A., & Mellow, M. A. (2000). Race, psychiatric diagnosis, and mental health care utilization in older patients. *American Journal of Geriatric Psychiatry*, 8, 301–309.

Kasiske, B. L., London, W., & Ellison, M. D. (1998). Race and socioeconomic factors influencing early placement on the kidney transplant waiting list. *Journal of the American Society of Nephrology*, 9, 2142–2147.

Lannin, D. R., Mathews, H. F., Mitchell, J., Swanson, M. S., Swanson, F. H., & Edwards, M. S. (1998). Influences of socioeconomic and cultural factors on racial differences in late-stage presentation of breast cancer. *Journal of the American Medical Association*, 279, 1801–1807.

Library Index. The impact of immigration on twenty-first century America—Black immigrants from africa differ from American Black population. Retrieved February

19, 2009, from http://www.libraryindex.com/pages/2463/Impact-Immigration-on-Twenty-First-Century-America-Black-IMMIGRANTS-FROM-AFRICA-DIFFER FROM-AMERICAN-Black-POPULATION.html.

Malat, J. R., Van Ryn, M., & Purcell, D. (2006). Race, socioeconomic status, and the perceived importance of positive self-presentation in health care. *Social Science & Medicine, 62*, 10, 2479–2488.

Mayberry, R. M., Mili, F., & Ofili, E. (2000) Racial and ethnic differences in access to medical care. *Medical Care Research and Review, 57*, 108–145.

Mechanic, D., & Meyer, S. (2000). Concepts of trust among patients with serious illness. *Social Science Medicine, 51*, 657–668.

Mukherjee, S., Shukla, S., Woodle, J., Rosen, A. M., & Olarte, S. (1983). Misdiagnosis of schizophrenia in bipolar patients: A multiethnic comparison. *American Journal of Psychiatry, 140*, 12, 1571–1574.

Myrdal, G. (1944). *An American dilemma.* Vol. 1. New York: Harper & Brothers Publishers.

National Diabetes Statistics. (2007). Retrieved June 12, 2009, from http://diabetes. niddk.nih.gov/DM/PUBS/statistics/al.

Naumburg, E., Franks, H., Bell, B., Gold, M., & Engerman, J. (1993). Racial differentials in the identification of hypercholesterolemia. *Journal of Family Practice, 36*, 4, 425–430.

Office of Minority Health. (2005). African American profile report. Retrieved June 12, 2009, from http://www.omhrc.gov/templates/browse.aspx?lvl= 2&lvlID=51.

Peterson, E. D., Shaw, L. K., DeLong, E. R., Pryor, D. B., Califf, R. M., & Mark, D. B. (1997). Racial variation in the use of coronary-revascularization procedures. Are the differences real? Do they matter? *New England Journal of Medicine, 336*, 7, 480–486.

Prussian, K. H., Barksdale-Brown, D. J., & Dieckmann, J. (2007). Racial and ethnic differences in the presentation of metabolic syndrome. *The Journal for Nurse Practitioners, 1*, 33, 229–240.

Read, J. G., & Emerson, M. O. (2005). Racial context, Black immigration and the U.S. Black/White health disparity. *Social Forces, 84*, 1, 181–199.

Reid, V. J. (1992). Ethnicity, interpersonal factors and pain expressions: Implications for physician patient interaction. In: *Dissertation abstracts international.* Ann Arbor, MI: UMI, 53:DA922505.

Rosenfield, S. (1984). Race differences in involuntary hospitalizations. Psychiatric vs. labeling perspectives. *Journal of Health and Social Behavior, 25*, 14–23.

Roy, M., & Affouf, M. (2006). Six-year progression of retinopathy and associated risk factors in African-Americans with type 1 diabetes: The New Jersey 725. *Archives of Ophthalmology, 124*, 1297–1306.

Saha, S., Arbelaez, J. J., & Cooper, L. A. (2003). Patient-physician relationships and racial disparities in the quality of health care. *American Journal of Public Health, 93*, 10, 1713–1719.

Saha, S., Komaromy, M., Koepsell, T. D., & Bindman, A. B. (1999). Patient-physician Racial concordance and the perceived quality and use of health care. *Archives of Internal Medicine, 159*, 9, 997–1004.

Salimbene, S. (2000). Providing culture-sensitive care to African Americans. In: *What language does your patient hurt in? A practical guide to culturally competent patient care.* Amherst, MA: Diversity Resources.

Sleath, B., Svardstat, B., & Roter, D. (1998). Patient race and psychotropic prescribing during medical encounters. *Patient Education and Counseling, 34*, 227–238.

Smedley, B. D., & Jenkins A (Eds.). (2007). *All things being equal: Instigating opportunity in inequitable times.* New York: The New Press.

Smedley, B. D., Stith, A. Y., & Nelson, A. R. (2003). *Unequal treatment: Confronting racial and ethnic differences in health care.* Washington, DC: Institute of Medicine.

Smith, C. (1999). African Americans and the medical establishment. *Mt. Sinai Journal of Medicine, 66,* 4, 280–281.

Stokes, L. G. (1977). Delivering health services in a Black community. In A. M. Reinhardt, & M. B. Quinn (Eds.), *Current practice in family centered community nursing.* St. Louis: Mosby.

Thom, D. H., & Campbell, B. (1997). Patient-physician trust: An exploratory study. *Journal of Family Practice, 44,* 169–176.

Todd, K. H., Samaroo, N., & Hoffman, J. R. (1993). The effect of ethnicity on physicians' estimates of pain severity in patients with isolated extremity trauma. *Journal of the American Medical Association, 269,* 12, 1537–1539.

Todd, K. H., Deaton, C., D'Adamo, A. P., & Goe, L. (2000). Ethnicity and analgesic practice. *Annals of Emergency Medicine, 35,* 11–16.

Underwood, S. M. (1999). Development of a cancer prevention and early detection program for nurses working with African Americans. *Journal of Continuing Nursing Education, 30,* 30–36.

US Census Bureau. (2008). Table 4: annual estimates of the Black or African American alone or in combination population by sex and age for the United States: April 1, 2000, to July 1, 2007. Source: Population Division, US Census Bureau. Release Date: May 1, 2008.

Van Ryn, M., & Burke., J. (2000). The effect of patient race and socioeconomic status on physicians' perceptions of patients. *Social Science and Medicine, 50,* 6, 813–828

Voils, C. I., Oddone, E. Z., Weinfurt, K. P., Friedman, J. Y., Schulman, K. A., & Bosworth, H. B. (2005). For the patient. Who trusts healthcare institutions? Results from a community-based sample. *Ethnicity & Disease, 15,* 1, 150.

Wallace, S. P., Levy-Storms, L., Kington, R. S., & Andersen, R. M. (1998). The persistence of race and ethnicity in the use of long-term care. *The Journal of Gerontology, 53,* 2, S104–112.

Whaley, A, L. (1998). Cross-cultural perspective on paranoia: A focus on the Black American experience. *Psychiatry Quarterly, 69,* 4, 325–343.

Woolfram, W. A., & Clark, H. (1971). *Black-White speech relationships.* Washington, DC: Center for Applied Linguistics.

World Health Organization. (2000). Female genital mutilation. Fact Sheet No. 241. Retrieved January 29, 2009, from www.who.int/mediacentre/factsheets/fs241/en/.

Chapter 6

Hispanics/Latinos

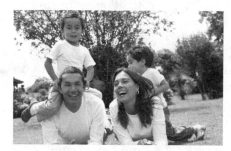

Source: © Andresr/ShutterStock, Inc.

Chapter Objectives

Upon completion of this chapter, the nurse will be able to:

1. Define and differentiate between the terms Hispanic and Latino.

2. Plan nursing care for Hispanic/Latino patients that considers and incorporates the ethnicity, traditional health beliefs, and biologic variations of these patients.

3. Consider the barriers to care that exist and plan for strategies to overcome these barriers.

Introduction

The information provided in this chapter is intended to serve as a guide with the intent to help the reader become more aware of the culture and values of patients from cultures different from their own. Be sure to question your patients about their individual beliefs and practices to provide individualized and culturally sensitive nursing care. It is important for the nurse to remember that not all people within a culture are the same. The nurse must always consider the uniqueness and individual characteristics of each and every patient.

Terminology: Latinos or Hispanics?

The terms Latino and Hispanic are not synonymous. The word "Latin" comes to us from a tribe in early Italy called the Latins. The Latins lived in Latium, whose capital city was Rome. Their language was called Latin as well. As the Roman Empire spread its dominance, the language Latin evolved into several other languages: Italian, Spanish, Portuguese, and French (these are often referred to as the "Romance" languages). Later, when the Romans invaded the Iberian peninsula, they found an existing city named Hispalis (Seville). The name Hispalis appears to be derived from Greek. The Romans annexed the Iberian peninsula, naming it Hispania. The Romans spent seven centuries in Hispania, leaving behind an extensive legacy. This legacy tied Hispania to the rest of the Latin world.

The term Hispano (Hispanic) later was used when referring to Spain; thus, Hispanic refers to people whose culture and heritage have ties to Spain (they may or may not speak Spanish).

The term Hispanic did not come into wide usage until the 1970s and 1980s. In the 1950s and 1960s, Hispanics tended to organize around their own national identities as Mexicans, Mexican Americans, Puerto Ricans, Cuban Americans, Central Americans, and South Americans. Today, the term Hispanic has emerged as an inclusive term that refers to all Spanish-speaking ethnic subgroups. Hispanics in the United States can be of any racial background: White, Black, Asian, American Indian, etc.

In the United States, the government used the term Hispanic in forms and to identify people with a Spanish heritage during the 2000 Census (US Census Bureau, 2008). Hispanic is not a race but an ethnic distinction and is translated from Hispania (Latin) and Hispano (Spanish). People from Latin America are all Latin(o) but not all are Hispanics. For example, Brazilians speak Portuguese, which makes Brazilians Latin but not Hispanic. To be inclusive, both terms will be used in this chapter of the textbook. It is also important to state that although Hispanics/Latinos are collectively grouped together in this chapter, each subgroup has differing dialects, foods, and traditions determined by the country of origin. Consideration needs to be given for personal differences, socioeconomic status, migration status, subcultures, and life experiences.

Background

According to the Office of Management and Budget federal guidelines on race, Hispanic or Latino people are Mexican, Puerto Rican, or Cuban; some may also indicate that they are of some other type of Spanish origin. Origin can be viewed as heritage, nationality group, lineage, or country of birth of the person or person's parents or ancestors before their arrival in the United States. According to Grieco and Cassidy (2001), people of Spanish origin can be of any race.

Some prefer the term Latino to describe the ethnic heritage because it is inclusive and because of its emphasis on geographical area. Others prefer Hispanic, which emphasizes the Spanish heritage and is consistent with the US Census (US Census Bureau, 2008). Hispanic/Latino is not a racial group but an ethnic grouping of people from 20 countries. As a result, many Hispanics/Latinos self-identify with their country of origin. Most Hispanics/Latinos are immigrants to the United States with a few exceptions that are granted refugee status (Cubans, some Columbians, El Salvadorans, Nicaraguans, and Guatemalans).

Statistics

Latino/Hispanics make up the largest minority in the United States (45,504,311 people according to 2007 Census estimates). The majority of Latino/Hispanics in the United States (as of July 2007) were males by more than 1.5 million. This is a tremendous increase of over 10 million people in only 7 years, as the number was 35,305,818 in the 2000 Census. The median age for both genders as of July, 2007, was 27.6 years of age. Nationally, 75% of Hispanic/Latino Americans are made up of Mexicans, Puerto Ricans, and Cubans (US Census Bureau, 2008).

According to the 2000 US Census data, the Latino/Hispanic population is growing rapidly in the United States. This minority group is the most prevalent, exceeding the number of African Americans. Latino/Hispanics now account for 12.5% of the US population. It is not clear if the change in labels used by the US Census in 2000 (inclusion of Latinos) is responsible for the increased numbers (US Census Bureau, 2008).

History of Hispanics in the United States

Having a historical perspective is helpful for the nurse to develop an understanding of the health status of Hispanics/Latinos. History provides perspective to the genetic, biologic, and environmental events and clarifies potential health behaviors that may be seen in practice.

In 1453, Constantinople fell to the Ottoman Turks, cutting off Europe's silk and spice trade with India and Asia. Thirty-nine years later, an Italian named Christoforo Colombo (Cristobal Colón in Spanish), or Christopher Columbus, sailing west for the Queen of Spain, first reached the New World thinking he had found a new route to the Orient. His first landfalls included Juana (Cuba) and the island of Hispaniola (known today as the Dominican Republic and Haiti).

The Conquistadors were committed to expansion of the Spanish empire and recovery of treasure for the crown. Spanish Catholic missions soon followed with the goal of winning new religious converts. Colonial administrators began spreading Spanish culture from Mexico across Central and South America. Spanish settlement of North America came early and included the first permanent European settlement of the New World at St. Augustine, Florida, in 1565. In 1598, Don Juan de Oñate colonized New Mexico.

Immigration was also impacted by US policies, such as Manifest Destiny and the Monroe Doctrine. The Spanish American War that brought Cuba and Puerto Rico under US administration in 1898 and various invasions of the Dominican Republic, Nicaragua, Honduras, and other parts of Central America caused waves of immigration following war, rebellion, and occupation. This process has continued as recently as the 1980s, when large numbers of Guatemalans, Nicaraguans, and Salvadorans fled to the United States to escape civil wars.

Mexican Americans

Mexican Americans are the largest group of Hispanics/Latinos. Mexican Americans are also referred to as Chicanos. The term Chicano is used solely to refer to people of Mexican descent. The term Chicano is controversial. Although it is an old word, many elderly Mexicans do not like the term because in the past it was a derogatory reference to Mexican peasants (peons). In the 1970s, the name "Los Chicanos" was taken by a militant group to make a political statement.

Mexico is a country in the southern part of North America. Mexico is the third largest Latin American nation, and it consists of 31 states and a federal district. In 1821, Mexico fought to win its independence from Spain. The Mexican American War was fueled by two major factors. The first was Manifest Destiny, which was the belief that America has a God-given right, or destiny, to expand its borders from the Atlantic to the Pacific oceans (or from sea to shining sea). This desire for expansion would result in tremendous negative impact on Mexicans as well as Native Americans and US citizens. The second was the Texas War of Independence. In the 1820s and 1830s, Mexico, newly free of Spain, needed settlers in its underpopulated northern parts. Anyone agreeing to take an oath of allegiance to Mexico and convert to Catholicism (the national religion) was permitted to settle in this area which was then known as the Mexican province of Texas. Many settlers became unhappy with the Mexican government and war broke out in 1835 when Texas revolted. In 1836, Santa Anna, the Mexican President, signed the Treaty of Velasco, granting Texas its independence. Many Mexicans refused to see the legality of the treaty because President Santa Anna was a prisoner at the time he signed the treaty. Border fights continued, often with savage fighting. This fighting resulted in some negative stereotypes regarding the Mexican people, some of which have persisted until today. As the conflict escalated, eventually full war broke out; the Mexican American War on April 25, 1846.

Following the Mexican American War, which ended in 1848, Mexico lost half of its northern territory to the United States. This change in the border has caused language and cultural obstacles that still exist today.

For the past 30 years, Mexico has been suffering with a significant financial crisis, which has resulted in high unemployment and the defaulting of the government in repaying foreign debts. The financial difficulty has been compounded by ongoing governmental and political conflict, which has contributed to many Mexicans deciding to leave Mexico and immigrate to the United States, both legally and illegally. The geographical closeness of Mexico to the United States as well as the extensive shared border, which is difficult to fully protect, has contributed to the ability of some Mexicans to move back and forth between Mexico and United States illegally. It is estimated that approximately one third of the undocumented aliens in the United States come from Mexico. Obviously, the lack of American citizenship presents a significant barrier to Mexicans who are in the United States illegally. Illegal aliens often suffer significant psychologic stress caused by fear of discovery and deportation back to Mexico. The implementation of laws requiring employees to present proof of US citizenship to employers often results in illegal immigrants to accept very low paying day work, such as picking crops. Despite the hardships the illegal immigrant is faced with in the United States, they are still motivated to leave Mexico because of the life-threatening poverty and political instability that is prevalent in that country. They hope that immigration into the United States will improve the economic conditions of themselves and their families. Immigration is often in response to the promise of employment, although most of the jobs are in low-paying agricultural and industrial labor positions. Mexican Americans often sacrifice being with their extended family back in Mexico in order to come to America with the hope of finding a job to support themselves and their families both in the United States and in Mexico.

There are also Mexican Americans who are descendants of the early Spanish settlers in what is today known as New Mexico. Over time, US citizens also began to settle into this formerly Mexican territory. These early settlers contributed greatly to the development of southwestern cities by sharing and teaching skills in mining, farming, and ranching with the newer settlers.

Today, Mexicans make up over 57% of the US Hispanic/Latino population and include at least 2 million seasonal migratory workers who spend part of the year in the United States and part in their native Mexico. This population group is least likely to have access to a regular source of healthcare services, most likely to underutilize the available healthcare services, and is least likely to have health insurance (National Alliance for Hispanic Health, 2001).

Definition of Health and Illness

The Hispanic/Latino culture views health from a synergistic point of view through the continuum of the mind, body, and spirit (espiritu). Symptoms of health and illness will present from the mind, body, and spirit connection.

Hispanics are far more emotionally expressive. They expect to be pampered when ill, as it is viewed as the way the family shows love and concern. They rely on their families, other relatives, and friends for support and help. They are not likely to accept or request the help from social workers or social services. This is a present-oriented society, and as such they may neglect preventive health care and may also show up late, or not at all, for appointments. Most Hispanics are Catholics, and birth control methods other than rhythm are unacceptable. Most Latin Americans see thinness as a problem and plumpness as the ideal. The nurse needs to consider this when counseling the patient or family on weight management issues as any advice that the patient receives recommending weight loss may not be followed because weight loss would result in a negative body image.

Curanderismo is defined as a medical system. It is a coherent view with historical roots that combines Aztec, Spanish, spiritualistic, homeopathic, and scientific elements. The *curandero* is a holistic healer; the people who seek help from him do so for social, physical, and psychologic purposes. Because the *curandero* has a religious orientation, much of the treatment includes elements of both the Catholic and Pentecostal rituals and artifacts: offerings of money, penance, confessions, lighting

---

Box 6-1

Pertinent Research Studies

Study #1

This study found that Hispanics who were treated for certain bone fractures at the University of California, Los Angeles (UCLA), Emergency Medicine Center were twice as likely as non-Hispanic Whites to receive no pain medication. The precise reason for this was not specified, but the investigators identified failure on the part of hospital staff to recognize pain in Hispanic patients as a possible reason for the discrepancy.

Source: Todd, M. D., Samara, N., & Hoffman, J. R. (1993). Ethnicity as a risk factor for inadequate emergency department analgesia. *Journal of the American Medical Association, 269*, 12, 1537–1539.

Study #2

For Spanish-speaking patients, having a language-concordant physician resulted in better outcomes for well-being and functioning. Monolingual Spanish-speaking patients were more likely to ask more questions and had a better understanding with physicians who also spoke Spanish.

Source: Pérez-Stable, E. J., Nápoles-Springer, A., & Miramontes, J. M. (1997) The effects of ethnicity and language on medical outcomes of patients with hypertension or diabetes. *Medical Care, 35*, 12, 1212–1219.

Study #3

Unfortunately, even when Hispanic patients have medical insurance and do seek medical services, they often must contend with a healthcare system that is not responsive to their needs. For example, a study of UCLA Emergency Medicine Center patients with long-bone fractures found that Hispanics were twice as likely as non-Hispanic White patients to be denied adequate pain medication (analgesia) in the emergency room. The study went on to find that ethnicity—not language, gender, or insurance status—was the main predicator for inadequate pain relief.

Source: Todd, M. D., Samaroo, N., & Hoffman, J. R. (1993). Ethnicity as a risk factor for inadequate emergency department analgesia. *Journal of the American Medical Association, 269*, 12, 1537–1539.

---

candles, wooden or metal offerings in the shape of the afflicted anatomic part, and laying on of hands.

Privacy is highly valued as it is felt that personal matters should be handled only within the family. Modesty is valued in Hispanic culture for all, not just for women. The nurse should recognize that the area between the waist and knees is considered particularly private. Privacy extends to childbirth. To attend a woman during delivery is viewed as the job of women; ideally, the job of the woman's mother and the midwife. In general, Hispanic/Latino women prefer that their mothers attend them during labor. Cultural tradition dictates that the husband does not see his wife or child until the delivery is over and both have been cleaned and dressed. Postpartum, the custom of lying-in may be followed. The lying-in period is designed to give a woman the period of rest between childbirth and returning to work. Traditionally in these cultures, women worked at hard physical jobs and required rest prior to resuming work.

Typically, Hispanics look down on people who are mentally ill. Patients with mental health concerns do not like to share this information with their relatives or friends and are shy of seeking professional help. Mental health problems and life stressors may appear as chest pain, shortness of breath, abdominal pain, sweats, and/or chronic illness (such as frequent headaches). These symptoms have traditional labels such as "de nervios" (stress). It is felt culturally that each has a specific cause and a nonmedication treatment. Mental health problems are often not validated within the culture and may carry a stigma as a sign of weakness.

Within the last century, health and illness have been approached through a variety of treatments, each with its own philosophical base. Some have been based on empirical science (mainstream medicine), some believe disorders linked to the musculoskeletal system can be corrected by physical manipulations (osteopathy), and some developed treatments based on the belief that minute doses of drugs that mimic diseases can be used to treat diseases (homeopathy). Still other approaches continue to base states of health on a purely spiritual belief system (Christian Science).

Combining respect for the benefits of mainstream medicine, tradition, and traditional healing, along with a strong religious component from their daily lives, Hispanic patients bring quite a broad definition of health to the medical encounter.

Health promotion and disease prevention strategies that focus on the mind-body-spirit connection would be culturally competent and would be more likely to meet with success. Keep in mind, however, that Hispanics/Latinos do not routinely seek out medical care unless they are ill. Seeking out preventive care is seen as an unaffordable luxury or odd. It is for this reason that participation in health screening by this population is low. The nurse should consider this and to use the mind-body-spirit focus when planning for and providing all patient education sessions. See Box 6-4 for more on this.

Traditional Healing Methods

The health and healing philosophy of Hispanics/Latinos is a result of a fusion of cultures. The Central and South American influences are a belief that the natural forces of the sun, moon, and the sea play an important role in an individual's health. Showing respect for these forces was viewed as the key to a healthy life. The Spanish influence is seen in the beliefs of the Catholic religion and Hippocrates' humoral theory of health. According to this theory, health is dependent on the proper distribution of the four humors of the body: blood, phlegm, yellow bile, and Black bile, which are further classified based on their physical properties as hot, cold, moist (wet), or dry. Illness was caused by an imbalance in the humors, and treatment was geared toward restoring balance.

Religion and faith are also considered important factors in health maintenance. Spiritual healing (curanderismo), magic (Santeria), and some herbal remedies were introduced by some African slaves, particularly in Brazil and the Caribbean.

In the Hispanic theory of disease, illness is a result between an imbalance between hot and cold. It is believed that exposure to extreme changes in temperature can cause illness; therefore, one must avoid extremes of hot or cold. Low metabolic diseases are "cold diseases," whereas "hot diseases" are highly metabolic. Specific conditions are classified as either hot or cold and the treatments are also classified as either hot or cold. See Box 6-5 for classification of common hot and cold disorders. The treatment recommended for any illness would have the opposite property of the illness. This means a "hot" illness would require a "cold" treatment. Because the female in the Hispanic/Latino culture is usually responsible for treating illness, it is usually the female who possesses the knowledge regarding alternative therapies. This information is usually handed down from a female relative to another female relative. The female will treat an illness until she feels it has progressed outside her area of expertise. Common illness is hardly ever brought into the formal healthcare system. It is at the discretion of the female caregiver if and/or when the patient will be brought into the formal healthcare system.

There are folk conditions that are culture bound as well. An "evil eye" (mal de ojo) is a spell that is cast as a result of someone looking at an infant and complimenting the child without physically touching the child. A susto (fright) is described as the experience of the spirit leaving the body as a result of a traumatic event and is associated with panic attacks. Ataque de nervios (attack of the nerves) occurs when a person is not able to deal with stress. Families may treat these folk conditions in more than one way. Some may do promesas (promises), let the hair grow long, dress the child or oneself in robes or White clothes, kneel-walk to church, or offer extra tidings to a specific church. Others may use amulets for good luck or to keep them healthy.

Although first-generation and new immigrants are more likely to hold traditional health beliefs, a significant number of Hispanics/ Latinos utilize at least one complementary/alternative modality either alone or in combination with conventional therapy. Today, there is an extensive practice of traditional medicine carried out by curanderas, espiritistas, or healers within the Hispanic/Latino community. In urbanized barrios, this tradition has been carried on, in part, by Hispanic pharmacists, familiar with both traditional treatments like té de manzanilla (chamomile tea), as well as placing a strong value on the use of modern prescription medicines such as antibiotics.

Alternative/Complementary Folk Medicine

It is possible that the Hispanic/Latino patient may be utilizing complementary/alternative medicine (CAM), specifically the use of herbal therapies that may be unfamiliar to you. The Hispanic/Latino population does utilize herbs that are unique from other groups. Some commonly used herbs are linden, sapodilla and star anise, brook mint, and passion flower.

CAM modalities are usually used to manage chronic conditions such as diabetes mellitus (DM), asthma, and hypertension. DM is considered a "hot disease." Home remedies for diabetes are usually administered in combination with traditional medicine. Nopal (cactus), aloe vera juice, and bitter gourd are three of the common home remedies used that may be unfamiliar to healthcare practitioners (Ortiz, Shields, Clauson, & Clay, 2007). The efficacy of these therapies is yet to be fully elucidated. Some published data suggest that nopal and bitter gourd may be helpful in reduction of blood glucose levels. Nopal may exert its effect as a result of high fiber content or have some insulin-sensitizing properties, and components of bitter gourd may have some insulin-like properties.

Hypertension is also a hot illness according to the Hispanic hot/cold theory. Anger (corajes), fear (susto), nervousness, and thick blood are thought to be the most common causes of hypertension in this belief system. Cold remedies are used to treat this condition including lemon juice, linden (tila) tea, passion flower tea (pasionara), and sapodilla (zapote blanco) tea. Minimal information is available about the safety or efficacy of these products, but all should be treated as pharmacologically active agents (Ortiz et al., 2007).

Asthma is considered a "cold" disease and remedies with "hot" properties, such as cod liver oil, oregano, lemon, and castor oil, along with massage, are the most popular modalities used as home remedies (Ortiz et al., 2007). A commercial product, called Siete Jarabes, is often used by Puerto Ricans to treat a cough (Ortiz et al., 2007).

It is important for the nurse to keep an open mind and to demonstrate acceptance toward the use of CAM. Hispanics/Latinos often do not inform healthcare professionals about their use of these practices. If a negative attitude is perceived, they will be even less likely to do so. Lack of knowledge about the use of these agents can put the patient in serious jeopardy. Whenever possible, and of course only if it is safe to do so, the nurse or nurse practitioner should encourage the use of CAM. This will result in improved adherence to conventional treatment and will help to gain the patient's trust. An easy way to do this would be to add the recommendation to a patient who must increase fluids to treat a cold or flu to use a natural tea drink or natural soup to facilitate the replacement of fluids and electrolytes (Ortiz et al., 2007).

Current Healthcare Problems Including Morbidity and Mortality

The use of the US healthcare system has been problematic for Latinos/Hispanics. There are several reasons for this. Lack of health insurance is a major problem for this group. There are many explanations offered for the lack of insurance including communication issues and a lack of understanding of a competitive healthcare system with the resultant understanding of the need for health insurance. Illegal or undocumented aliens do not qualify for Medicare or Medicaid, which has contributed to a lack of willingness to treat uninsured, indigent people. Another reason for Latinos/Hispanics not utilizing the US healthcare system is lack of access or transportation concerns. A third reason may be that the Mexican American group strives hard to maintain its cultural uniqueness and resists becoming absorbed into the dominant American culture. This desire to retain a cultural identity is often cited as a reason why Mexican Americans have experienced discrimination in education, jobs, and housing.

The median age for Hispanics/Latinos is much lower than for other ethnic groups (26.3 years compared to 36.6 years for the non-Hispanic White population), and this impacts the top causes of death for this group. The top 10 causes of death for Hispanics/Latinos of all age groups, according to the National Alliance for Hispanic Health (1996), are:

1. Heart disease
2. Malignant neoplasms
3. Accidents and adverse effects
4. Human immunodeficiency virus infection (HIV)
5. Homicide and legal intervention
6. Cerebrovascular diseases
7. DM
8. Chronic liver disease and cirrhosis
9. Pneumonia and influenza
10. Certain conditions originating in the prenatal period

Impact of Communication

The most common language spoken by Latinos/Hispanics is Spanish. A majority of Hispanics/Latinos in the United States are bilingual and likely to retain their Spanish language skills as their communities are replenished with new Spanish speaking immigrants. Although only 24% of Hispanics were born outside the United States and the Commonwealth of Puerto Rico, 77% report Spanish as their primary language and the language they speak at home.

Interfacing with Hispanics, appreciation of the Spanish language, and appreciating the different accents, idioms, and meanings within different Spanish-speaking subgroups are crucial to becoming culturally competent. Language is a communication tool by which cultural meaning is transferred and its complexity understood. When understanding language from this perspective, it is important to differentiate its layers. In its simplest form, each word has a meaning. The combination of words within a particular context takes on a specific cultural meaning.

The initial stage of language development is direct translation of words with their literal meaning. However, this level of language may not be effective in communicating health beliefs, core values, or a description of symptoms. As a result, language differences and the width of the gap pose a challenge to both the patient and provider in healthcare communication. To fully understand the complexities of language and culture, one has to examine the layer of language development. Primary language development, the first learned language, provides relational meaning to words and phrases that reflect culture. Secondary language development, or learning a second language, may not provide the speaker with the idiomatic expressions or cultural meanings specific to location and ethnicity. One can learn to speak a language without learning how to use the language to reflect culture. Although it is a difficult proposition, the message is that we should try to bridge any language differences because quality health care can be achieved and language differences overcome, even in the most extreme situations. Cultural competency is not necessarily indicated by the nurse's ability to speak the patient's language, but a patient/provider that do not share any language knowledge will have more challenges to quality care than those who have learned the other's language.

Language differences can have a major impact on diagnosis for the nurse practitioner who follows the medical model. Subjective diagnosis or assessing which modality to test for in determining a medical diagnosis is influenced by the patient's description of the symptoms. What the patient says and how they say it is essential to establishing the appropriate diagnosis. Without the element of communication, quality care can be obtained, but it is a challenge. The patient can become frustrated, does not return, or is unable to comply with treatment. Language discordance can result in misdiagnosis and incorrect patient treatment as well as contribute additional costs to patient care.

There is a growing number of healthcare professionals who care for America's multiethnic, multiracial, and increasingly multilingual society. According to the Census Bureau, at least 14% of the nation's population now speaks a language other than English in their home. In major cities including New York, Los Angeles, Miami, Honolulu, Newark, and El Paso, Texas, the figure is over 40%. More alarmingly, there are approximately 7 million persons in the United States who

Box 6-2

Seven Approaches for Bridging Language Barriers

1. **Bilingual/Bicultural Professional Staff**
   - Recruit and retain bilingual/bicultural staff at all levels of the organization.
   - Provide significant additional compensation for bilingual ability.

2. **Interpreters**
   - Establish minimum standards for interpreter training, competency, and other continuing education efforts.
   - Make a concerted effort to increase and foster medical interpreter training through national conferences, information clearinghouses, technical assistance, and start-up grants.
   - Provide courses designed to train providers to work with interpreters.
   - Use only trained medical interpreters.
   - Reimburse for interpreter services.

3. **Language Skills Training for Existing Staff**
   - Support the development of bilingual skills for all staff members.
   - Establish clear goals and realistic expectations for Spanish language courses, including idioms.
   - Offer classes in medical Spanish to all staff.
   - Utilize training programs that have a demonstrated track record in increasing the bilingual level or the interpretation quality of services provided.

4. **Internal Language Banks** (Only as a back-up measure)
   - Hire supervisors to assess the language and interpretation capabilities of language bank members, to provide minimal interpreter training, and to regularly assess the quality of the language bank program.
   - List interpretation as a secondary responsibility of language bank members so that supervisors of these staff members understand why they may spend time away from their regular duties.
   - Compensate language bank members who do a significant amount of interpretation.

5. **Phone-Based Interpreter Services** (Emergency back-up measure for brief follow-up questions only.)
   - Inform healthcare providers that phone-based interpreters may not be proficient in medical terminology.
   - Use simple or common terms when using phone interpreters.

6. **Written Translators** (Emergency stop-gap measures, never as the sole means of communication)
   - Develop mechanisms to promote the sharing of bilingual written materials, such as consent forms and patient education pamphlets.

7. **Cultural Mediators**
   - In addition to medical interpreting, the cultural mediator interprets the cultural and social circumstances that may affect care.
   - This enables providers to gain a more comprehensive understanding of patients needs and to negotiate culturally appropriate plans of care.

*Two common approaches to resolving language differences are so detrimental that they require "*Do not Statements.*"

Do not use patient's relatives, especially those who are younger in age as interpreters.

Do not use support staff whose primary job is NOT translation.

Source: National Alliance for Hispanic Health. (2001). *Quality health services for Hispanics: The cultural competency component.* Washington, DC: US Department of Health and Human Services.

do not speak English well, if at all. Spanish is the second most common language spoken in the United States after English and is the language spoken by half of the non-English speakers in the United States (US Census Bureau, 2008).

Language diversity in the Spanish language exists in terms of pitch, vocabulary, accent, pronunciation, dialect, and grammar rules depending on the country of origin. There are over 50 different languages and dialects in Mexico and over 15 in Central and South America. People from the Caribbean have a higher pitch and different accent compared with the people in Central and South America. Puerto Ricans do not pronounce the last "s" and pronounce the double "r" with guttural sounds; Spaniards pronounce the "c" with a "z" sound. One word can be benign in one country and considered rude or offensive in another. The nurse must be careful when using Spanish (if not her first language) when communicating with a patient. Other difficulties are verb tenses and pronoun construction, which are very different than those used in the English language.

Many Hispanics/Latinos speak with their hands and become very animated when expressing emotion or giving emphasis to their words. Nodding the head does not indicate agreement with what was said, just that it was heard. This is a very important concept for the nurse to remember when communicating with Hispanic/Latino patients.

It is important to be aware that not all Latinos/Hispanics are Spanish speakers. Although Brazil, Belize, and Haiti are all considered Latin American countries, the official language of Brazil is Portuguese, English is the official language of Belize, and French or Creole are the primary languages used in Haiti. Literacy, in any language, should not be assumed. It also should never be assumed that all communication between Spanish speakers will be understood by all other Spanish speakers. This is because there are many words and phrases that have different usages and meanings in different countries. This is important for the nurse to consider when dealing with the use of an interpreter who is not of the same ethnic group as the patient.

There have been six identified approaches for bridging language barriers. The six approaches are listed in order from most to least effective (for more information on these six approaches see Box 6-2):

1. Bilingual/bicultural professional staff
2. Interpreters
3. Language skills training for existing staff
4. Internal language banks
5. Phone-based interpreter services
6. Written translators

Ten tips that the nurse can follow to have successful patient interactions across cultures are listed in Box 6-7, and Box 6-8 includes five tips for working with interpreters.

Impact of Time

Mexican Americans have a present orientation to time and are often unable or reluctant to consider the future when planning. The Mexican custom of the siesta comes from this present orientation to time. It is believed that the present need for rest takes priority over safeguarding the future through the generation of more work/income.

It is felt that a present time orientation, or elasticity, is responsible for the lack of social upward mobility in Mexican Americans as well as a barrier to assimilation and integration into the mainstream American culture. This focus on the present to the exclusion of the future may result in missed appointments or being late for appointments. This is a result of the concern for a present activity and not for the activity of planning ahead to be on time. The concept of elasticity implies that present activities cannot be recovered if lost or missed, whereas future activities can be recovered.

It is important for the nurse to consider the present orientation to time when planning for patient education. Focusing on long-term effects (such as what could occur if medication is missed or discontinued) will not be as beneficial as focusing on any potential short-term problems that could occur.

Impact of Space and Touch

Mexican Americans value physical contact and having a close physical space with family members. As a group, they demonstrate togetherness. A pattern of socialization begins in childhood when parents are permissive, warm, and caring with all of their children. In later years, girls remain much closer to home and are protected and guarded, whereas boys are allowed to be with other boys in informal social groups to develop machismo. Although Mexican Americans are comfortable with physical touching among their social group, a female nurse should always assist a male physician in examining a female client to preserve modesty. Male patients may refuse a complete physical examination because of modesty factors. Females prefer caregivers of the same gender. Nursing care may be resisted if the Mexican American feels that the caregiver is different from the patient. Details are important as both space and touch influence the patient encounter. The nurse should consider maintaining a close personal space—close enough where a handshake would be possible without moving closer. Eye contact and touching are also important components to an effective interaction. For more on cultural nuances that govern social interactions, see Box 6-3.

Impact of the Environment

Mexican Americans have an external locus of control. This is the belief that the outcome of circumstances is controlled by external forces. They believe that life is under the constant influence of God (or divine will). There is also a reliance on fatalism. This is the belief that one is at the mercy of the environment and has little control over the environment or what occurs. It is felt that personal efforts are unlikely to influence a situation's outcome. This means that Mexican Americans do not believe that they are personally responsible for any future successes or failures. This can be especially impactful when asking the Mexican American patient to participate in screening or health maintenance activities because failing to see any value will not encourage participation.

The environmental health status of Hispanic communities is poor and is a major source of health problems. Among their high-risk exposures are ambient air pollution, worker exposure to chemicals in industry, pollution indoors, and pollutants in drinking water. In terms of exposure, Hispanics consistently face the worst exposure levels, or levels that represent significant threats to health. Nurse practitioners and nurses should consider environmental sources in diagnosing and treating a variety of conditions that affect their Hispanic/Latino patients.

Biologic Variations

Several diseases occur with high incidence in Mexican Americans. The incidence of diabetes is five times the national average with a higher rate of complications. There is an increased tendency toward decreased insulin action in peripheral tissues, skeletal muscle, and also in the liver. The incidence may also be a result of increased abdominal obesity, and there may also be abnormalities in beta-cell function (this is not yet well understood), which, in combination, may lead to more problems. Thirty-six percent of Mexican American women and 28% of Mexican American men have metabolic syndrome (this diagnosis requires at least three medical abnormalities from the following disorders: high fasting plasma glucose, high triglycerides, low high-density lipoproteins cholesterol, high blood pressure, or increased abdominal obesity). Sixty-five percent of Hispanic women are overweight and 62% of Hispanic men are overweight.

There are cultural aspects that influence diabetes care that are specific for the Hispanic/Latino population. The following have been identified as factors that may influence diabetes care: family orientation, fatalism, faith/religion, body image, nutrition/physical activity, acculturation, language, and myths. In the Hispanic/Latino culture, the family is the primary unit—this is referred to as "familisimo." The family's needs are placed above an individual's needs. They also place a strong emphasis on "respecto." Respecto dictates deferential behavior toward others based on their position of authority, social position, gender, and economic status. Hispanic/Latino patients expect their healthcare providers to engage in nonhealth-related conversation. The attitude of the healthcare provider is also analyzed by the patient. It is important for the nurse to realize that a neutral attitude can be perceived as negative by the Hispanic/Latino patient.

When caring for Hispanic/Latino patients, it is important to try to win their "confianza." This is done by showing a respect for their culture. Being open and warm with the patient will help to develop confianza. The development of a therapeutic relationship will be difficult, if not impossible, if confianza has not been achieved. Fatilismo is a significant threat to providing effective nursing care. Fatilismo is the belief that you cannot change your destiny or fate. Thus, fatalismo acts as a barrier to self-care, something that is held in high esteem by nurses and all healthcare professionals who are trained in the Western biomedical model.

When providing for patient education regarding DM with the Hispanic/Latino patient, the nurse should recognize that a preference has been found for listening to stories over reading printed materials. In a study conducted at the Latino Diabetes Initiative at the Joplin Diabetes Center by Dr. Caballero (2005), patients learned more and retained more information when it was presented in an audio-based manner rather than with printed material. Culturally appropriate resources are available from the American Diabetes Association, National Diabetes Education Program, and the National Institute of Health and nutritional information is available from the National Dietetics Organization. The Joslin Diabetes Center Web site (www.joslin.org) is an excellent resource because it has initiatives for the African American, Asian American, and Hispanic/Latino cultural groups. Another study by Caballero (2006) found that one out of three Hispanics/Latinos believe that insulin causes blindness. The belief in this myth was found to be highly correlated with decreased adherence to the diabetes management plan and highlights the need to address pertinent myths, such as this, when providing patient education.

Hypertension is also found with an increased prevalence among Mexican Americans, as this group is slightly more likely to have high blood pressure than non-Hispanic Whites. The onset of pernicious anemia, which is most often seen in the elderly, has been shown to occur in those of Latin American origin at a younger age than in White patients.

Approximately 85% of the health problems common to Mexican Americans involve communicable diseases, including respiratory tract infections, diarrhea, and skin disorders (National Center for Health Statistics, 2002). The risk of contracting tuberculosis (TB) among Hispanics/Latinos is more than four times the risk among non-Hispanic Whites. Among Hispanics, TB is most prevalent in young adults aged 25–44 years. Evidence suggests that the HIV epidemic is, in part, responsible for the recent increases in TB. TB also appears to be a significant problem for migrant workers. This is a group that would benefit from TB screening.

The prevalence of HIV is a major concern. By 1997, Hispanics/Latinos made up 12% of the total US population yet accounted for 21% of the new acquired immunodeficiency syndrome (AIDS) cases, and HIV diagnoses have gone up 10% in this group, whereas other ethnic groups, such as African Americans, have seen a decline. The primary mode of exposure is heterosexual sexual activity with an intravenous drug abuser.

AIDS strikes Puerto Ricans the hardest, followed by Cubans, probably, in part, because Puerto Ricans and Cubans are concentrated in East Coast cities where AIDS has taken a high toll. Mexican Americans seem less affected by the epidemic. Overall, Hispanic men are nearly twice as likely as White non-Hispanic men to die from AIDS, and Hispanic women are nearly five times as likely to die from the disease as White non-Hispanic Women (National Alliance for Hispanic Health, 2001).

Malignant neoplasms are the second leading cause of death in the United States among both Hispanics and non-Hispanic Whites, although Hispanics have a slightly lower rate. This trend continues with cardiovascular disease. Although it is the leading cause of death for Hispanic/Latinos, the incidence is less than found in Whites or African Americans, despite the fact that Hispanics/Latinos have a higher prevalence of conditions, such as obesity and DM, that increase the risk for coronary heart disease.

Hispanic/Latino men are more likely to have undiagnosed and untreated hypertension than the national average. Although Hispanic/Latino women are more likely than men to be aware of the diagnosis, they are more unlikely to have it be controlled or treated. It appears that race is a significant factor in hypertension. There also appears to be a genetic link to DM as the incidence of noninsulin-dependent DM appears to be highest in Mexican Americans who have a substantial Pima Indian heritage.

Impact of Social Organization

It is not possible to make accurate generalizations about an area as large and diverse as Latin America. There are many different kinds of Latinos/Hispanics. The intent of this section of this chapter is to provide some background on Latino/Hispanic family life and to acknowledge the impact the struggle for economic survival experienced by many in this group has caused. The prevalence of economic hardship and the increase number of children in this group has resulted in poverty being the way of life for most Latino/Hispanic children. Childbearing is still the highest social status available to Latino/Hispanic women. High costs place marriage out of reach for many poor, and for those who are unhappily married, divorce is often financially out of reach.

According to 2000 US Census data, 70.2% of Mexican American families were married couple families, whereas 21% were female-headed households. Thirty-one percent of Mexican American households had five or more people making up the household compared with 12% among non-Hispanic Whites. Latinos/Hispanics are a rapidly growing group. They are a younger population with 35.7% aged 18 years old or younger. The mean age for this group is 25.8 years, and Mexican Americans are the youngest group among all Latinos/Hispanics (US Department of Commerce, 2000).

The family is the most valued institution and the main focus for social identification. Elders have a prestigious status in the Hispanic family because of their experience. Family members look to elders for advice. An individual who becomes sick will turn first to family members, especially elders, for support, comfort, and advice. They may recommend safe, simple home remedies.

In the traditional household, the man is the head of the family and makes all major decisions. There is a strong sense of paternalism what most Westerners call "male dominance," but the female's role is equivalent and she is the maternal powerhouse in her home. The truth is that the female is sacred and revered, often protected, not because she cannot handle herself or has no voice, but because the solidarity of the family unit depends on her well-being. The nuclear family is strong, but there also commonly exists many extended families of three or more generations. Men are the authority figure and women tend to maintain traditional roles. The Hispanic/Latino family is usually patriarchal; however, the mother cares for the children and older relatives and possesses power within the family. Mothers within the Mexican American community enjoy a high social status. Mexican American women consider motherhood a desirable role and are likely to leave a career during pregnancy to care for self and the pregnancy and to remain out of work to care for their children as they grow. Many Mexican American mothers rate their role as a mother as second in importance only to God. It is felt that personal behavior has the potential for increasing community respect for the family.

An important concept for Mexican Americans is familism. Familism is a model of social organization, based on the prevalence of the family group and its well-being being placed against the interest

Box 6-3

Common Cultural Nuances for Hispanics in the United States and Its Impact on Nursing Care

Disclaimer: It is always important to note that there can be individual variation from any cultural norm.

La Familia (Family)

Hispanics include many members in their extended family. Family involvement often is critical in the care of the patient. For many, several family members and extended family members such as commadres, compadres, or padrinos (godparents) will accompany patients to medical visits. Often, family members include the very young and very old. They will want to hear what is being said and participate in the interactions. This may be in violation of institution rules that may limit the number of patient visitors to only two at a time. Hispanic families also traditionally emphasize interdependence over independence and cooperation over competition, and are therefore far more likely to be involved in the treatment and decision-making process for a patient. This level of involvement may not always be possible but should be encouraged and supported by the nurse if at all possible. Flexibility is required of the nurse. The patient may not be the one responding to the provider's questions or even the one asking questions because he or she may defer to someone in the familial group. The person conversing with the provider may be a spouse, the eldest family member, son or daughter, or friend. Often, the spokesperson will be the person who has the most respect and power in the family. Most often, the speaker is the matriarch/patriarch or, in many cases in the United States, it is the more acculturated children.

If it is the children, the nurse needs to be aware that this will cause a disruption in the family dynamics. The nurse must be respectful and inclusive of the elders even though the younger family members may be the key communicator. The nurse must understand the collective nature of this interaction to realize the patient may not be the key decision maker for symptom descriptions, treatment options, or compliance. Getting the whole family on board with any treatment decisions offers the best chance for a positive outcome.

Respeto (Respect)

Respeto dictates appropriate deferential behavior toward others based on age, sex, social position, economic status, and authority. This means that elders expect respect from younger people, men expect it from women, and employers from their employees. Nurses, by virtue of our education and calling toward healing, are afforded much respeto from Hispanic/Latino patients. A sign of respect from a Hispanic/Latino patient to the nurse would be the avoidance of eye contact. On the other hand, it would be considered disrespectful for the nurse not to maintain eye contact with the patient, even if another is translating for the patient. Often, the nurse will exclude the patient or focus on the translator, which is felt to be very disrespectful by the patient.

If the patient feels that the nurse is being disrespectful, they may terminate the therapeutic relationship. The nurse needs to be sensitive when asking essential history questions and consider a different approach when dealing with the Hispanic/Latino patient. Avoid asking direct questions about things that would be considered too personal or information that should stay within the family (such as alcohol intake, incidence of domestic or substance abuse, sexual activity, or family history of mental illness). Directly asking for this information may be viewed as challenging and disrespectful to the practice of keeping such things within the family. A better approach is to ask for the essential information in a more nondirect manner.

Pearls for the nurse to follow to maintain respect from Hispanic/Latino patients:

1. If you are younger than the patient, you should use formal titles and more formality when communicating with the patient to convey respect to the patient because they are your elder. The formal title can be spoken in either English or Spanish. The Spanish terms are *señor* (Mister), *don* (Sir), *señora* (Missus), or *doña* (Madam).

2. Even if you do not speak Spanish, offering an opening Spanish phrase at the beginning of the interaction (such as "buenos dias," which means good morning) suggests that you have respect for the Spanish language and the patient. Make sure to use formality when speaking Spanish.

3. Encourage the patient to ask questions. Often out of a sign of respect, the Hispanic/Latino patient will avoid asking questions that may appear to be challenging and instead will just not follow the treatment plan or end medical care totally. There is a cultural taboo against expressing negative feelings directly. Nurses need to take seriously the responsibility and respeto (respect) conferred on them by many Hispanic patients. The nurse needs to explain all medical procedures and treatments thoroughly, and to ascertain through careful questioning whether the patient has fully understood the explanations and instructions he or she has received.

Personalismo (Personal)

Hispanics expect health providers to be warm, friendly, and personal, and to take an active interest in the patient's life. The nurse should offer the patient a personal greeting that will put the patient at ease prior to any needed intervention. The Hispanic/Latino patient often develops loyalty to their primary care provider and other regular caregivers, which can have significant implications for continuity of care. When assigning nursing staff to care for a Hispanic/Latino patient and his or her family, keeping the same nursing assignment (if at all possible) during the course of the admission will be very helpful toward establishing personalismo. The nurse should also recognize that Hispanics/Latinos prefer a close personal space. The standard 2-ft-away space traditionally utilized during history taking can be perceived as the nurse being uncaring, uninterested, or detached from the patient. This can be overcome if the nurse leans forward, sits closer, or uses other body language cues (such as patting the patient's hand) that indicate the nurse has a personal interest in the patient as a human being.

Confianza (Trust)

Respecting the patient's culture and showing interest in the patient can, over time, result in the development of confianza. This means that the patient believes that the nurse has the patient's best interest at heart. Unfortunately, in today's healthcare system where time with our patients is extremely limited, achieving this level of trust is rare. The nurse should still strive to establish this level of trust because it will result in increased compliance on the patient's part, which will improve the patient's health outcome.

and necessities of each one of its individual members. It is part of a traditional view of society and highlights loyalty, trust, and cooperative attitudes within the family group. There are positives and negatives associated with familism. Familism provides a source of collective pride which is a strong positive. Familism has also been identified as a major cause of resistance to change and it is felt to be a contributor to the lack of collective and individual progress found in this group.

Impact of Faith and Spirituality

The vast majority of Latinos/Hispanics are Catholic with an increasing presence of Pentecostals. In addition to spirituality, the Catholic religion also has a powerful influence on the perceptions of norms and behaviors, beliefs about social interaction, and spiritual ideas regarding fate and faith. The Catholic Church and Catholic religion provide a powerful source of support, hope, and strength within the Latino/Hispanic community. Health is a gift from God and should not be taken for granted. The prevention of illness is an accepted practice that is accomplished with prayer, the wearing of religious medals or amulets, and keeping relics in the home. Visiting shrines, offering medals and candles, offering prayers, and the lighting of candles is a frequently observed practice. Many homes have shrines with statues and pictures of saints. The candles are lit here and prayers are recited. Many believe that illness is a result of God's will and that fate controls life and health. Spirituality can be manifested as a fatalistic feeling in which individuals are seen as having little control over their lives and health or by the optimistic belief that divine faith and trust can overcome any possible adverse event. Family and faith are the two most important sources of strength

---

Box 6-4

Body-Mind-Spirit Focus for Patient Education

Body
1. Do not smoke.
2. Limit alcohol.
3. Eat healthy meals.
4. Exercise regularly.
5. Listen to your body.

Mind
1. Set limits.
2. Learn to relax.
3. Worry less.
4. Give yourself time for pleasure.
5. Nurture healthy relationships.

Spirit
1. Do good acts.
2. Think good thoughts.
3. Have quiet time to yourself.
4. Pray.
5. Have lots of family and friends around to listen and talk with.

---

to Hispanics/Latinos. Most will not have living wills or advance directives caused by the belief that it is God's decision as to when it is your time to die and that no one should make that decision on their own. They believe that they possess a spirit and a soul and that their spiritual needs must be given attention.

The Protestant religion is gaining some Latino/Hispanic followers. The grass root efforts of the Protestant Evangelical Movement are making inroads as an organizing force for Latinos/Hispanics.

Many Mexican Americans (as high as 72% in a study by Kalish & Reynolds, 1981) believe that whatever the cause of death, it is God's will. This compares with just 56% of Anglo Americans (Kalish & Reynolds, 1981).

Puerto Ricans

Puerto Ricans are the second largest Hispanic/Latino group in the United States. Puerto Ricans are American citizens who possess a different language and culture. The island is located about 1000 miles east-southeast of Miami. The geography of the island, which encompasses 3425 square miles, is diverse and includes a central mountain range, northern coastal plains, low eastern mountains, and the El Yunque rain forest.

The island was claimed for Spain by Christopher Columbus in 1493. Columbus found the island was populated by Taino Indians who were living in small villages. The Spanish colonizers who arrived in 1508 were welcomed by the Taino. The port of San Juan (today the capital of Puerto Rico) became a very important military outpost in the Caribbean for Spain.

Under the leadership of Governor Juan Ponce de Leon, extremely brutal treatment came to the Taino Indians. A fixed number of Indians were distributed to officials and colonists to provide forced (wage free) labor.

Those that come to the mainland are in a unique position; they are technically neither natives nor immigrants. Despite the fact that Puerto Ricans are American citizens, there is a general lack of knowledge that it is a poor island and the culture is also not well known or understood by the many Americans. When many Puerto Ricans come to the mainland, they bring with them problems from the island such as poor health and poor socioeconomic status. Most migrate to the East Coast with the largest number living in New York City and New Jersey. They come to the mainland in search of a better life or to join family members already here. Unemployment is very high on the island.

According to the US Census Bureau, there are 3 million people living on the US mainland and 3.2 million living on the island of Puerto Rico. Nine percent of the Hispanic population is made up of Puerto Ricans (US Census Bureau, 2008).

Puerto Rico was discovered by Columbus in 1492 and conquered by Ponce de Leon in 1508. The natives who lived there, the Taino and Arawak Indians were killed off through starvation and forced labor. Yoruba African slaves were then brought to the island to work in the sugar cane fields. Eventually, the slaves were freed and intermarried, which resulted in the two cultures and beliefs being incorporated into a new culture. In 1815, more Spanish settlers came to the island and attempted to establish themselves as the elite, which caused tension between the groups. In 1897, Puerto Rican nationalists declared themselves independent from Spain. A year later during the Spanish American War, the US landed in Puerto Rico and maintained its claim to the island. In 1917, Puerto Ricans were made US citizens under the Jones Act. In 1952, Puerto Rico was declared a commonwealth of the United States.

Economic underdevelopment on the island has resulted in a large number of Puerto Ricans coming to the mainland of the United States, which has resulted in large Puerto Rican communities in New York and throughout the Northeast and Chicago. Because of the relationship between the United States and Puerto Rico, Puerto Ricans can easily move back and forth freely between the mainland and the island. It is for this reason that they are unlike other Hispanics/Latinos in that they can maintain many cultural, family, and social connections with their island home even after many years of living in the mainland of the United States.

Traditional Health Beliefs

Many people from Puerto Rico share similar health beliefs as other Hispanics/Latinos and are most similar to the beliefs held by Mexican Americans. There are, however, important differences in how health and illness are perceived by Mexicans and Puerto Ricans. They classify their diseases as hot or cold, like the Mexicans, but they have three categories for treatments: hot (caliente), cold (frio), and cool (fresco). Cold illnesses are treated with hot treatments, and hot diseases are treated with either cold or cool remedies. The goal is to maintain the proper hot–cold balance in the body. In addition, some Puerto Ricans also practice Santeria.

Santeria is a form of magic that has a very structured system. It was first practiced in Nigeria by the Yorubas. Many Yorubas were brought to America as slaves, and in time, the practice has been handed down through the generations. There is a reliance on storytelling to promote coping with life. The traditional religion brought from Nigeria was, over time, combined with Catholicism. The Yoruba gods (orishas) were identified with Christian saints, so the saints were invested with supernatural God-like powers.

Box 6-5	
Disease Classification Based on the Hot/Cold Theory	
Disease or Condition Classification	
Arthritis	Cold
Common cold	Cold
Constipation	Hot
Diarrhea	Hot
Fever	Hot
Indigestion	Cold
Menstrual pain	Cold
Muscle spasm	Cold
Pregnancy	Hot
Rash/hives	Hot
Stomachache	Cold
Ulcer	Hot

Box 6-6

Pain Response in Hispanics/Latinos

To most Hispanics/Latinos, pain is accepted as part of life, a fate that one is obligated to endure. Accepting pain without complaint is a sign of courage and strength. Pain may also signify immoral behavior, a punishment from God. Pain can also represent disharmony between the person and the environment and, therefore, must be managed in order to restore balance. When Hispanics/Latinos describe pain, they do with emotional terms that may not be easy to quantify, such as terrible, doloroso, or fatal. Because of machismo, some males may exhibit a high tolerance for pain and not complain. Studies have shown that Hispanics/Latinos are less likely to receive pain medication or to have their pain acknowledged by medical staff than are White ethnic groups.

There is a hierarchy in Santeria. Certain people claim to have facultades which provide them with the ability to practice. It is believed that the facultades was given to the healer from the Catholic saints. The head is a man, the babalow; second is the presidente who is the head medium; and third are the santeros. Novices to Santeria are called believers. Santeria can be and is practiced anywhere—even in some college dormitories. Santeros wear special beaded bracelets so they can be identified by other believers. They wear White robes during the conduction of ceremonies.

Mental health is also viewed somewhat differently by Puerto Ricans. They have a higher tolerance for what others may consider odd or unique behaviors. They make a very sharp distinction between what would be odd behavior versus being "loco." To be loco is considered to be dangerous or evil and will result in the loss of all social status. As such, Puerto Ricans who seek mental health treatment are ostracized and criticized by their community. It is acceptable to seek help from a santero; the symptoms are accepted because they are not attributed to the patient but to spirits outside the body which are causing the mental illness. The santero also will maintain confidentiality so the patient has no worry about being labeled or judged—or more importantly, worry that his confidence will be violated. Culturally competent mental health providers need to recognize the prevalence of santero when dealing with the mentally ill Puerto Rican, as the reliance on santero in that situation can be frequent. The inclusion of a belief in God and the benefit of prayer will also be an important cultural component of the treatment plan.

Impact of Communication

Both Spanish and English are the two official languages of Puerto Rico, despite the fact that many Puerto Ricans do not speak English well or at all. An attempt was made, because of political pressure, to pass a bill to make Spanish the only official language of the island. Equal status was restored to both languages shortly after that, and today, Spanish tends to be the language spoken at home and in schools, whereas English is used for all federal matters, is spoken in major Puerto Rican tourist sites, and is taught as a second language in most schools. Of all Puerto Ricans, those from large cities are more likely to read, understand, and speak at least some English.

Puerto Rican Spanish is unique and differs from the Spanish from other cultures, which may present a problem when the use of

---

Box 6-7

Ten Tips for Improving the Cross-Cultural Patient Interaction

1. Let the culture of the patient determine how you treat the patient.

   The Golden Rule of doing unto others does NOT work across cultures. We are all not the same and our responses are also individual. Culture determines the rules for what is considered appropriate nursing care.

2. Formality is best.

   The use of first names as a means of communicating respect and equality is unique to the United States. In most countries, a respectful distance is maintained between patient and nurse. Unless the patient is a child or young adult, it is best to use the patient's last name when addressing the patient unless and until told otherwise.

3. Be aware of how the patient may be showing you respect as it may be negatively impacting them.

   Our cultural group determines how we show respect. Patients want to show you respect as the nurse for your knowledge and position. In many countries, it is disrespectful to look directly at another person (especially one in authority) or to contribute to the authority figure losing face by asking questions. Encourage the patient to ask any questions that they may have.

4. Determine the patient's views on how they maintain health, causes of illness, and methods to prevent or cure illness. Do not assume.

   Perform a cultural assessment by asking questions that will help you determine the patient's beliefs about health and illness.

5. Do not discount your patient's beliefs.

   Allow the patient to be open and honest with you in regard to their traditional health beliefs or the use of alternative or complementary medicine practices.

6. Consider that the patient may have supernatural beliefs.

   The patient may believe that their illness is caused by bewitchment or the casting of a spell or the evil eye as a punishment for something they may have done. Ask the patient about their beliefs.

7. Use indirect questioning when asking about supernatural beliefs.

   An indirect approach is more likely to be successful.

8. Determine the value of including the entire family in the treatment plan.

   In many cultures, medical decisions are made by the entire family. Inclusion of the family increases the likelihood of gaining patient compliance.

9. Use restraint when discussing bad news or potential complications—do not exceed the amount of information that the patient can handle.

   The "need to know it all" is an American custom. In some cultures, placing yourself in your provider's hands is the ultimate sign of trust. The nurse should watch for signs that the patient has learned as much as they are able to deal with.

10. If not contraindicated, incorporate the patient's traditional health beliefs into the plan of care.

    The inclusion of the patient's health beliefs will encourage the development of trust and compliance in the treatment plan.

Source: Salimbene, S. (2000). Providing culture-sensitive care to African Americans. In: *What language does your patient hurt in? A practical guide to culturally competent patient care.* Amherst, MA: Diversity Resources.

an interpreter is required. When an interpreter lacks the cultural and linguistic background in Puerto Rican Spanish, the meaning of the words may change from one culture to the next and the translation may be inaccurate. Nonverbal communication and symbolism are conveyed with hand gestures and facial expressions and are a critical component of the message being sent. A close distance is maintained by Puerto Ricans when talking, and they may feel slighted if the nurse were to move away, even slightly, during a clinical encounter. The use of titles to show respect is also valued as is saving face. A Puerto Rican patient who speaks limited English may be hesitant to ask the nurse for even basic clarification or to slow down the speed of her speech. They have a tendency to be sensitive especially if they interpret an action as being a rejection of them. In addition, tone of voice is unique in that it is typically melodic and peaceful. A tone of voice that is considered high in pitch and inflection may be perceived as confrontational and the nurse should consider this when communicating with Puerto Rican patients.

Impact of Social Organization

The family, and especially children, is highly valued, and the patient may rely on the advice and guidance of older adults and elders. In some families, it is the eldest son or daughter who has the final decision-making authority for health-related matters; if the patient is married, the wife will typically consult her husband. This may vary depending on the age of the family members and the patient, so the nurse should establish who has decision-making authority on an individual basis.

Impact of Faith and Spirituality

The vast majority of Puerto Ricans are Catholic (estimated at 85%), whereas the remainder are made up of Protestants and agnostics/atheists. Despite the separation of church and state in Puerto Rico, religion plays a highly public role. Many Christians may also practice espiritismo (spiritualism) which is a blend of Indian, African, and Catholic beliefs. This is the belief that both good and bad spirits are present and can be influenced through the use of herbs and rituals.

There are important cultural beliefs related to death and dying for this cultural group that the nurse must be aware of. In some Hispanic families, there is a code of silence which means the patients are not informed that they are terminally ill. In this situation, the family will wish to provide a constant vigil and the family's spiritual leader should be with the patient at the time of death. The nurse should then notify the appointed family spokesperson for the news to then be communicated to the rest of the family members. The family may wish private time to say final goodbyes and this may include touching and kissing of the loved one's body. Organ donation is often supported in this culture as a way to help others, but the nurse must handle this matter very delicately. On the other hand, autopsies are not supported as it is viewed as invasive and a violation to the body. If an autopsy is required, the reason must be clearly communicated to the family spokesperson and consent obtained.

Biologic Variations

It appears that health and quality of life for Puerto Ricans are affected by a multifaceted combination of biology, demographics, and socioeconomic status. Lower income is associated with decreased quality of life and increased illness, whereas the opposite is true with a higher income. When counseling patients about a healthy body, it is important to recognize the value that is placed on excessive body weight in the Puerto Rican culture. Being thin or underweight is viewed negatively as it is associated with poor health and illness, whereas being overweight is associated with good health and an economic advantage. This belief must be considered and incorporated into the nurse's patient teaching plan. This is especially important when providing nutritional counseling for the diabetic Puerto Rican patient. As with other Hispanic/Latino groups, type 2 diabetes is a major health problem.

Cuban Americans

Cuban Americans make up about 4% of the Hispanic/Latino population in the United States. Cuba is only 90 miles from Key West, Florida. It was colonized by Spain in 1511 and all of its native people were killed. Cuba and its capital port of Havana became a major shipping and transportation hub. It was a key port in the trade of rum, sugar, cod, and slaves. Because all of its native people were killed, Cuba's population was made up of European settlers and African slave laborers. In 1902, the United States granted Cuba its independence but maintained a major influence over the island, which became a popular resort destination for the next 50 years until the Cuban Revolution of 1959.

The Cuban Revolution of 1959 that overthrew the regime of Fulgencio Batista and brought Fidel Castro to power drove close to half a million upper- and middle-class refugees to south Florida. Between 1965 and 1978, many Cuban immigrants came directly from Cuba, whereas others came through Spain, Mexico, and Jamaica to the United States. In the late 1970s and early 1980s, Cubans came to America when Castro allowed political prisoners to meet their families. The last large group arrived in the early 1980s and was referred to as the "Marielitos," because they left from the Mariel port in Havana, Cuba. This group of immigrants was of a lower socioeconomic status, some had criminal records, some were less educated, and they all were more likely to live in poverty.

Central Americans

Since its early settlement, Central America has had a history of turmoil. People from Central and South American countries including Colombia, Nicaragua, Guatemala, and Venezuela, have come to the United States over the last 25 years because of political instability, civil wars, as well as natural disasters such as landslides, earthquakes, and tropical storms. The economies of Central American countries tend to be unstable because of their dependence on a few agricultural export crops such as coffee, sugar, bananas, and cotton owned by a very small segment of society. Because of the political and economic struggles that the nations of this region have endured, many Central Americans have immigrated to the United States, often in search of refuge from violence and economic instability created by civil wars and other conflicts.

Central Americans have settled in different parts of the country. Salvadorans have settled mainly in Los Angeles and Washington DC; Guatemalans in Los Angeles, San Francisco, and Houston; and Nicaraguans in San Francisco and Miami. Many suffer from post-traumatic stress problems, relating to their countries' civil wars. Communication can be complicated by the large number of languages and dialects spoken in both Central and South America (estimated to be over 15). Diseases that are endemic to Central and South America include leprosy, cholera, yellow fever, and malaria.

Dominican Americans

Discovered by Columbus in 1492, the island of Hispaniola later divided following a slave rebellion and the establishment of the independent nation of Haiti. The remaining eastern two thirds of the island would eventually become the Dominican Republic, a predominantly agricultural Spanish-speaking nation.

Since the US invasion of the Dominican Republic during a period of civil unrest in 1965, over half a million Dominicans and their descendants have settled in the United States, with 70% of them located in New York City and adjacent parts of New Jersey.

South Americans

Several hundred thousand Colombians have also settled in the United States, mainly in Florida and New York. Smaller numbers of Hispanics have come to the United States from Venezuela, Ecuador, and other Latin American nations. Although there are various reasons for South American immigration to the United States, two key causes include political instability in certain instances and the search for economic opportunity or prosperity in others.

Consequences of Immigration to the United States for Hispanics

When dealing with the Hispanic/Latino groups, it is important for the nurse to recognize the tremendous range of historical experiences that exist within this group. Each nationality has its own perspective on how they view themselves within the context of living in the United States and how they have been treated as an immigrant in this country. How they entered the country (whether legally or illegally, as a refugee, or for economic reasons) will impact on them as well.

Summary

Hispanics/Latinos are a heterogeneous group with many similarities but also many differences. Each patient must be assessed within the context of their unique circumstances, the role of their family, and membership in subgroups or subcultures. The degree of acculturation exhibited along with the level of education, socioeconomic status, and country of origin all must be considered when planning for care delivery in the Hispanic/Latino patient population.

Case Study 6-1

Hispanic/Latino Patient in Pain

Tomas is a 42-year-old Hispanic male construction worker who presents with sudden onset low back pain for the past 2 days to the emergency room. Tomas is slightly obese and developed sharp, right-sided low back pain that has worsened over the last 2 days. The pain began immediately after Tomas tried to life a 50-pound bag of concrete. He has no paresthesias or bowel or bladder dysfunction. His past medical history is negative, he has no known drug allergies, and he is not taking any medication other than the occasional over-the-counter acetaminophen for the back pain. Family history is positive for type 2 DM in his mother and hypertension in his father. He is a nonsmoker and does not drink alcohol. Tomas denies any substance abuse. Physical examination is within normal limits except that the flexion of the right great toe is weaker than on the left side. Radiograph reveals slight narrowing of the L5-S1 disc space. He is diagnosed with lumbar disk herniation impinging on the L5 nerve root. Because this is a relatively recent onset, and the patient does not demonstrate any muscle weakness or loss of bowel or bladder control, a conservative treatment course is warranted. In the acute phase, the patient will benefit from a combination of physical and pharmacologic treatment. Bed rest for 24 hours only (because there is a disk herniation), a course of physical therapy modalities such as moist heat, ice, and massage, later attendance at "back school" once he is stable is also appropriate. For pain management, a nonsteroidal anti-inflammatory drug (NSAID) was prescribed. The patient was also counseled on the benefits of weight loss for back health.

The nurse questions the order for the NSAID for pain management. The nurse is concerned because earlier in the same day, the same physician prescribed an opiate pain medication for a patient with the same diagnosis except that patient was a 48-year-old White male. She is aware of the study (Pletcher, Kertesz, Kohn, & Gonzales, 2008) that examined treatments for more than 150,000 pain-related visits to US hospitals between 1993 and 2005. This study found that 31% of Whites received opioid drugs compared with only 23% of Blacks and 24% of Hispanics. About 28% of Asians received opioids. In contrast, nonopioid pain relievers (such as was the case with Tomas) such as ibuprofen were prescribed much more often to non-Whites (36%) than to Whites (26%). According to Dr. Mark Pletcher, the study's lead author, "studies in the 1990s showed a disturbing racial or ethnic disparity in the use of these potent pain relievers, but we had hoped that the recent national efforts at improving pain management in emergency departments would shrink this disparity; unfortunately, this is not the case." Based on the results of this study, the nurse feels empowered to advocate on behalf of Tomas and discusses Tomas' need for pain management with the emergency department-attending physician.

Box 6-8

Five Tips for Improving the Effectiveness in the Use of Interpreters

1. Brief the interpreter in advance. Summarize the key information that needs to be communicated. Do not be afraid to repeat yourself or to restate important information.

2. Keep it short. Avoid long or complicated sentences.

3. Do not interrupt and do not be impatient. Take as much time as is needed.

4. Position yourself so that you, the patient, and the interpreter are visible to each other. Look for signs of comprehension or confusion.

5. Do not underestimate the impact of culture.

   Culture may cause even a professional interpreter to modify what the nurse or the patient may say. The nurse should clarify with the interpreter whether it is appropriate or comfortable to discuss sexual or other delicate subjects and ask for input from the interpreter on the best approach to take to increase patient comfort during interpretation.

Source: Salimbene, S. (2000). Providing culture-sensitive care to African Americans. In: *What language does your patient hurt in? A practical guide to culturally competent patient care.* Amherst, MA: Diversity Resources.

Case Study 6-2

The Use of Family Member as Interpreter for a Female Hispanic/Latino Patient

The importance of the use of a qualified interpreter and the need to avoid the use of family members as interpreters is quite clear from this case study.

Gabrielle is a 36-year-old Hispanic woman who was asked to sign an informed consent for a hysterectomy. Gabrielle only speaks Spanish but she was accompanied by her bilingual son, Jose, who is an adult aged 18 years old. The hospital was not able to find a qualified interpreter, so the son was asked to serve in that role. When the son explained the procedure to the mother, he appeared to be translating accurately and indicating the proper body parts. His mother signed the consent form willingly. The next day, after the surgery was completed, when she learned that her uterus had been removed and she could no longer bear children, she became very angry and threatened to sue the hospital.

What went wrong? Because it is inappropriate for a Hispanic male to discuss his mother's private parts with her, the embarrassed son had explained that a tumor would be removed from her abdomen and pointed to the general area. He did not tell her that her uterus would be removed as he was uncomfortable to discuss or describe the sexual organ with his mother. Gabrielle became quite angry and upset because a Hispanic woman's status is derived, in large part, from the number of children she produces. She was very upset because she was not yet finished with childbearing.

When selecting an interpreter, it is always best to avoid the use of family members. Even if a potential interpreter can speak the same language, it is not always sufficient. Cultural rules often dictate who can discuss what and with whom. In general, it is best to use a same-sex interpreter when translating matters of a sexual or private nature with this cultural group.

References

Caballero, A. E. (2005). Diabetes in the Hispanic or Latino population: Genes, environment, culture and more. *Curr Diab Rep*, 5, 3, 217–225.

Caballero, A. E. (2006). Building cultural bridges: Understanding ethnicity to improve acceptance of insulin therapy in patients with type 2 diabetes. *Ethnicity and Disease*, 16, 2, 559–568.

Grieco, E., & Cassidy, R. (2001) Overview of race and Hispanic origin. Census 2000 Brief, C2KBR/01-1. Washington, DC: US Census Bureau.

Kalish, R. A., & Reynolds, D. K. (1981). *Death and ethnicity: A psychocultural study* (2nd ed.). New York: Baywood.

National Alliance for Hispanic Health. (1996). *Delivering preventive health care to Hispanics: A manual for providers*. Washington, DC: US Department of Health and Human Services.

National Alliance for Hispanic Health. (2001). *Quality health services for Hispanics: The cultural competency component*. Washington, DC: US Department of Health and Human Services.

National Center for Health Statistics. (2002). Chartbook on trends in the health of Americans. Retrieved June 14, 2009, from http://www.cdc.gov/nchs/data/hus/hus02.pdf.

Ortiz, B. I., Shields, K. M., Clauson, K. A., & Clay, P. G. (2007). Complementary and alternative medicine use among Hispanics in the United States. *The Annals of Pharmacotherapy*, 41, 6, 994–1004.

Pletcher, M. J., Kertesz, S. G., Kohn, M. A., & Gonzales, R. (2008). Trends in opioid prescribing by race/ethnicity for patients seeking care in U.S. emergency departments. *Journal of the American Medical Association*, 299, 1, 70–78.

Todd, M. D., Samaroo, N., & Hoffman, J. R. (1993). Ethnicity as a risk factor for inadequate emergency department analgesia. *Journal of the American Medical Association*, 269, 12, 1537–1539.

US Census Bureau. (2008). Table 4: Annual estimates of the Black or African American alone or in combination population by sex and age for the United States: April 1, 2000, to July 1, 2007. Source: Population Division, US Census Bureau. Release Date: May 1, 2008.

US Department of Commerce. (2000). Overview of race and Hispanic origin. Census 2000 Brief. Retrieved June 14, 2009, from http://www.census.gov/prod/2001pubs/cenbr01-1.pdf.

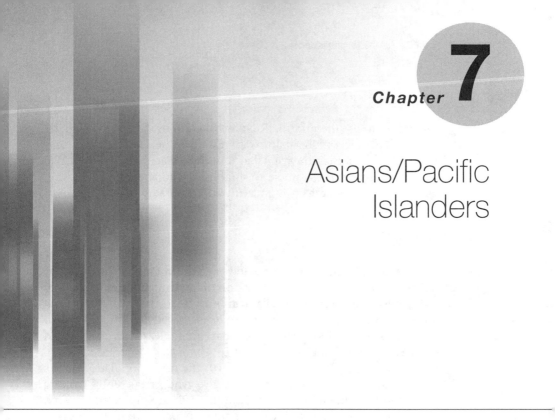

Chapter 7

Asians/Pacific Islanders

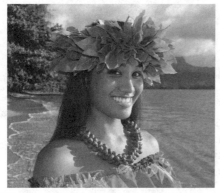

Source: © Christian Kieffer/ShutterStock, Inc.

Chapter Objectives

Upon completion of this chapter, the nurse will be able to:

1. Describe the illness behaviors of Asians/Pacific Islanders (Chinese Americans, Japanese Americans, Korean Americans, Vietnamese Americans, Cambodians, Laotians, Filipino Americans, and Pacific Islanders).

2. Provide a plan of care that considers the cultural needs of Asians/Pacific Islanders.

3. Identify the biologic variations of Asians/Pacific Islanders.

Introduction

Remember to use the information contained in this chapter as a guide only as all people within a culture are not the same. Developing awareness and an understanding of Asian American/Pacific Islander (AAPI) cultures will permit the nurse to establish a therapeutic relationship and to deliver more effective, individualized nursing care.

Background

The year 2000 census data revealed that the members of the AAPI groups made up 3.6% of the population of the United States. According to the most recently available data from July 2007, the Asian population alone was 13,366,154, and the number increased significantly when the Asian alone and in combination data was released as that totaled 15,165,186 (US Census Bureau, 2008).

According to Healthy People 2010, the AAPI population is the fastest growing of all of America's ethnic groups. Currently making up about 4% of the total US population, AAPIs are projected to reach 41 million US residents (11% of the total US population) by the year 2050 (Ghosh, 2003).

AAPIs have roots in at least 29 Asian countries and 20 Pacific Islander cultures. Members of this group speak over 100 languages and belong to numerous religions; most (95%) are of Asian origin, whereas the rest (5%) are Pacific Islanders. The 1990 census shows the largest of the AAPI subpopulations to be Chinese Americans (23%), followed by Filipino Americans, Japanese Americans, and Asian Indian Americans. The 2000 census states that Chinese Americans and Filipino Americans remain the first and second largest subpopulations, followed by Asian Indian Americans and Korean Americans (Fig. 7-1). It is somewhat problematic comparing data from the 1990 and 2000 censuses because of the change in categorizing AAPIs. The 2000 census divides the "Asian origin" category into the numerous Asian ethnicities, which allows for a much more detailed and accurate count of these particular populations (US Census Bureau, 2008). According to the Office of Management and Budget (1997) Federal Guidelines on Race, Asians are persons having origins in any of the original people of the Far East, Southeast Asia, or the Indian subcontinent including China, India, and the Islands of the Philippines. Native Hawaiians and other Pacific Islanders include people who have origins in any of the original peoples of Hawaii, Guam, Samoa, or other Pacific Islands.

There were slightly more than 12 million people who were considered Asian according to the 2000 census; that number has now increased to over 15 million people based on 2007 estimates. The reason for

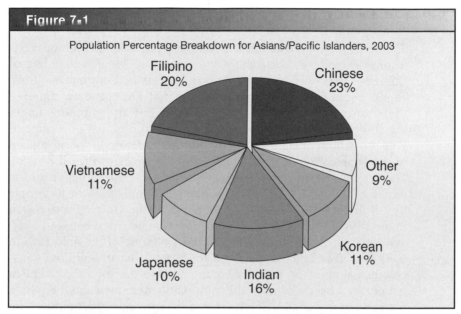

Figure 7-1

Population Percentage Breakdown for Asians/Pacific Islanders, 2003

Filipino 20%

Chinese 23%

Vietnamese 11%

Other 9%

Korean 11%

Japanese 10%

Indian 16%

Source: Ghosh, C. (2003). Healthy People 2010 and Asian Americans/Pacific Islanders: Defining a baseline of information. *American Journal of Public Health, 93*, 12, 2093–2098.

number variability is that Native Hawaiians and other Pacific Islanders were listed as a separate category in the 2000 census (US Census Bureau, 2008). This change in data collection complicated and contributed even more diversity to an already diverse group. The ranks of Asians are rapidly growing, and they represent the third largest minority group. There are more than 30 different languages spoken and many unique cultures exist. It is helpful to note that much of the health and illness beliefs and practices of AAPIs are derived from Chinese traditions. Having a strong understanding of Chinese health and illness beliefs will provide a foundation or starting point when striving to provide health care for AAPIs. The nurse should consider utilizing a Chinese frame of reference when planning for or providing care to Pacific Islanders because less is known about this group. This is because this group is so small, health data is not reported separately. It is for these reasons that AAPIs will be discussed as one grouping in this chapter.

Statistics

The largest group of Asians is Chinese with a total of 2.7 million, closely followed by Filipinos with 2.4 million. Close to half of the Asian born population in the United States lives in one of three metropolitan areas: Los Angeles, New York, or San Francisco (US Census Bureau, 2008).

Chinese Americans

The People's Republic of China has the world's oldest continuous civilization extending more than 4000 years. The People's Republic of China is often referred to as Mainland China or Communist China. Taiwan became a Chinese province in the mid-1680s and was annexed to the Japanese in 1895. After World War II, Taiwan again came under the control of China in the form of a noncommunist government, which is still in effect today. Hong Kong was returned to the control of the People's Republic of China after 150 years of British control. The People's Republic of China is the most populated nation in the world with over 1.3 billion inhabitants; yet, only 13% of its people live in urban areas. Chinese immigration to the United States began in the 1800s. A rapid increase in immigration occurred between 1850 and 1880 (from 1000 to over 100,000) because of the gold rush in California. This resulted in a need for cheap labor to build the transcontinental railroads. The Chinese intended to stay for a short time as temporary workers. Most of the immigrants were men and they clung to their customs and beliefs and stayed close to their communities. Life was difficult and, other than work on the railroads, jobs were hard to find—in fact, many were closed to them because they were not White. This caused a large number of immigrant workers and their families to return to China before 1930. There was a 20% decline in the population of Chinese living in America between 1880 and 1930. The Chinese that remained in the United States left the West and moved eastward to cities where there were more employment opportunities, such as running laundries and restaurants. The Chinese settled in tight knit groups in urban neighborhoods called, "Chinatown." In Chinatowns, they were able to maintain their ancient traditions. Because of hard work, they were able to survive on menial jobs.

US immigration laws and political problems in China have greatly impacted the Chinese population in the United States. Many men were left alone without the possibility of their family ever joining them. By 1965, a large number of refugees who had relatives in the United States were able to come here to join them, causing the Chinese population to grow. The new immigrants joined their relatives in the urban Chinatowns. Since 1965, the population rate of increase has been 10% per year. The newer immigrants were better educated professionals and specialists. This change in the type of immigrants coming from China has resulted in a great deal of cultural and linguistic diversity among Chinese Americans. The majority of Chinese Americans today are immigrants from Taiwan, Hong Kong, and mainland China. A total of 66% of Chinese Americans live in five states: California, New York, Hawaii, Illinois, and Texas (Harris & Jones, 2005).

Chinese Americans maintain high educational standards but have a poverty rate of 14% (compare this with 13% for the general US population). The majority (65.9%) participate in the workforce (Harris & Jones, 2005). In the United States, the educational levels of Chinese are divided between the highly educated and poorly educated. It is important to recognize that not all Chinese Americans are poorly educated or have service-oriented occupations (garment industry, restaurant work). The failure of Chinese Americans to return to China once they have been educated in the United States has been viewed as a detriment to China and has resulted in much tighter control over immigration today.

The majority of Chinese Americans are immigrants from Taiwan, Hong Kong, and mainland China. Chinese Americans are the majority group of Asian Americans, totaling 2,314,537 according to the most recent census data (Harris & Jones, 2005). This is a 47.5% growth rate from 1980 to 1990, and now Chinese Americans residing in the United States represent 0.7% of the total US population (Harris & Jones, 2005).

Chinese culture is dominated by Confucianism. This encourages people to strive for piety, righteousness, decorum, and wealth. A harmonious relationship with nature and other people is stressed. The emphasis is on accommodation and not confrontation, and the individual should submit to the interest of the group if conflict is present. Public debate is not socially acceptable and a person is expected to be very sensitive and gracious to others, so as not to make them "lose face."

As we shall see, Chinese Americans are a very diverse group in terms of economics, healthcare behaviors, and modernization. As always, a disclaimer is important: While possessing knowledge of the dominant Chinese values, as is true of all of the AAPI values and culture, is extremely helpful, it should only be used as a guide.

Chinese Definition of Health and Illness

Health is a state of spiritual and physical harmony with nature. Most beliefs come from old philosophies, most especially Taoism. To live according to the Tao, one must adapt to the order of nature. In Chinese culture, physical problems are hard to distinguish from psychologic or spiritual concerns. Illness may be attributed to typical scientific causes, but it may also be seen as being caused by spirits, emotions, or taboo behaviors. Disability carries a stigma in Chinese culture. At a minimum, the onset of disability may be seen as bad luck, or it may be seen as a result of inappropriate behavior by the birth mother if disability occurs in the newborn.

The Chinese believe that each being has a function within the universe. No one thing can exist without the other with the goal to achieve harmonious balance. Violation of harmony results in illness. The underlying belief is that people must adjust themselves within the environment and that five elements can both create and destroy each other. The five elements are wood, fire, metal, water, and earth.

The holistic concept is an important idea for preventing and treating disease. A holistic view is one that considers that pathologic changes are always considered in conjunction with other organs of the body as well as the integration of the human body with the environment.

The Chinese have made tremendous contributions to medicine. The first known description of how blood circulates, including the oxygen-carrying powers of blood, was Huang-ti Nei Ching's *Yellow Emperor's Book of Internal Medicine*, which was published in the 1200s. This book also defined the two basic principles of yin and yang, which are powers that regulate the universe and human beings. Yin represents the female, a negative energy such as the force of darkness, cold, and emptiness. Yang represents the male, a positive energy source that produces light, warmth, and fullness.

According to the yin and yang theory, everything in the universe contains these two aspects, which are in opposition and in union. When yin and yang are in disharmony, illness will result. The pulse is controlled by both yin and yang. If yin and yang are not balanced, the person's life will be short. Half of the yin force is depleted by age 40, and it is for this reason that it is believed a person becomes sluggish at age 40. At age 60, the yin is totally depleted and the body then begins to deteriorate. See Table 7-1 for more on yin and yang.

It is felt that alertness at the time of near death is important for spiritual reasons. It is for this reason that the patient or his family may refuse medications that may impair consciousness. As a general rule, Chinese do not report discomfort. Death is a topic that is not readily discussed. Family members may not tell the patient that he is dying, and they also may not discuss it among themselves. This is less

Table 7-1	
Components of Yin and Yang	
Yin	**Yang**
Inside of the body	Outside of the body
Front part of the body	Back of the body
Gall bladder, stomach, large intestine, small intestine, bladder, lymphatic system	Liver, heart, spleen, lungs, kidneys
Diseases of winter and spring	Diseases of summer and fall
Stores the vital strength of life	Protects the body from outside forces

common in younger generations of Chinese Americans as they may be more open to talking about the illness and the patient's prognosis. A great deal of importance is placed by the family on being present with the loved one at the time of death. There is also ritual associated with the care of the body and how the body is dressed. The women in the family prepare special funeral clothing. Funerals are carried out in an extremely traditional manner.

Food, illness, and medications are classified as "hot" or "cold," according to the perceived effects on the body. Health is believed to be a balance of positive (yang) and negative (yin) energy in the body. Many Chinese people will assume a "sick role" when they are ill where they depend heavily on others. If a healthcare provider seems demanding, they may be viewed as uncaring by the Chinese patient. To appear caring, the nurse should speak sympathetically, take an interest in the patient, and verbally encourage them.

The use of hospitals and healthcare professionals is avoided in the Chinese culture. When health care is sought, a doctor of the same sex is preferred, especially by female patients. Most Chinese people will expect to be given a prescription when they go to the doctor, so going to the doctor when they are not sick, such as for health prevention or health promotion, might be considered strange. A nurse will have cultural awareness of the Chinese if he or she remembers the Chinese cultural norms of lack of eye contact, shyness, and passivity. Assertiveness may be mistaken or interpreted by the Chinese patient as aggressive or even hostile behavior. Because of the cultural norm of shyness, it is important for the nurse to realize that the Chinese will be reluctant to talk to them—an outsider about their health and psychosocial problems. Finally, many Chinese believe that saying no is impolite so the nurse must be cautious not to mistake silence for agreement.

Traditional Healing Methods

Nutrition is essential to health. There are strict rules governing food combinations and timing of ingestion especially in relation to monumental life events such as childbirth and surgery. Daily exercise is important and many Chinese participate in tai chi.

"Congee" is a rice porridge often given to sick children. The nurse should consider that many Western foods may be foreign to the patient as the Chinese prefer to eat traditional foods.

Acupuncture is an ancient practice, older than 5000 years, that is believed to cure disease or relieve pain (Xinnong, 1987). The body is punctured with special needles at precisely predetermined sites known as meridians and is considered a "cold" treatment. Acupuncture is used when there is an excess of yang (Xinnong, 1987). According to traditional Chinese medicine, health is achieved by maintaining the body in a "balanced state"; disease is caused by an internal imbalance of yin and yang. This imbalance leads to blockage in the flow of qi along pathways known as meridians. Qi can be unblocked by using acupuncture at certain points on the body that connect with these meridians. Sources vary on the number of meridians, with numbers ranging from 14 to 20. One commonly cited source describes meridians as 14 main channels "connecting the body in a weblike interconnecting matrix" of at least 2000 acupuncture points (Acupuncture, 2009). It is believed that the way to treat internal problems is to puncture the meridians, which are also categorized as yin or yang, with the goal of treatment being restoration of yin and yang. Through the years, acupuncture has gained some legitimacy within Western medicine, and non-Asians are seeking treatment. According to the 2002 National Health Interview Survey—the largest and most comprehensive survey of complementary and alternative medicine (CAM) use by American adults to date—an estimated 8.2 million US adults had ever used acupuncture, and an estimated 2.1 million US adults had used acupuncture in the previous year (Barnes, Powell-Griner, McFann, & Nahin, 2004). Relatively few complications from the use of acupuncture have been reported to the US Food and Drug Administration when the fact that millions of people are treated each year and the number of acupuncture needles used is taken into consideration. Still, complications have resulted from inadequate sterilization of needles and from improper delivery of treatments. Practitioners should use a new set of disposable needles taken from a sealed package for each patient and should swab treatment sites with alcohol or another disinfectant before inserting needles. When not delivered properly, acupuncture can cause serious adverse effects, including infections and punctured organs.

Moxibustion is another ancient treatment. Moxibustion is a traditional Chinese medicine technique that involves the burning of mugwort, a small, spongy herb, to facilitate healing. Moxibustion has been used throughout Asia for thousands of years; in fact, the actual Chinese character for acupuncture, translated literally, means "acupuncture-moxibustion." The purpose of moxibustion, as with most forms of traditional Chinese medicine, is to strengthen the blood, stimulate the flow of qi, and maintain general health. It is used in diseases in which there is an excess of yin. It is performed by applying it directly to the skin along certain meridians; although, it cannot be applied to all of the meridians that are used for acupuncture. Mugwort, also known as *Artemisia vulgaris* or "ai ye" in Chinese, has a long history of use in folk medicine. Research has shown that it acts as an emmenagogue, that is, an agent that increases blood circulation to the pelvic area and uterus and stimulates menstruation. This could explain its use in treating breech births and menstrual cramps. Moxibustion is most commonly used during labor and delivery. In Western medicine, moxibustion has successfully been used to turn breech babies into a normal head-down position prior to childbirth. A study published in the *Journal of the American Medical Association* in 1998 found that up to 75% of women suffering from breech presentations before childbirth had fetuses that rotated to the normal position after receiving moxibustion at an acupuncture point on the bladder meridian compared to 48% in the control group (N = 260) (Cardini & Weixin, 1998).

Other studies have shown that moxibustion increases the movement of the fetus in pregnant women, and may reduce the symptoms of menstrual cramps when used in conjunction with traditional acupuncture. A Cochrane review published in 2005 found that there is evidence, although limited, suggesting that moxibustion may be useful for turning babies from breech presentation (bottom first) to a cephalic presentation (head first) for labor (Coyle, Smith, & Peat, 2005).

Cupping refers to an ancient Chinese practice (over 3000 years old) in which a cup is applied to the skin and the pressure in the cup is reduced (by using change in heat or by suctioning out air), so that the skin and superficial muscle layer is drawn into and held in the cup. In some cases, the cup may be moved while the suction of skin is active, causing a regional pulling of the skin and muscle (the technique is called "gliding cupping"). Cupping is applied by acupuncturists to certain acupuncture points, as well as to regions of the body that are affected by pain (where the pain is deeper than the tissues to be pulled). In ancient times, cups were made of animal horn, bamboo, or, for the wealthy, brass. Since the 20th century, the cups are made of glass. In ancient times, the name for cupping was horning. When the cups are moved along the surface of the skin, the treatment is somewhat like *guasha* (literally, sand scraping), a folk remedy of southeast Asia that is often carried out by scraping the skin with a coin or other object with the intention of breaking up stagnation. Movement of the cups is a gentler technique than *guasha*, as a lubricant, allows the cup to slide without causing as much of the subcutaneous bruising that is an objective of *guasha*. Still, a certain amount of bruising is expected both from fixed position cupping (especially at the site of the cup rim) and with movement of the cups. In some cases, a small amount of blood letting (*luoci*, or vein pricking) is done first, using a pricking needle, and then the cup is applied over the site. The pricking is usually done with a three-edged needle that is applied to a vein, and it typically draws 3–4 drops of blood (sometimes, the skin on either side is squeezed to aid release of blood). A standard thick-gauge acupuncture needle or plum blossom needle may be used instead. Generally, the cup is left in place for about 10 minutes (typical range is 5–15 minutes). The skin becomes reddened because of the congestion of blood flow. The cup is removed by pressing the skin along side it to allow some outside air to leak into it, thus equalizing the pressure and releasing it. Some bruising along the site of the rim of the cup is expected.

Today, cupping is mainly recommended for the treatment of pain, gastrointestinal disorders, lung diseases (especially chronic cough and asthma), and paralysis, although it can be used for other disorders as well. It is frequently used to treat lung congestion. The areas of the body that are fleshy are preferred sites for cupping. Contraindications for cupping include areas of skin that are inflamed; cases of high fever, convulsions or cramping, or easy bleeding (i.e., pathologic level of low platelets); or the abdominal area or lower back during pregnancy. Movement of the cups is limited to fleshy areas: The movement should not cross bony ridges, such as the spine.

Cupping is said to promote blood circulation, remove stasis, and alleviate swelling and pain. It is employed especially when there is a toxic heat syndrome and for a variety of acute ailments. Cupping is used to draw blood and lymph to the body's surface that is under the cup, which increases the local circulation. Cupping is used to remove cold and damp from the body and to assist with blood circulation. Cupping is also frequently applied after treatment by acupuncture, blood letting, or plum blossom treatment. Cupping is not only traditionally practiced in China and Japan; it is also a traditional healing method in Arab cultures where it is called Al-hijamah.

Dermabrasion and cupping, both of which can leave marks or bruising, can easily be mistaken as signs of physical abuse that is very important for the nurse to be aware of.

Alternative and Complementary Folk Medicine

CAM represents a group of diverse medical and healthcare systems, practices, and products that are not presently considered to be part of conventional medicine. Complementary medicine is used together with conventional medicine, and alternative medicine is used in place of conventional medicine.

Some Chinese prepare amulets that are used to protect health by preventing evil spirits. The amulet is hung over a door or on a curtain or wall, worn in the hair, pinned on clothing, or carried in a red bag. Jade is considered the most precious of all stones and when worn, it is believed to bring health. Jade is so valued that in Chinese contests, jade is awarded for first place, followed by gold for second, and ivory for third place. It is believed to be the closest mineral form of the yin and yang and it is used to speak to heaven. It is also believed that the jade stone can prevent harm and accidents and can keep children safe. Jade is also seen as the "giver of children," health, immortality, wisdom, power, victory, growth, and food. It is important that the jade stone be maintained for it is believed that if the stone turns dull or breaks, the wearer will have misfortune.

Figure 7-2

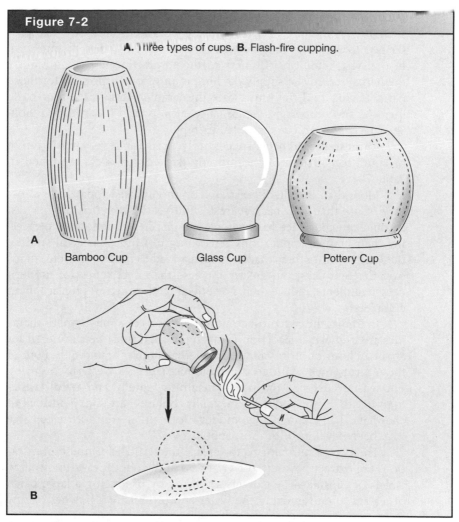

A. Three types of cups. **B.** Flash-fire cupping.

Bamboo Cup   Glass Cup   Pottery Cup

A

B

Source: Dharmananda, S. Cupping. Retrieved August 27, 2009, from http://www.itmonline.org/arts/cupping.htm.

Acupuncture is among the oldest healing practices in the world. As part of traditional Chinese medicine, it aims to restore and maintain health through the stimulation of specific points on the body. In the United States, where practitioners incorporate healing traditions from China, Japan, Korea, and other countries, acupuncture is considered part of CAM.

Medicinal herbs are still widely used in the practice of Chinese healing. Herbs used in Chinese medicine are derived from plant, animal, and mineral substances. Although plant-derived herbs, such as ginseng and ginger, are the most common, minerals and animal parts such as oyster shells, deer antlers, and bear gallbladder are also prescribed. In China, herbs in powder form are boiled and made into a tea. In the West, traditional Chinese medicine practitioners often premix the herbal remedy or supply the herb in pill form, especially for those patients who find the bitter taste intolerable. Herbs have four basic qualities and properties: nature, taste, affinity, and its primary action. See Table 7-2 for more on herbal therapy.

Chinese medicine is successfully used for a very wide range of conditions. The more commonly treated disorders are listed in Table 7-4.

More than 300 herbs that are commonly used today have a history of use that goes back at least 2000 years. Over that time, a vast amount of experience has been gained that has gone toward perfecting their clinical applications. According to Chinese clinical studies, these herbs, and others that have been added to the list of useful items over the centuries, can greatly increase the effectiveness of modern drug treatments, reduce their side effects, and sometimes replace them completely.

In China, the two most common methods of applying herb therapies are to make a decoction (a strong tea that must be simmered for about an hour or more) and to make large honey-bound pills. Both of these forms meet with considerable resistance in Western countries. The teas are deemed too time-consuming, smelly, and awful-tasting to justify their use, and the honey pills (boluses) are sticky, difficult to chew, and bad tasting. Thus, modern forms that are more acceptable have been developed for most applications.

The two popular forms to replace the standard Chinese preparations are extract powders (or granules) and smooth, easy-to-swallow tablets or capsules. The extracts are made by producing a large batch of tea and then removing the water and producing a powder or tiny

---

Table 7-2
Herbal Therapy

Nature: An herb's nature is often described as cooling or heating, but it can also be described as moistening, relaxing, and energizing. The peppermint herb, for example, has a cooling energy, and is used to lower the metabolism or reduce gas and bloating.

Taste: Herbs are categorized by five tastes—**sour**, **bitter**, **sweet** or **bland**, **spicy**, and **salty**—and herbs representing different tastes are used to treat different conditions. Dandelion and goldenseal are two bitter herbs used for their drying properties in treating upper respiratory conditions.

Affinity: This property refers to the affinity that an herb has for a particular organ network.

Primary action: This property refers to the effect of a particular herb. An herb may be used to dispel (move), astringe (restrain), purge (expel), or tonify (strengthen).

pellets; the resulting material is swallowed down with some water or mixed with hot water to make a tea. Tablets and capsules contain either powdered herbs or dried extracts or a combination of the two.

Arguably, the most important Chinese herb is ginseng. Ginseng (renshen) has long been valued as a disease-preventive. It is purported to calm the spirit and help one gain wisdom. Modern usages include normalizing blood pressure, regulating blood sugar, resisting fatigue, increasing oxygen utilization, and enhancing immune functions. Traditionally, the root is cooked in a double boiler to make a tea, used either alone or with several other herbs. Today, ginseng is much easier to ingest. A tea can be made quickly and there are tablets and other formulations to ease consumption. Typical ginseng dosage is 0.5–3.0 g. Higher doses may be used over the short term for specific therapeutic actions: in China, 30 g is recommended to treat shock (sudden hypotension). As with all herbs, there is concern that they are not regulated by the US Food and Drug Administration; purity of herbs can be an issue as well. Use caution when recommending the use of herbal preparations for yourself or your patients. Although herbs such as ginseng are considered safe, be aware that excessive consumption of ginseng can lead to nervousness and may produce hormonal imbalances in women.

Current Healthcare Problems Including Mortality and Morbidity

The four leading causes of death for Chinese Americans are identical to those for White Americans. They are heart disease, cerebral vascular disease, cancer, and chronic respiratory disorders (National Center for Health Statistics, 2002). The fifth leading cause of death is pneumonia. The rate of suicide found in Chinese Americans, especially females, is an area that is under further investigation. Suicide ranks ninth as a cause of death for Chinese Americans and eleventh for White Americans (National Center for Health Statistics, 2002). Mortality data reveals that the four leading causes of death for Chinese Americans is the same as those for European Americans.

There is a stigma among the Chinese and Chinese Americans regarding mental illness. Many believe that mental illness indicates inabilities to solve problems or out-of-control behavior and that it brings shame to the individual and the family. Further study is required to determine if the lower rates of psychiatric hospitalization among AAPIs is caused by this stigma or prevalence.

Impact of Communication

In China and Taiwan, the official language is Mandarin, which is based on the Northern Beijing dialect and is spoken by more than 70% of

Table 7-3

Comparison of Health Beliefs Among Asians/Pacific Islanders

Group	Health Beliefs	Traditional Healing Methods
Cambodian	Comfortable with Western medicine but will resort to traditional healing first. They are reluctant to complain. Tend to focus on symptoms, not the cause. May view symptom remission as a cure and stop medications too early.	Coin rubbing Cupping Massage Herbs
Korean	The Kior Chi Force is the life force of the body. Withdrawing blood, sweating, and sex reduce the kior chi force. Illness if often seen as fate. Hospitalization is seen as a sign of impending death. Illness is attributed to disharmony. Illness can have spiritual causes. Treatment is through the use of the opposite force to achieve balance. Traditional healing can be provided by family members or healers. They do believe in do not resuscitate orders. They do not wish to discuss terminal status as it is viewed as unacceptable. Organ donation and transplantation are seen as a disturbance in integrity of the body. Most patient care is provided by the family. Physician is seen as powerful and trustworthy.	Herbs Acupuncture Cupping Moxibustion
Vietnamese	Expect to be cured immediately. Seek out Western medicine to relieve symptoms. May view symptom remission as a cure and stop medications too early. Feel medicines are too powerful for them and may adjust dosage down. Fear loss of blood to lab studies is harmful to health.	Coining Cupping Balm Acupuncture Massage Herbs
Laotian	Illness may be attributed to the loss of one of the 32 spirits thought to inhabit the body and maintain health. Health is related to ability to eat and sleep. Will look to family and community for treatment first. Traditional treatments may be tried first—last resort is Western medicine. Often will continue traditional healing with Western medicine in combination. Obtaining a health history is difficulty because of desire for privacy. Patient is concerned about confidentiality and will benefit from reassurance that confidentiality will be maintained. The entire family will want to present for a patient's last days. Respect for the patient and his culture is essential. The head of the body is sacred. Avoid touching the head and the shoulder unless absolutely essential. Modesty is highly valued, especially among women.	Coining Pinching—rubbing the temples, pulling forward to the eyebrow and nose and pinching the nose—is used to relieve headache. Cupping Massage Traditional Chinese medicine. Ceremony—if the cause of illness is thought to be a result of a spirit, a special ceremony may be performed. Mental illness is attributed to spirit loss. In Laos, if a person exhibits symptoms that we may think of as mental illness, such as hallucinations, they will simply be left alone as long as they are viewed as not dangerous to others. If they consider mental health a problem, they are more likely to go to a monk for a ceremony to treat it. Here in the United States, some Laotians have learned about the value of treatment for mental health problems and will accept help. They are not likely to understand, however, why some medications have side effects that sometimes make a person feel worse.

Group	Health Beliefs	Traditional Healing Methods
		Laotians are not likely to seek treatment from a traditional mental health source unless there is a long-standing or very serious problem, or unless specifically referred for treatment.
Japanese	Believe body is as holy as the mind. View the mind and body as one. Concerns with medical diagnosis of "brain death" and organ donation. Organ donation violates oneness of body and soul, and receipt of organs can cause anxiety in Japanese recipient. Individual assertion is highly discouraged so may not ask questions during health teaching. Silence may be away of avoiding conflict. Healthcare providers should avoid prolonged eye contact to show respect. Patience is an important skill when dealing with Japanese. Avoid physical touching, which can cause anxiety.	
Asian Indians	Most Indians in the United States accept and understand Western medicine. The traditional philosophy and science of medicine in India is called "Ayurveda." "Ayur" means longevity and "veda" means science. This promotes a routine where one's health and daily routine, body, and the five elements of the universe are in sync. The five elements are water, fire, earth, wind, and ether. When elements are in balance, the body is healthy, and imbalance results in illness. Foods have properties that determine if they are "hot" or "cold" (it is not based on temperature of the food or the spiciness of the food) and it is believed that proper food balance is essential for temperature regulation. Consuming certain foods can cause a temperature imbalance. Examples of "cold" foods are yogurt, fruit, and rice and "hot" foods are teas, chicken, garlic, and cloves.	Most Indians feel that blood is precious and not to be wasted. Expect reluctance on the patient's part for any blood drawing. Colostrum is perceived as bad for newborns. Newborns are fed sugar water until the third day postpartum. On the third postpartum day, the new mother has a ritual bath and then will commence breastfeeding. Honey is often given to newborns, which is potentially dangerous because of bacterial contamination. Smiling is only done in informal situations and then only shared between people of an equal social status. Although there is a public health system in India, Indians who can afford it will use a fee-for-serve private system. There is no health insurance in India. Three of the five elements correspond to the human body. Bile corresponds to fire, phlegm to water, and gas to wind. Balance equates with health. Most Indians are vegetarians. Most Hindus follow dietary restrictions, which prohibits ingestion of beef. Muslims do not ingest pork or pork products. Second-generation Asian Indians may not follow these food taboos. Fasting is common with Hindus and Muslims during certain times of the year.

Table 7-4

Systems and Disorders Treated with Chinese Herbs

System	Associated Disorders
Integumentary	Eczema, psoriasis, acne, rosacea, urticaria
Respiratory	Asthma, bronchitis, and chronic coughs, allergic and perennial rhinitis and sinusitis
Gastrointestinal	Irritable bowel syndrome, chronic constipation, ulcerative colitis, hepatitis C
Gynecologic/genitourinary	Premenstrual syndrome and dysmenorrhea, endometriosis, infertility, chronic cystitis
Endocrine	Diabetes (treatment and prevention)
Psychologic	Anxiety, depression
Rheumatologic	Osteoarthritis, rheumatoid arthritis, chronic fatigue syndrome

the population. Nearly all Chinese are bilingual, speaking the national language as well as a native dialect. The major dialects are Cantonese and Shanghaiese. Chinese who immigrated from Hong Kong and Southeast China speak Cantonese. Because these native dialects are so different, many groups cannot understand one another verbally although the written language is the same. It is important for the nurse to recognize that all dialects of spoken Chinese share the same written language of Mandarin. Mandarin in the written form can be used as a way to ensure effective communication among all Chinese patients. Written Chinese consists of characters that represent an object or idea. Each Chinese character consists of only one syllable. Tones within the language change the meaning of a syllable or word. The Chinese language has a limited number of verbs, does not have tenses, and does not use plurals. The Chinese rely on a highly contextualized language where the nonverbal communication is just as important as the verbal. Eye contact is minimal as too much eye contact is viewed as rude. Few words are used to express a thought; they value silence highly and strive for intuitive understanding. Individuals endeavor to conduct themselves with restraint and speak in a moderate-to-low volume of voice. To raise one's voice is viewed as a loss of control.

Also of note is the avoidance of the use of the word "no." In China, one usually avoids saying "no" out of respect to the other person. Remember that the Chinese typically communicate more with the use of nonverbal language and may be saying "yes" when they really mean "no." Do not forget to ask for assistance from an interpreter, especially if you note a disconnect between the verbal and nonverbal communication. An interpreter is also very helpful in interpreting the meaning of silence during a conversation. Silence in Chinese culture can mean respect, interest, anger, or even disagreement, so clarification of the meaning of the silence is very important. The Chinese American may also be uncomfortable with discussing family-related problems with strangers as it is viewed as disrespectful. Rapport building by the healthcare provider is essential.

Impact of Time and Space

Asians typically prefer a greater amount of physical space than we may be accustomed to. Physical touching or displays of affection are uncommon. The nurse should consider carefully the appropriateness of touching an Asian patient as it would be considered inappropriate to hug or console a Chinese adult or child with touch.

Timing may be an issue with appointments. Chinese Americans are often polychromic (adhering less rigidly to time as a distinct and linear entity, focusing on the completion of the present, and performing more than one activity at the same time) (Hall, 1963). The US healthcare system has a monochromic orientation, which emphasizes schedules, being on time, synchronization with clocks, and standardization of activities (Hall, 1963), which can cause clashes. Some Chinese Americans have a more modern view of time, especially if they have been in the United States for a prolonged period of time or are a second-generation immigrant. This modern view emphasizes the importance of being on time and lateness is viewed as a serious act of disrespect. These Chinese Americans will arrive on time and will expect others to do the same. It is important for the nurse to not cause the Chinese American to lose "face," which occurs in Chinese culture if you make a high-ranking person wait for you, both of you have then "lost face." Chinese Americans value the past as evidenced by the value placed on elders and also an appreciation for the future by stressing education in the younger generation.

Environment

Harmony with nature is stressed. Some Chinese Americans ascribe to feng shui (wind and water). Feng shui is an effort to achieve harmony and balance through the art of location and design of physical structures. Positive feng shui wards off evil spirits, promotes good health, and brings prosperity. Others have beliefs related to colors and numbers. Certain numbers are considered to bring good or bad luck. The number 4 is bad luck, whereas the number 8 is good luck. The birth date of the patient can be perceived as being either lucky or unlucky depending on the numbers utilized. A person born in August (the eighth month) on the eighth day of the month in a year beginning or ending in eight would be considered extremely lucky. Colors also are lucky or unlucky. White, the color of mourning, is considered bad luck. This can be upsetting to the Chinese American when dealing with many members of the healthcare team who traditionally wear white coats, scrubs, or uniforms.

Biologic Variations

Chinese Americans tend to be shorter at all ages and tend to complete growing earlier when compared with White ethnic groups, although there are some Chinese who are taller than 6 ft in height. The Chinese are more prone to fractures and osteoporosis because their bone density is lower than White Americans. Most Chinese do not have much facial or body hair and the hair on the head is usually black and straight.

There are three genetic diseases found in the Chinese: adult lactose intolerance, alpha-thalassemia, and glucose-6-phosphate dehydrogenase (G-6-PD) deficiency. Lactose intolerance causes gastrointestinal disturbances after milk or dairy products (cheese is often tolerated) containing the sugar lactose are ingested. There are two types of thalassemia, which is a hemoglobin abnormality characterized by a high rate of red blood cell destruction. The first type usually does not have a major effect on health status and is characterized by an increase in red blood cells. The second type is more serious as it is associated with an early death and requires frequent blood transfusions. G-6-PD also causes fragility of the red blood cells and makes patients prone to anemia.

Drug metabolism is an issue. Studies have revealed that Asians require lower dosages than Whites for several psychiatric medications (antidepressants, lithium, neuroleptics). There is an increased sensitivity to alcohol; often, Chinese demonstrate facial flushing and vasomotor responses when drinking, which may explain the low alcoholism rate among the Chinese (Overfield, 1995). This information is especially important for the nurse to consider as the Chinese are of the belief that medications are too potent for them and, while this may be true of some medications (such as the psychotropic agents), it is important that the patient not self-adjust medications but have an open dialogue with their prescriber.

Infectious diseases, including tuberculosis (TB), are a major health threat to the Chinese immigrant. Complicating the diagnosis of authentic TB from false-positive on the Mantoux test is the widespread exposure of Southeast Asians to the bacilli-Calmette-Guérin vaccine against TB in childhood. Other infection risks include parasites, hepatitis and malaria.

Cancer is a major burden for all AAPIs. Cancer is the leading cause of death for AAPIs aged 25–64. This is startling because cancer does not become a leading cause of death for Whites until they reach the age range of 45–64 (Chen, 2000). Cancer death rates have increased at much higher rates for AAPIs than for any other racial or ethnic group

(Chen, 2000). Part of the blame may be a result of the high rate of cigarette smoking among male AAPIs (US Department of Health and Human Services, 1998). Smoking is the single most important preventable cause of death, including death from cancer.

Diabetes is an emerging disease in Asian Americans, particularly those who have lived in the United States for several years. If you compare the prevalence of diabetes for Japanese living in Tokyo with Japanese Americans living in Seattle, WA, the rates for diabetes are four or five times higher for that population in the United States. The data is similar for Chinese in China versus Chinese Americans and Vietnamese in Vietnam versus Vietnamese Americans. Reliance on the use of body mass index (BMI) as a screening tool to identify patients at risk for diabetes has not been found to be effective as there is difficulty in defining obesity in this population using BMI. People in the Asian American population may develop insulin resistance and type 2 diabetes at much lower BMI levels than would be found in other population groups. BMI criteria for being overweight is between 25 and 30 kg/m^2, whereas a BMI above 30 kg/m^2 is considered obese. For the Asian American population, the numbers need to be lower: probably between 23 and 25 kg/m^2 to be considered overweight and anything above 25 kg/m^2 as obese. Another screening tool is waist circumference, but this also must be modified based on population group. The International Diabetes Foundation (IDF) has suggested that for Caucasians, the waist circumference should be less than 37 inches in men and 31.5 inches in women. For South Asians (Chinese and Asian Indian populations), the waist circumference in men should be less than 35 inches and less than 31.5 inches in women. In the Japanese, the waist circumference should be less than 35 inches in men and in women, it should be less than 33.5 inches. According to the IDF, when dealing with sub-Saharan Africans, eastern Mediterranean, and middle-east (Arab) populations, it is acceptable to use the Caucasian data for now. For South Americans and Central Americans, use the South Asian recommendations for now.

Impact of Social Organization

Family is the foundation of Chinese society. The family includes multiple generations and also includes ancestors in daily life. The most treasured values of Chinese society are family relationships, loyalty, obligation, obedience, cooperation, interdependence, and reciprocity. The father is typically the family spokesperson and decision maker, whereas the mother is the manager of the house and finances and is responsible for childrearing. There is frequent use of the "family bed" as children may sleep with their parents in one bed until school age. Early toilet training is valued (and is often completed by age 1), but breastfeeding is continued until age 2 or even longer.

Maintaining face is very important to the Chinese and is accomplished by adhering to the rules of society. Chinese believe in status and do not feel that true equality is possible based on Chinese history. Decisions are made based on group consensus with deferral usually given to the oldest members. The individual must strive not to bring shame and not cause another to lose face. Status is acquired through age, job, marriage, and wealth. The concept of privacy is negatively viewed. Privacy is not highly valued or viewed as a luxury by the Chinese people. This is helpful because the majority of Chinese reside in urban areas where privacy is difficult to achieve.

Impact of Faith and Spirituality

Older generations of Chinese may be influenced by a blend of Buddhism, Taoism, and Confucianism. A small minority of Chinese are Muslim or Christian. Many Chinese state that they have no particular religion affiliation or tradition, although they may be very active spiritually.

Korean Americans

Prior to World War II, Korea was impacted by Japanese culture during the 35 years the country was under Japan's control. During World War II, Japan sided with Nazi Germany, and the Japanese government forced the Koreans to support the war effort. When Japan attacked Pearl Harbor, Hawaii, on December 7, 1941, bringing the United States into World War II, the Korean provisional government finally had an opportunity to take a stand against Japan. The provisional government declared war on Japan and formed the Restoration Army to fight alongside the Allies in the Pacific theater.

At the end of World War II in 1945, the United States and the Soviet Union divided the peninsula along the 38th parallel into two zones of occupation—a Soviet-controlled region in the north and an American-controlled one in the south. The peace that Koreans envisioned did not come, however. The Soviets occupied the north and the United States stationed troops in the south. In the months that followed the end of World War II, postwar international decisions were made without the consent of the Korean people. The Soviet Union set up a provisional Communist government in northern Korea, and the United States created a provisional republican government in the south. In 1948, the Republic of Korea was founded south of the 38th parallel, followed by the establishment of the Democratic People's Republic of Korea in the north. Both governments claimed authority over the entire peninsula and tempted fate by crossing the border at various points along the 38th parallel.

On June 25, 1950, North Korea launched a surprise attack on South Korea, beginning a costly, bloody, 3-year struggle known as the Korean War. It was perhaps the most tragic period in modern history for the Korean people. In the end, neither side achieved victory. On July 27, 1953, in the town of Panmunjom, the two sides signed an armistice designating a cease-fire line along the 38th parallel and establishing a surrounding 2.5-mile-wide (4-kilometer-wide) demilitarized zone, which remains the boundary between the two Koreas. The war left the peninsula a wasteland and a divided country that still exists in the 21st century.

Korean emigration was discouraged by the South Korean government after World War II, and North Korea forbade any kind of emigration. The quota system created by the United States Office of Immigration in the 1940s allowed between 105 and 150 immigrants from each of the Asian nations into the country. This law favored immigrants with postsecondary education, technical training, and specialized skills. Most of the Koreans allowed to immigrate were women with nursing training. The War Brides Act of 1945 also helped women and children obtain papers to immigrate.

More women who had married American soldiers were allowed into the United States after the Korean War. By this time, Koreans and all Asians in America were able to acquire citizenship through naturalization as a result of the McCarran-Walter Act of 1952. Foreign adoption of Korean babies also began at the end of the Korean War. The war had left thousands of children orphaned in Korea. Over 100,000 South Korean children have been adopted abroad since the war, and roughly two thirds of these children have been adopted by American families. An estimated 10,000 Korean children have been adopted by Minnesota families alone. Criticized by other countries for running a "baby mill," the South Korean government began to phase out the practice in the 1990s. Although adopting children is traditionally frowned upon in Korean society, social workers are attempting to encourage domestic adoption.

In 1965, the US Congress passed the Immigration and Naturalization Act. The quota system was replaced with a preference system that gave priority to immigration applications from relatives of US citizens and from professionals with skills needed by the United States. Thousands of South Korean doctors and nurses took advantage of the new law. They moved to America and took jobs in understaffed, inner-city hospitals. Koreans with science and technological backgrounds also were encouraged to immigrate. These new immigrants came from middle- and upper-class families, unlike the earlier immigrants. The portion of the law informally known as the "Brothers and Sisters Act" has also been a factor in the dramatic increase in the Korean American population. In 1960, 10,000 Koreans were living in the United States. By 1985, the number had increased to 500,000. According to the US Department of Commerce's

1990 Census of Population, 836,987 Korean Americans had settled in the United States. The 1991 Statistical Yearbook of the Immigration and Naturalization Service states that 26,518 Koreans were admitted to the United States in 1991, making up 1.5% of the total number of immigrants arriving in America that year (US Census Bureau, 2008).

Statistics

Nearly 78% of the US Census Bureau estimated 1.077 million Koreans who live in this country are foreign-born. Despite the changes in immigration law that permitted educated Koreans to enter the United States, problems with language have consequences (US Census Bureau, 2008).

A lack of command of English remains a major setback in the work and social arenas. It is for this reason that some Koreans choose to work in family-owned businesses, which permits them to hold on to their customs and native language. There is a strong desire to maintain a sense of community. Korean culture is maintained within Korean American communities through church organizations, Korean schools, and Korean culture camps. Most Korean immigrants are active Christians and that connection has held strong during migration to the United States. Since the beginning of this century, Korean Protestant churches have offered classes in Korean culture and language. This link between the church and the community has resulted in an easier acculturation for Korean Americans than for other Asian Americans. Today, approximately 1 million Korean Americans live in the United States, and 19% of those live in the South.

Korean Americans' Traditional Health Beliefs

Koreans often avoid entering the US healthcare system because they fear being a burden because of language difficulties. They also fear the unknown, fear being taken advantage of, or fear accruing a large medical bill because of the lack of health insurance.

Koreans are very private people who do not like to seek medical attention. The language barrier also impacts on the seeking out of traditional health care. The act of asking for help from a stranger is considered bold in the Korean culture. The desire to stay within their own cultural group is another barrier as Koreans prefer to seek help only from members of their own social group. Self-expression is not counted as a virtue among Koreans and, therefore, many Koreans feel that medical problems should be kept to oneself. Furthermore, Koreans do not like to discuss things that are distressful in nature; they would prefer to go without necessary health care.

Endurance of pain without complaint is a measure of a person's maturity, and emotions are not freely expressed. Although it is not culturally acceptable to complain of sadness or emotional pain, it is acceptable to utter somatic complaints and seek treatment for indigestion, insomnia, or abdominal pain. Women are more likely to complain of physical symptoms and seek care; men are more likely to seek relief in alcohol.

In general, no restrictions exist that prevent healthcare providers from delivering care to the opposite gender. However, some women may prefer a female physician for gynecologic and obstetric problems.

Impact of Communication

The Korean alphabet consists of 14 consonants and 10 vowels. The degree of formality that exists during communication is dependent on social status and age. In order to gauge a person's age during conversation, the Korean American may ask questions (such as what year did you graduate from high school) to help determine the age of the person with whom they are communicating, and hence the degree of formality that is required. Age is the most important factor in determining the degree of respect a person should be given. It is traditional to bow when greeting elders and to use titles such as "Nurse" in greetings and communication to convey respect. Men may shake hands in greeting but the shake will be done lightly with eyes averted.

Gestures and nonverbal methods of communication are very important in Korean culture. Eye contact is minimal as prolonged eye contact is considered to be rude. Koreans, when needing to point to an object, will use the entire hand or the middle finger—not the index finger. Men do not shake hands with women, and women will usually offer a nod in greeting. Any public displays of affection between genders, such as hugging and kissing, are considered inappropriate. It would be considered appropriate for two members of the same gender to walk down the street holding hands, but not for a male and female couple to do so. It is considered impolite to enter a home or room without knocking or removing one's shoes.

Impact of Time and Space

Time is a loose construct in Korean culture. Even in the school setting, the submission of assignments or schoolwork is not guided by a deadline. The priority is on work completion, not its timeliness. Education is highly valued, however. Korea has the world's highest ratio of PhDs to the general population, as well as one of the lowest illiteracy rates.

Impact of Environment

Food is very important to this culture. Korean food is very unique and highly valued. Garlic is the primary flavoring utilized. Because generally there are far fewer Korean restaurants than Chinese or Japanese, many

Koreans eat in those restaurants or they prepare their own food at home. Larger cities that have a Koreatown or a high number of Korean immigrants may have some Korean restaurants. Korean cuisine is similar to that of the Chinese and Japanese.

Biologic Variations

In the Korean culture, a son or daughter of a cancer survivor or patient might be considered less marriageable because of the concern that there is an "inferior" gene in the family. Mental illness also carries a stigma in Korean culture and should be approached with sensitivity. Koreans are reluctant to talk about psychologic issues or share emotion-laden issues. Stress and depression can affect an older Korean immigrant who is isolated by the language barrier and insulated by social customs.

Impact of Social Organization

Family provides a very important social structure in Korean culture. The family is male-led as the male is the decision maker for the family unit. Individualism is not considered a virtue, and the use of discipline of children within the family may be considered strict when evaluated by other cultures. Education is highly valued and no expense is spared for this. A Korean child's first birthday is considered an event of great importance. Until recently, the infant mortality rate for children younger than the age of 1 was very high in Korean children. As a result, the first birthday is celebrated with prayers and feasts. This celebration, a major milestone in a child's life, is called Tol.

Korean social class is determined by educational level, family background, and financial status. There are a large number of Korean American business owners. Twenty percent of all dry cleaning businesses in the United States are Korean-owned. Although business people may have a higher income than professionals (physicians, attorneys, etc.), the professional, based on his educational level, would be considered to possess the higher social status in the Korean culture.

Korean culture is based on a vertical concept of respect, which is different from the horizontal concept found in the United States. Koreans adhere to a vertical concept of respect in which hierarchical relationships determine to whom you give respect. The mannerisms used and the formality of the language are all based on this vertical concept of respect.

Impact of Faith and Spirituality

Ethnic churches serve as social networks and opportunities for health-care professionals to provide education and programs relating to physical and mental health.

Although many Koreans have a Buddhist heritage, Christianity has become very popular and most Korean immigrants to the Unites States are Protestants.

Cambodian Americans

Cambodia is part of Southeast Asia. Although mainly known as a small agricultural country, Cambodia has a rich artistic and musical tradition. Cambodia was deeply affected by the conflict in Vietnam and was the target of many attacks. The conflict forced many Cambodians to escape to refugee camps in Thailand, and many have made their way to the United States. In addition, there was a terrible genocide in Cambodia called the Khmer Rouge Holocaust. This occurred in the 1970s after the US supported government in Cambodia was overturned in 1975. The Khmer Rouge slaughtered millions of Cambodians in an attempt to establish a new government. Former supporters of the United States within Cambodia were targeted for elimination, as were intellectuals and the upper classes. Education is viewed as a route for advancement. Others, such as rice farmers once driven from the land, made their way to refugee camps in nearby countries and then eventually to the United States.

This forced immigration caused a tremendous amount of stress, which led to psychologic and physical problems in many immigrants. Also, because many Cambodian immigrants were rice farmers with limited education and financial resources, employment opportunities were and continue to be severely limited. Some have found work in factories or have developed trades, such as jewelers or mechanics. With the recent downturn in the US economy, many have lost their positions and are having difficulty finding a new job that would permit reentry into the US workforce.

Cambodian Traditional Health Beliefs

Cambodians believe that imbalance can cause illness. This imbalance may be caused by natural forces or changes in the environment. Cambodians also believe that illness can have spiritual causes. They are likely to use traditional herbs that they purchase at Asian markets, and the traditional Khmer rely on spiritual healing practices.

Traditional healing may be performed by family members or traditional healers and is preferred. Cambodians are fairly comfortable with Western medicine, but they are likely to try more traditional methods of healing first. This means Cambodians are not likely to enter the health-care system for most illnesses, and they practice few if any preventative measures. Normally, they will only seek treatment when experiencing serious injury or illness. Cambodians are usually reluctant to complain or express negative feelings, so it may be difficult for a physician to identify the problem. There is acceptance within the culture of illness and discomfort. Because the illness or discomfort is accepted, the result may be not to seek out care or it can result in a delay in seeking treatment. Cambodians traditionally tend to focus on the symptoms rather than the cause of an illness or disease and, therefore, may stop using medicines after symptoms disappear. They do not place an emphasis on preventive health. Cambodians do not normally value adult immunizations, early disease detection, or health screenings, but they do believe in childhood immunizations. One practice that may be employed is coining. Coining is the practice of firmly rubbing a coin repeatedly on an ill person. The nurse should be careful to consider this healing practice as a possibility when suspecting abuse or physical punishment. Coining has been mistaken for child abuse in some instances.

Impact of Communication

Khmer is the ethnic term for most people from Cambodia, as well as the name of their most commonly spoken language. Other languages, such as English, French, Thai, and Chinese, are also sometimes utilized in schools and business settings. Immigration to the United States has resulted in most second-generation Cambodians being fluent in English. Some first-generation Cambodians may only speak Khmer and require the use of an interpreter.

Impact of Time and Space

Because most Cambodian refugees were farmers, time orientation has its routes in an agricultural paradigm. In the morning, they would head to the fields to work and in the fields, they would stay until the sun went down. This lack of reliance on the use of a clock has resulted in many Cambodian immigrants missing or being late for scheduled appointments.

Be mindful of spacing and avoid prolonged eye contact. It is considered highly inappropriate to stare. Children and youth are expected to approach adults with respect. If an elderly person is seated, children should not walk in front of them or stand up higher than them without bowing the head. Girls should not whistle and must sit with their legs tightly closed. It is considered very disrespectful for a male to approach a female to start a conversation.

Impact of Environment

Cambodians choose to live in close proximity or to have several generations of family all under one roof. The traditional Cambodian diet is healthy as it is rice- and vegetable-based. Some immigrants have adapted their diet to be more American (including fast foods), which has resulted in the development of preventable diseases such as diabetes mellitus and obesity.

Biologic Variatons

Excessive alcohol ingestion is becoming a problem with the Cambodian immigrant population. Drinking alcohol is viewed as a very American activity. The use of alcohol is frowned upon in Buddhist tradition and access to alcohol in Cambodia was nearly impossible. Many drink in excess because the lack of access to alcohol has not permitted them the ability to drink moderately or to become social drinkers.

Excessive alcohol use may be in response to the tremendous stress that the Cambodian immigrant is experiencing. There is a very high incidence of mental health issues, especially posttraumatic stress disorder. Although many Cambodian immigrants have been exposed to traumatic situations prior to entering the United States, which has resulted in significant mental health issues, there is a tremendous reluctance to seek help from Western mental health services.

Impact of Social Organization

A high value is placed on the family unit. Elderly family members are cared for in the home (placement of an elderly family member in a nursing home or assisted living facility is extremely rare). Family needs always take top priority. The male is the head of the household, providing income and making the important decisions. The female is to keep house and rear the children. Because of the Khmer Rouge holocaust, there are more females than males. This has resulted in the development of some female-headed households (where the female is separated from her spouse or widowed). The shortage of Cambodian men has resulted in some cross-cultural arranged marriages, but this is not generally accepted within the majority Cambodian culture. Children are treated differently based on gender. The role of the girl child is to stay home and help her mother, whereas boys are allowed more freedom and can participate in activities outside the home. Marriages are generally arranged but disagreement over this practice is causing conflict among second- or third-generation Cambodian immigrants and their families. Gambling and betting are activities that have been traditionally enjoyed.

Impact of Faith and Spirituality

The primary religion in Cambodia is Buddhism. There are a small number of Cambodians who are Muslim or Christian. Most Cambodian immigrants follow Buddhist practices, recognize Buddhist holidays, and actively participate in Buddhist rituals.

Table 7-5

Cultural Nursing Implications When Caring for Asian/Pacific Islander Patients

Group	Nursing Implications
Laotians	Avoid touching the head or shoulders during assessment. Always provide for modesty, especially with female patients. Respect for the patient, family, and culture is essential. Ensure confidentiality. Remember the patient will be reluctant to share health information. It may take some time to establish a rapport before the patient may feel comfortable to share personal or health information. Laotians, in general, prefer to avoid conflict and are unlikely to show signs of anger even when displeased or annoyed. If they are not satisfied with their nursing or health care, they will not complain but will go elsewhere. When asked a question to answer or given a command to follow, they may say "yes" even if they really mean "no." It is helpful to use open-ended questions that cannot be answered with a simple "yes" or "no" in order to ensure accuracy. One of the most important things that the nurse must do is always offer respect. This is demonstrated by being polite, courteous, friendly, and having good manners.
Japanese	The patient will listen attentively to patient education but will not ask clarifying questions. Remember that silence does not mean agreement. When providing education, remember that the Japanese believe that illness is out of their control. Therefore, they do not place an emphasis on personal control and may not be open to lifestyle modification for disease prevention. They greatly value guidance from the nurse and other healthcare team members regarding health-related issues—not a proponent of patient autonomy. Avoid physical touch as it may result in role confusion and cause the patient anxiety. They prefer formality and structure. The nurse should keep this in mind when planning for nursing interventions. Avoid intense or prolonged eye contact. Patience is an important skill to utilize when providing nursing care.
Vietnamese	Ensure that patient education stresses the importance of compliance with all prescribed interventions, especially with medications and antibiotic therapy as the patient may not complete the dose and store the medication for later use. They may also self-adjust medication doses downward because of the belief that the medications are "too strong" for their body build. There is the concern that oral medications can throw the body out of "balance." Anticipate fear and resistance to cooperating with laboratory and diagnostic testing. They believe blood loss can exacerbate the illness and cannot be replaced because of the illness. Surgery is particularly feared and will only be considered as a last resort.
Koreans	Prolonging life is seen as unacceptable, so do not resuscitate orders are not considered. Discussing terminal status is unacceptable. Organ donation and transplantation are seen as a disturbance in the integrity of the body. Kimchi is considered the national dish and is served at virtually every meal. Made from cabbage, turnips, radishes, or cucumber, kimchi can be prepared many ways, from mild to very spicy. If dietary restrictions permit, allow the patient's family to bring this to the patient. Korean Americans are often comfortable with silence, according to Confucius' belief that "silence is golden." Small talk could appear senseless and insincere. In the Korean culture, the physician's social role can be extremely powerful. Families trust the physician and do not question other options. The sharing of thoughts, feelings, and ideas is very much based on age, gender, and status in the Korean society. The Korean American community might value age over youth, men over women, and the group over the individual.

Group	Nursing Implications
Chinese	The patient may be reluctant to disclose the use of alternative treatments. Many Chinese will assume the "sick role" and rely on others for care/assistance. To appear caring, the nurse should stand close to the patient, speak sympathetically, take an interest in the patient, and verbally encourage them. Do not mistake silence for agreement. There is a reluctance to say "no." The Chinese are shy and will be reluctant to talk to an outsider about their health or psychosocial problems. Try not to be too assertive. Assertiveness can be interpreted as aggressive or even hostile. Avoid touching the head unless absolutely essential. If it must be done, inform the patient first and ask for permission. Avoid touching children, as "careless" touching is believed to be damaging. Again, the nurse should request permission and explain the reason why touch is required.

Vietnamese Americans

Vietnam is a part of Southeast Asia, making up approximately half of the Malay Peninsula. There was a protracted military conflict in Vietnam. In 1975, the communist troops invaded most of Southeast Asia (Vietnam, Cambodia, and Laos). The United States began to admit refugees from these three countries. The need to depart suddenly may have resulted in psychologic stress, trauma, and physical complaints. The Vietnamese comprises the largest population of Southeast Asian refugees that have settled in the United States. There was a large influx of Vietnamese boat people in the late 1970s, which resulted in the passage of the Refugee Resettlement Act of 1980.

It is interesting to note that there are cultural differences between North and South Vietnam. A region of Vietnam was once part of Cambodia, so many of its inhabitants are ethnic Cambodian and speak Khmer. Other ethnic identities exist, including the Cham, a Muslim group, and the tribal people of the Southern Highlands (the Montagnards) who maintain a separate cultural identity from the Vietnamese.

Vietnamese Traditional Health Beliefs

The diagnosis of illness is frequently attributed to three different models. The Vietnamese believe illness can come from spiritual causes, an imbalance (similar to the yin and yang in Chinese culture), and Western medicine (concept of diseases being caused by germs). Traditional Vietnamese medicine is based on the premise of air, fire, water, earth, and metal, with associated characteristics of cold, hot, wet, and dry. Elements must be kept in balance similar to Chinese traditions of yin/yang and hot/cold. A sweet rice porridge is often given to the ill. Dermabrasion is often used to treat a cough. Cupping is used as a treatment for fever reduction and balance, and it may leave marks on the skin that can be mistaken as abuse.

The Vietnamese view Western medicine or American health care as a way to relieve symptoms. When seeking medical care, the expectation is they will be prescribed something to cure their illness immediately. The Vietnamese frequently discontinue medicines after their symptoms disappear because they feel that if they do not experience any symptoms, there is no illness. This can make chronic disease management very difficult. Patient education must place an emphasis on the need to continue therapy, that chronic disease requires long-term medication management, and that symptom remission is not equivalent to a cure. Another safety concern is the fact that it is quite common for Vietnamese patients to save large quantities of half-used prescription drugs for another use. This can be extremely dangerous with infection management. Patient education must stress the importance of completing the full course of prescribed antibiotics. Medicines are viewed as causing imbalance, which may also be another barrier to compliance. The Vietnamese prefer traditional alternatives like a balm, which may better meet the patient's needs while incorporating their cultural values. The Vietnamese have concerns about Western medicine believing that it was developed for Americans and Europeans and not Asians. They feel the dosages are too strong and often will self-adjust the prescribed dosage downward to compensate for this belief.

The Vietnamese hold great respect for those with education, and this is especially true of physicians. The physician is considered the expert on health. The expectations of health restoration are difficult to achieve because they desire a diagnosis and treatment to just take one visit and they do not want much time spent on physical examination or any time spent on laboratory or other diagnostic procedures. Laboratory procedures involving the drawing of blood are feared and even resisted by Vietnamese, who believe that blood loss will exacerbate their illness and that their body cannot replace what was lost. Surgery is particularly feared for this reason and will be agreed to only as a last resort.

In conclusion, Vietnamese people will combine all treatment elements—both traditional healing and Western medicine—in order to achieve maximum benefit. The culture is strongly influenced by China.

Impact on Communication

The Vietnamese language is shared by most people from Vietnam except for isolated minorities such as Montagnards. Dialects vary between north and south and also between rural and urban areas.

Communication is subtle and repetitive. Courtesy is important, and smiling is common. Laughing is not reflective of something being funny or humorous but rather a reflection of disharmony or conflict. Pointing and gesturing can be interpreted as rude.

It is important to not publicly criticize or correct a Vietnamese American as this can cause them to lose face.

Impact of Environment

Many distinguishing cultural factors have been lost to the passage of time since the huge influx of Vietnamese refugees in the 1970s. Today, some Vietnamese Americans are third generation. Earlier immigrants were factory workers but since then, many Vietnamese have moved into technology, education, and business. Prevalent Vietnamese businesses include restaurants, grocery stores, video stores, nail salons, and gift shops.

Biologic Variations

Many Vietnamese Americans are Amerasians, children born in Vietnam to Vietnamese women and American men during the Vietnam War. More than 100,000 immigrants were Amerasians. There is not much focus on exercise, but a healthy diet is the norm. A large part of the diet consists of meat, fish, vegetables, and rice.

Social Organization

Family is the primary social organization. Families often live in multi-generational or extended housing and great respect is provided to the elders. The eldest male is the head of the household. While handshaking is acceptable, elder Vietnamese prefer to bow the head.

Impact of Faith/Spirituality

Many of the early Vietnamese refugees were Roman Catholic and well-educated because they worked closely with the government of the United States. Later refugees were more diverse.

Buddhism, especially Mahayana Buddhism that is heavily influenced by Chinese tradition, is the prevalent religion of the country. The Buddhism of the Khmer is different and is part of the Theravada tradition connected to India. Roman Catholicism, although a minority religion, has also been influential because of the history of colonialism by the French and the political structures that grew out of that. Another popular religion is Cao Dai, prevalent primarily in regions of South Vietnam.

The Lunar New Year is known as Tet Nguyen Dan. It occurs at the beginning of the year between January and February, and it is usually treated as a community celebration regardless of religious affiliation or faith commitment. Another important celebration is Tet Moon. It is celebrated usually around September and its significance is to remind children to be obedient and honest.

Asian Indian Americans

India is a peninsula and is the most populous country in South Asia. The population of approximately 900 million is second only to China. It is populated by a diverse group of ethnicities, languages, and religions.

Most Asian Indians migrated to the United States for educational or economic reasons. In general, the more educated or affluent Indians are the ones that visit or immigrate to the United States. Effort is spent on maintaining close ties with family and loved ones who remain in India.

Impact of Communication

In India, there are more than 17 languages. The most common is Hindi, which is understood by about 71% of the population, followed by English, which is understood by approximately one third of the population. There are hundreds of dialects in India. The English language is commonly used for national and commercial needs. Because India was ruled by Great Britain for more than 100 years (British control was relinquished in 1947), the English spoken is "British English." Some of the vocabulary is different from "American English." India is a multilingual country with over 300 dialects. About 24 of these dialects are spoken by over 1 million people. This diversity is reflected in the Asian Indian community in America. First-generation Indians continue to speak their native language within the family—with spouses, members of the extended family, and friends within the community. Most also speak English fluently, which has made the transition to American society easier for many Indian immigrants.

Regional differences are prevalent. Hindi is spoken mostly by immigrants from northern India and is generally not spoken by South Indians. Immigrants from the states of southern India speak regional languages like Tamil, Telegu, or Malayalam. A substantial number of immigrants from western India, particularly those from the state of Gujarat, continue to speak Gujarati, whereas those from the region of Bengal speak Bengali. Most second- and third-generation Asian Indians understand the language spoken by their parents and extended family, but tend not to speak it themselves. Many Indians are multilingual and speak several Indian languages.

Impact of Faith and Spirituality

Two sovereign nations developed at the end of British rule of British India: India and Pakistan. This was a result of the irreconcilable differences between the Hindu and Muslim religions. India became the land

Box 7-1	

Characteristics of the Religions of Asian Indians

Religion	Characteristics of Religion
Hindu	Functionally polytheistic, but philosophically monotheistic.
	Less formally organized than other religion as prayer meetings can be held in individual homes.
Muslim	Islam means submission to God.
	Believe in the prophet Muhammad who the angel Gabriel ordered to spread the word of God in 610 AD.
	Muhammad recorded the revelations in the holy book, the Koran.
	There are five pillars (requirements) of Islam: (1) confess that there is "no god but God," and Muhammad is the messenger of God; (2) pray five times daily; (3) give of alms; (4) fast in daylight hours for the Muhammadan month of Ramadan; and (5) pilgrimage to Mecca at least once in a lifetime.
Sikh	Sikhism is different from Hinduism in its belief in one God.
	Sikhs follow the teachings of Guru Nanak, the founder of the religion, and worship in temples called Gurudwaras (Gurudwaaras). Services in Gurudwaras are held about once a week as well as on religious occasions. Tenets of the Sikh religion include wearing a turban on the head for males and a symbolic bangle called a Kara around their wrists. In addition, Sikh males are required not to cut their hair or beards. This custom is still followed to by many in the community; others choose to give up the wearing of the turban and cut their hair.

of the Hindus and Pakistan the land of the Muslims. Today's India is a secular nation; although, there is growing political unrest and a push to restore India as the land of the Hindus (Pavri, 2000).

The two primary religions are Hinduism (approximately 82%) and Muslim (approximately 12%) with a small number of followers of Christianity, Sikh, Buddhism, Jainism, Zoroastrianism, and Judaism. Jains follow the doctrine of ahimsa (nonviolence), which causes them to be vegetarian because of the refusal to kill animals. For more on traits of the different religions of Asian Indians, see Box 7-1.

Religion plays a part in burial and funeral rites. After priests offer prayers, the Hindu dead are cremated. In India, the cremation traditionally takes place on a wooden pyre, and the body, which is often dressed in gold-ornamented clothing, burns over several hours. This is in contrast to electric cremation in the United States. Asian Indian Muslims are buried in cemeteries according to Islamic tradition and Christians in accordance with Christian tradition.

Impact of Social Organization

Family is an important construct, and Indian families tend to be large. Extended family may all live together in the same house or in close proximity and rely on each other for childcare. Public displays of affection are avoided as love and affection are only expressed in private. Problems in communication can occur because Indians may shake their head from side to side (indicating "no") to mean "yes." Other body language of interest is that pointing is considered rude and to beckon someone, the palm should be turned down.

Asians Indians are divided into castes, and a child belongs to the caste of his parents. The caste placement has implications for everything: social standing, education, career, and marriage. Marriage is influenced by region and religion in addition to the caste system and is often arranged. Despite the discrimination associated with a caste system, tolerance and diversity are central to Indian culture. India is considered the largest democracy in the world.

Asian Indians are an extremely ethnically diverse group. The subgroups trace their roots to different regions or states within India, each of which speak different languages, eat different diets, and follow unique customs. On festive occasions, you may expect to see female Asian Indians wearing the traditional sari (yards of colorfully embroidered or printed silk or cotton wrapped around the body) or a bindi (a dot placed on the forehead), which may indicate that the woman is married but it may also be worn at celebrations. Jewelry is also valued in the culture. Indians are very fond of gold jewelry, and many women wear simple gold ornaments like rings, earrings, bangles, and necklaces daily, and more elaborate ones at special occasions. Jewelry is often passed down through the generations from mother to daughter or daughter-in-law.

Asian Indians Traditional Health Beliefs

Most Asian Indians accept the role of Western medicine and pay careful attention to health matters. Despite this, ayurvedic medicine continues to have many adherents.

Ayurveda emphasizes spiritual healing as an essential component of physical healing and bases its cures on herbs and natural ingredients such as raw garlic and ginger. Ayurveda also focuses on preventive healing. Homeopathic medicine also has adherents among Asian Indians in the United States. Some members of the Asian Indian American community practice yoga. The ancient practice of yoga dates back several thousand years. It combines a routine of exercise and meditation to maintain the balance between body and mind.

There is a stigma associated with mental health disorders, and Asian Indians are less inclined to seek out assistance for mental health problems than they are for physical health problems. The traditional Indian belief has been that mental problems will eventually take care of themselves, and that the family rather than outside experts should take care of the mentally ill.

Japanese Americans

Japan is a country of islands located in the Pacific Ocean. Japan is composed of four large islands and approximately 4000 small islands. There was a ban on immigration for all Asians between 1924 and 1950. In addition, there was a tremendous injustice perpetrated against Japanese Americans as a result of World War II. In 1942, anyone of Japanese ancestry living on the Pacific Coast was placed in a relocation camp. Descendents of the survivors of this internment may have psychologic issues. Many Japanese who seek out health care may be in the United States temporarily studying or working for Japanese-owned corporations.

Japanese Health Beliefs

The Japanese believe that the body is as holy as the mind. In fact, Japanese tradition views the mind and body as one. Japanese people are very reluctant to accept the diagnosis of being brain dead. Stating that the person is "dead" could be viewed as disrespectful.

Organ donation can be a very difficult topic to broach because many Japanese are unwilling to alter the dead body of a person who they feel could influence their lives in the future. Agreeing to donate one's organs could cause concern that the oneness of body and soul might be destroyed. The issues are not only related to donation of the organs but also to accepting a transplant. There is also concern about whether the patient would benefit from an organ transplantation. Accepting the organs of a dead person could be seen as disrespectful by some Japanese and could trigger anxiety.

Japanese individuals will probably listen well during health education, but they may be reluctant to ask a question or add a comment since individual assertion is highly discouraged in their culture. They may be reluctant to bring up anything they believe would cause a conflict and would not share a differing opinion. Be careful not to assume that silence means agreement with the plan of care as it just may be the patient's way of avoiding a conflict.

Japanese culture does not place an emphasis on personal control, so they will be more likely to view an illness as something outside their own control. Therefore, healthcare providers will need to keep this in mind when educating Japanese Americans about risk factors for a particular disease (such as a fatty diet being a risk factor for heart disease).

US healthcare delivery is based on the premise of patient autonomy and patient choice. Patient choice is not a value of the Japanese. It is for this reason that the Japanese patient will greatly require and appreciate guidance from physicians, nurses, and other healthcare team members.

Impact of Touch

Nurses and other healthcare professionals should avoid physical touching, which may cause anxiety in the Japanese. Because the Japanese view health professionals as authority figures, physical touching may cause role confusion. Careful explanation of all interventions, especially when touch is required, should always be provided. The nurse should also consider the amount of eye contact they are providing. To show respect, the nurse should avoid intense or long-term eye contact. Patience is an important skill and will be helpful when dealing with the Japanese.

Filipino Americans

Filipino Americans now rank as the second largest Asian group in the United States with over 1.8 million individuals reported in the 2000 census. The 2000 census reveals a tremendous growth in the Filipino American population from earlier census studies. There was a 32% increase from the 1980 census, and a 137% increase from the 1990 census. It is felt that this tremendous growth is caused by the search of Filipinos for economic opportunity and the political relationship between the governments of the United States and the Philippines (US Census Bureau, 2008).

Immigration from the Philippines to the American continent began with the Manila–Acapulco Galleon Trade. From 1565 to 1815, Filipinos were forced to work as navigators and sailors on Spanish ships. In 1587, Filipino sailors claimed Morro Bay, California, for the Spanish King. In 1763, the first permanent settlement occurred in the bayous of Louisiana. These early settlers, called "Manilamen," settled in Louisiana after jumping ship to escape the brutality they had experienced from the Spanish masters. They built houses on stilts along the gulf ports of New Orleans, Louisiana.

In Philippine society, Pilipino or Tagalog is the national language, and English is the second official language. Although about 80–100 ethnic languages are spoken in this country of 7000 islands, English is used to conduct internal and global business. Among Filipino Americans, a combination of English/Tagalog or "Tag-Lish," a hybrid language, is spoken by many and is used extensively. More than two thirds of households speak a non-English language.

Health Status

It is difficult to determine the health status of Filipinos because of the limited number of studies that have been conducted. Often, Asians are grouped together or there are other inconsistencies in coding for race or ethnicity. Therefore, it is not always possible to distinguish Filipinos from the rest of the AAPI sample. Moreover, it is difficult to generalize research findings because the sample size is too small, only one study has been done, or the only populations studied are in California or Hawaii. Finally, in some cases, data are just not available. For these reasons, the information contained in this section of the chapter is based on an estimate of Filipino American health status based on the limited data available.

The National Health Interview Survey (conducted between 1992 and 1994) revealed that 37% of the Filipino respondents described their health as excellent, 32% as very good, 24% as good, and 7% as fair or poor. These results are very similar to those for other APPIs (Kuo & Porter, 1998).

It does appear that high blood pressure is an issue for Filipino Americans as Filipinos living in the Philippines tend to have lower blood pressure. It appears that the excessive sodium intake associated with the American diet may be responsible. In addition to hypertension, Filipino immigrants are also considered at high risk for coronary artery disease, adult (or mid-life) onset diabetes mellitus, gout, and cancer. High rates of hyperuricemia and gout are found among men, particularly in low to middle income groups in the Philippines.

Filipino women have been shown to have a high rate of gestational diabetes. Filipino mothers born outside of the United States are significantly more likely to have diabetes during pregnancy. Very low birth weight (500–1499 g) and moderately low birth weight (1500–2499 g) was more likely among Filipino women than Whites.

Cancer is the second leading cause of death among Filipino Americans (Hoyert & Kung, 1997). The prevalence of some cancers seems to vary depending on place of birth.

Rates of primary liver cancer were higher for foreign-born Filipino men than American-born Filipino men (11% to 7%), and both were higher than Whites (3%).

Filipino women born in the Philippines had 3.2 times the rate of thyroid cancer of US-born White women, whereas US-born Filipino women were not at any increased risk than White women. For other cancers, prevalence does not seem to depend on place of birth.

Ovarian cancer incidence among US-born Filipino women is comparable to foreign-born Filipino women (8.1 versus 11.0 per 100,000), and lower than White women (15.6 per 100,000). Breast cancer incidence was the same for US- and foreign-born Filipino women, and 40% lower than breast cancer incidence of US-born Whites.

There are other disparities in cancer prevalence. The incidence of liver cancer in Filipino populations is higher than among Caucasians.

Filipino men born in the Philippines had 2.6 times the rate of thyroid cancer of US-born White men, whereas US-born Filipino men had 1.5 times the risk of White men.

Breast cancer is a concern and there appear to be regional differences in incidence. Filipino women in Hawaii had the lowest risk at 29 per 100,000 (Goodman, 1991), whereas women 40 years and older in the San Francisco Bay Area had an age-adjusted risk of 119, much higher than Black, Chinese, and Japanese women, but lower than Whites (Northern California Cancer Center [NCCC], 1993b). Filipino women had the lowest survival rate of the five groups except Blacks. Bay Area Filipino women had higher overall age-adjusted cancer incidence for all sites than the other groups except Whites (NCCC, 1993b). Rates in the Bay Area Filipino men for age-adjusted incidence of cancer in all sites are lower than most of the five groups compared, but higher than Chinese and Japanese (NCCC, 1993a). Liver cancer among Filipino men and women was second only to the Chinese and three times higher than among Whites (NCCC, 1993a,b).

The Philippines is reported to have the highest incidence of TB in the world. Filipino World War II veterans were permitted a rapid entry into the United States in the 1990s, which waived the need for a physical examination. It is felt that this may explain the increased incidence of TB in this population. Infectious diseases are a major health issues for AAPIs as AAPIs have greater incidence rates of TB and hepatitis B than any other ethnic or racial group.

Impact of Social Organization

The Filipino values of interdependence and social cohesiveness may have evolved from the group orientation necessary to live in an archipelago of 7000+ islands, located in the ring of fire, where only 1000 islands are habitable. This may partly explain the existence of hundreds of Filipino American organizations across the United States.

Impact of Faith and Spirituality

An estimated 80% of Filipinos are Catholics, some are members of Protestant churches, and others the Aglipay, a church whose origin is in the Philippines. Filipino Muslims originate primarily from Mindanao and Sulu, the southernmost region of the country where successful resistance to Spanish colonization led to preservation of their culture and traditions. Collectively, the sociocultural, psychologic, economic, and political legacy of the precolonial Filipino tribes was congruent with those of Islander people in the Pacific Rim.

Pacific Islander Americans

In reality, there is no such thing as one AAPI composite, especially when there are more differences than similarities between the many groups designated by the federally defined categories of "Asian American" and/or "Pacific Islander." Although there are varied and historical reasons for reporting these groups under one umbrella, it is critical for nurses to recognize that there are numerous AAPI ethnicities, many historical backgrounds, and a full range of socioeconomic spectra, from the poor and underprivileged to the affluent and highly educated. There is no simple description that can characterize AAPI patients or communities as a whole.

Statistics

In the 2000 census, a total of 861,000 people, or 0.3% of the total population, reported that they belonged to the Native Hawaiian and other Pacific Islander population. Three groups—Native Hawaiians (with over 100,000 people), Samoans, and Guamanians—together accounted for 74% of the Pacific Islander population (US Census Bureau, 2008).

In 2000, 78% of all Pacific Islanders 25 years and older had completed high school or beyond, and 14% had a bachelor's degree or more education. The corresponding rates for the US population were 80% and 24%, respectively (US Census Bureau, 2008).

Pacific Islanders were most likely to hold sales and office jobs (29%), whereas management, professional, or related occupations were most common (34%) for the total population.

Of the Pacific Islander population, 17.7% lived below poverty in 1999. This was higher than the 12.4% poverty rate for the US population. Among the detailed Pacific Islander groups, Marshallese had the highest poverty rate at 38.3%. Native Hawaiians, Guamanians, and Fijians had the lowest poverty rates among the detailed Pacific Islander groups (US Census Bureau, 2008).

Summary

AAPIs are one of the fastest growing ethnic groups. The nurse will encounter patients from this group. Because of the variety and complexity of cultural values and health beliefs, the nurse must strive to learn about these values and beliefs and then strive to provide individualized patient care. The nursing care should be formulated to consider the impact of barriers to care such as communication, time and space, social organization, and biologic variations. Comprehensive and holistic care can only be delivered when the cultural values and beliefs of the patient are incorporated and considered.

Case Study 7-1

Vietnamese Woman with Complaint of Dizziness

A 70-year-old Vietnamese woman presented to the emergency room, accompanied by her two adult children, with a complaint of dizziness. The emergency room physician during the examination noted deep red welts running up both of the patient's arms. Alarmed, the physician requested that the nurse contact social services with a suspicion of elder abuse. Luckily, the nurse has had cultural competency training and was familiar with the Vietnamese custom of coin rubbing. When the nurse questioned the patient's son, he told the nurse that he had rubbed his mother's body with a coin in an attempt to heal her. The woman was properly diagnosed with labyrinthitis and because the coin rubbing is not harmful to the patient, it was included in the treatment plan. The patient was discharged home where she recovered.

Rationale: The patient's family was practicing a traditional form of healing known as coin rubbing. There are several variations, including heating the coin, but they all involve vigorously rubbing the body with a coin. This produces red welts, which can distract medical staff from the real problem or be mistaken for elder or child abuse. It is important for the nurse to recognize and become familiar with this practice, and not to be distracted from the real problem or mistakenly make accusations of abuse.

Asians rubbing their children, their elders, or themselves with coins is not abuse as it is an attempt to heal an illness, and it is often effective.

Case Study 7-2

Critically Ill Korean Patient

A 27-year-old Korean man was visiting extended family in the United States when he became very ill. He was brought to the emergency room by his concerned family. The patient was diagnosed with renal and respiratory failure and an order was written for strict bed rest to limit his exertion. The patient speaks very little English and the family only a minimal amount of English. This made communication difficult for all involved. Frequently, conflict would erupt when a staff member would find the patient, with assistance from his family, standing over a bedpan attempting bowel elimination. The staff would interrupt and tell the patient and his family that the patient was not permitted out of bed and that the bedpan was to be used in the bed. This was difficult to convey because of the language barrier and the patient and his family would become very upset. The nurse educator for the hospital was consulted as she had expertise in cultural competency. She explained to the staff that the patient was using the bedpan in the only way that he knew because in most Asian countries, toilets are holes in the ground. To eliminate from the bowels, the Asian squats over the hole, just like the patient was attempting to do with the bedpan. The nurse called the nurse practitioner who changed the order to permit the patient out of bed for bathroom privileges as needed with assistance. The patient and his family were much happier and cooperative as a result.

Rationale: In Asian culture, bowel elimination is unclean and should not be done in bed. The patient and his family were trying to maintain standards of cleanliness and decency. Knowledge of cultural practices permitted the treatment plan to be safely modified so that the patient and his family could manage this bodily function in an appropriate manner.

References

Acupuncture. Natural Standard Database. Retrieved March 6, 2009, from http://www.naturalstandard.com.

Barnes, P. M., Powell-Griner, E., McFann, K., & Nahin, R. L. (2004). Complementary and alternative medicine use among adults: United States, 2002. *CDC Advance Data Report, 27, 343,* 1–19.

Cardini, F., & Weixin, H. (1998). Moxibustion for correction of breech presentation: A randomized controlled trial. *Journal of the American Medical Association, 280,* 1580–1584.

Centers for Disease Control and Prevention. (2007). Reported Tuberculosis in the United States, 2007. Retrieved March 28, 2009, from http://www.cdc.gov/tb/statistics/reports/2007/default.htm.

Chen, M. S. (2000). Launching of the Asian-American Network for Cancer Awareness Research and Training (AANCART). *Asian American and Pacific Islander Journal of Health, 8,* 1, 1–3.

Coyle, M. E., Smith, C. A., & Peat, B. (2005). Cephalic version by moxibustion for breech presentation. *Cochrane Database of Systematic Reviews, 2,* CD003928.

Ghosh, C. (2003). Healthy People 2010 and Asian Americans/Pacific Islanders: Defining a baseline of information. *American Journal of Public Health, 93,* 12, 2093–2098.

Goodman, D. S. (1991). *China in the nineties: Crisis management and beyond* (with Gerald Segal). New York: Oxford University Press.

Hall, E. T. (1963). A system for the notation of proxemic behavior. *American Anthropologist, 65,* 1003–1026.

Harris, P. M., & Jones, N. A. (2005). *We The People: Pacific Islanders in the United States. Census 2000 Special Reports.* Washington, DC: US Department of Commerce, Bureau of the Census.

Hoyert, D. L., & Kung, H. C. (1997). *Asian or Pacific Islander mortality, selected states, 1992. Monthly Vital Statistics Report.* Hyattsville, MD: National Center for Health Statistics.

Kuo, J., & Porter, K. (1998). *Health Status of Asian Americans: United States, 1992–94. Advance data from vital and health statistics; no. 298.* Hyattsville, MD: National Center for Health Statistics.

National Center for Health Statistics. (2002). Health, United States, 2002 with urban and rural chartbook. Hyattsville, MD: National Center for Health Statistics.

Northern California Cancer Center. (1993a). Average annual age-adjusted incidence rates for selected sites, 1986–1990, for men in the San Francisco Bay Area. Unpublished paper. Union City, CA: Author.

Northern California Cancer Center. (1993b). Average annual age-adjusted incidence rates for selected sites, 1986–1990, for women in the San Francisco Bay Area. Unpublished paper. Union City, CA: Author.

Office of Management and Budget. (1997). Revisions to the standards for the classification of federal data on race and ethnicity. Retrieved September 14, 2009, from http://www.whitehouse.gov/omb/rewrite/fedreg/ombdir15.html.

Overfield, T. (1995). *Biologic variations in health and illness.* Reading, MA: Addison-Wesley.

Pavri, T. (2000). Asian Indian Americans. *Gale encyclopedia of multicultural america.* New York: Gale Group.

US Census Bureau. (2008). Table 4: Annual estimates of the Black or African American alone or in combination population by sex and age for the United States: April 1, 2000, to July 1, 2007. Source: Population Division, US Census Bureau. Release Date: May 1, 2008.

US Department of Health and Human Services, (1998). Tobacco use among US racial/ ethnic minority groups - African Americans, American Indians and Alaska Natives, Asian Americans and Pacific Islanders, and Hispanics: a report of the surgeon general. Atlanta, GA: US Department of Health and Human Services, Centers for Disease Control and Prevention, National Center for Chronic Disease Prevention and Health Promotion, Office on Smoking and Health.

Xinnong, C. (1987). *Chinese acupuncture and moxibustion*. Beijing: Foreign Languages Press.

Chapter 8

Native Americans

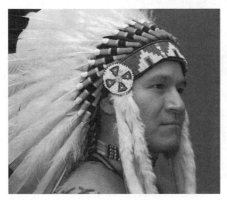

Source: © Elena Loachim/ShutterStock, Inc.

Chapter Objectives

Upon completion of this chapter, the nurse will be able to:

1. Describe the traditional health beliefs of Native Americans.

2. Develop a plan of care that incorporates those traditional health beliefs within the American healthcare delivery system.

3. Be familiar with the history of Native Americans in relation to its impact on current health status of Native Americans.

Introduction

There are at least two ways of learning about Native American culture. The first would be to commit to learning everything about one or two different tribes. This will limit the nurse's knowledge to only those tribes, and the nurse must understand that he or she cannot transfer that knowledge and apply it to another tribe. The second option, and the strategy employed in this chapter, is to learn general aspects of Native American culture that apply to more than one tribe's culture with the understanding that the knowledge possessed will only be at a very superficial level. The degree of acculturation into the dominant American society and its culture will also impact each and every individual Native American. There will be numerous exceptions to this knowledge from Native American culture to culture.

Historical Background

Native Americans had lived throughout the North American continent for thousands of years before European settlers came to America in the 15th century. Although still theoretical, most scientists agree that North America was populated by travelers who crossed a land bridge (Beringia) that once spanned the Bering Sea and connected Northeastern Asia to North America. The reasons or motivations for the migration are not known. The first travelers arrived over 10,000 years ago, just prior to the last Ice Age. Others, including some Native Americans and scholars, believe that the ancestors of Native Americans originated in the Americas. This belief is based on oral history that has been passed down through the ages and some gaps found in archaeological records.

What is not under dispute is the amazing ability of Native Americans to adapt to the climates and terrains of America and the ability to use natural resources. Over many thousands of years, many cultures developed across North America. Culture development and practices were suited to the local environment associated with the distinct geographic region. Each geographic region is made up of the climate, landforms, and natural resources. In the Northeast, Native Americans used the forests to build houses, canoes, and tools. Those living in the Pacific Northwest relied on the abundance of fish and other sea life for food. In the desert of the Southwest, corn was grown and housing developed from adobe (sun-dried brick). In the bitter arctic, adaptation continued and many survived by developing skills in hunting and fishing.

There were several hundred different Native American groups that settled in North America, many of whom still exist and have maintained their distinct culture. Each group has its own unique political structure, social systems, clothing styles, type of shelter and foods, art and musical style, language, education, and spiritual and philosophical beliefs. There are also many similarities including a strong tie and connection to the Earth and nature.

There is a clear distinction between American Indians and Alaska Natives. The term Native American is intended to apply to tribes residing in the continental United States (and does not include Canadian tribes such as Inuit). One should not consider that all American Indians reside on reservations in rural areas, as this is not correct. An equal number live in urban areas (cities) mainly in Oklahoma, California, New Mexico, and even Alaska (US Bureau of the Census, 2002).

It is believed by many that the term Indians resulted from the belief that the early settlers, under Christopher Columbus, were in Asia. Asia in Spanish is "the Indies" and the native people were called "indios," which meant people of the Indies. Later, that was translated to Indian. Others believe the early natives were called "In Dios," which means "Of God." The term Native American became popular in the 1960s, but critics feel that it really is too broad a term as it could also pertain to Hawaiians, descendents of immigrants, or to anyone born in America.

In many ways, the history of health disparities in the Native American population follows that found in the African American population. The arrival of European settlers to the new world resulted in many consequences. The Native American population was drastically reduced because of a wide range of communicable diseases that were brought to America from the crowded European cities that were home to the settlers. Because the Native Americans had no immunity, the diseases spread quickly and lethally. The spread of infection (i.e., measles, smallpox, typhoid) was so profound that infection could spread to a Native American and annihilate an entire Native American community before they had even seen a European settler. Once the European settlers had contact with the natives, sexually transmitted infections also became a huge infection problem. From the 16th century and up to the 20th century, epidemics and pandemics decimated the Native American population; for example, the Pueblo population (residents of the Southwest) fell by an estimated 90 to 95% in the 75-year period between 1775 and 1850.

Other consequences of European settlement were warfare, relocation, and removal of Native Americans from their homeland and the destruction of traditional Native American ways of life. Barriers to access to their land for hunting and farming resulted in starvation and malnutrition, which increased the likelihood of infection becoming lethal because of a greater susceptibility to disease. Relocation often resulted in the placement of one tribe on the land of another and hostilities often broke out.

Although Native Americans have not suffered the ignominy of slavery, there have, nonetheless, been abuses leveled against them by our government. In 1830, America passed the Indian Removal Act. This act permitted the forcible removal of Native Americans from their homelands in Florida, Mississippi, Georgia, and Alabama to reservations in the Oklahoma territory. The trail that these native Americans were forced to travel is referred to as the "Trail of Tears." Thousands of Cherokee Indians were killed on the Trail of Tears while being forced westward. After many different battles, the Indians were finally forced, on January 31, 1876, onto reservations. Today, many Native Americans continue to live on reservations, whereas many others do not. There are currently 563 reservations, most of them located in the western states. The reservations are exempt from US laws.

Some natives learned to live together with the European settlers by setting up trade and adopting some European ways. Many more faced turmoil and upheaval that lasted for many generations as Europeans and later Americans and Canadians took the land and attempted to extinguish their way of life. During the 20th century and beyond, many Native American tribes started to regain control and are experiencing a cultural resurgence. The population levels also began to increase. It is felt that the population increase is caused by decreased mortality rates, declining disease rates, improved fertility, and more people who are self-identifying as Native American on census forms. For the 2000 census, 2.48 million people identified themselves as American Indian, which was a significant increase from 1.8 million during the 1990 census (US Bureau of the Census, 2000).

Over the years, many treaties were signed between the Native Americans and the American government which promised education and healthcare services. Provision of health care fell to the US Army, which was not equipped to handle this responsibility. In 1955, the Indian Health Service was established.

The Indian Health Service falls under the jurisdiction of the US Department of Health and Human Services and coordinates federally mandated health-related services for Native Americans and Alaska Natives. The 1975 Indian Self-Determination Act allows tribes to manage health services independently if desired.

One of the most important cultural values that have been identified in Native Americans is resiliency and collaboration. Collaboration provides a force to work with or against the White nonnative populations. Native Americans have proven the ability to work with and reside in different environments and with different people. This ability permitted them to learn the ways of the settlers (White people) so they could use this knowledge to guide their interactions. Resiliency is evidenced by, for example, clinging to their native language to overcome linguistic oppression.

Despite these strengths of resiliency and collaboration, today, Native Americans are the poorest, least educated, and most neglected minority group in the United States. By any mathematical standard, reservation-dwelling Native Americans are on the lowest socioeconomic rung in the United States. At least half of reservation dwellers fall under the federal poverty level and continue to survive only through the utilization of government programs, such as food stamps, welfare, and Medicaid. How desperate are the economic circumstances? According to the US Census Bureau (2005), the median household income for Native Americans was $32,866 compared with a median household income of $43,318 for the overall US population.

Throughout the United States, numerous reservations have turned to gaming operations as a source of economic opportunity. In 1988, the US Congress passed the Indian Gaming Regulatory Act, which permitted tribes to negotiate with individual states to set up casinos. By 2001, approximately one third of federally recognized tribes owned a total of about 300 casinos in 29 states. Much of the revenue and the jobs go to non-Indian investors, overhead, and taxes, so despite the generation of revenue in the billions, only a few Native American communities have seen these large profits, which means the economic situation continues to be bleak for many Native Americans. Only an estimated 25% of gaming industry jobs is held by Native Americans.

Statistics

We must begin by stating that proper terminology usage is difficult as there is no consensus. Even the definition of what constitutes an Indian is subject to debate. Should the label be Indian or Native American? Many older American Indians prefer the term "Indian" to "Native American," believing that anyone born in the United States is a "Native American," and that the term "Indian" reflects the language used in treaties with the federal government. There is no one legal definition for the term "Indian." This lack of consensus has resulted in the courts establishing the following two-part definition: (1) the person must have some identifiable Indian ancestry, and (2) that the Indian community must recognize this person as an Indian. At the tribal level, each tribe determines the criteria for enrollment. This is further complicated because of intermarriage. The US census category includes anyone who self-identifies as "Indian."

Another determinant used is the amount of "Indian blood" possessed. Tribes have varying measures that must be met for tribe inclusion and enrollment (e.g., one-half, one-quarter, or one-eighth Indian blood). Finally, the Cherokee Nation accepts anyone whose ancestor's name appears on any one of several rolls, including the Dawes Roll. The Dawes Roll is a list that was drawn up by the federal government during the Allotment Era of Indians receiving a 160-acre "allotment" of land as their portion of the Indian Territory in Oklahoma.

According to the most recent population estimates from the US Census Bureau that were released on May 1, 2008, there are 2,938,436 American Indian and Alaska natives in the United States. More than 300 American Indian tribes are recognized by the federal government. The American Indian population is confined to 26 states, according to census data, with the vast majority residing in the Western part of the country because of the forced migration westward of the tribes by the government. According to the 2000 census, 43% of American Indians reported living in the West, 31% in the South, 17% in the Midwest, and 9% in the Northeast. In addition, there are at least another 1.6 million who are of a mixed heritage that includes American Indian or Alaska native (US Bureau of the Census, 2000). Most Native Americans prefer to be identified by their tribal affiliation, and the most common collective terms used are Native American or American Indian.

According to 2000 census data for Native Americans, the largest American Indian nations were Cherokee, Navajo, Latin American Indian, Choctaw, Sioux, and Chippewa (Ogunwole, 2002). The largest Alaska Native group was Eskimo (Ogunwole, 2002).

Variables Impacting Degree of Acculturation

There are many variables that impact the degree of acculturation of a Native American patient. Some of the most impactful variables identified are life experience such as geographic area of birth (on reservation versus off reservation or urban versus rural), previous exposure to traditional Native American health beliefs, military service, intertribal marriage, presence or absence of health benefits, as well as the types of health benefits possessed (Indian Health Service, Medicaid, tribal contract/compact, health maintenance organization, etc.).

Definition of Health and Illness

Although it would be impossible to include information on each and every one of the hundreds of Indian tribes in the United States, there are common themes regarding health and illness that provide general beliefs and practices that the nurse can become familiar with in order to deliver culturally appropriate care to Native American patients. Many Native Americans consider illness as a result from an imbalance in mind, body, and spirit.

Unlike other minority groups, the federal government is required by law and by treaty to provide healthcare services through the Indian Health Service. Conflict can occur because in Western medicine, the provider often asks the patient for their impression of what may be wrong. Asking this question of a Native American may result in them thinking the provider is ignorant not only of their culture but also of how to care for them as a patient. Support of the sick role in this culture is also not acceptable. Instead, support is directed at assisting the person to regain harmony with nature and with others. It is felt that people with illness have done something to place themselves out of harmony or have had a curse placed on them. This is especially the view with regard to mental illness or mental disorders. Mental illness is viewed as resulting from witching (the placing of a curse) on a person. Treatment requires the expertise of a specialized Native American healer. The degree of nonacceptance of the sick role, for any disorder, is so strong that even a seriously ill elderly Native American will continue to work even if that will result in further illness or a poor outcome. A great deal of encouragement for the patient to rest will be required without guarantee of success.

Specific Nursing Considerations

It is important for the nurse to approach patient care with an appreciation and basic understanding of common factors that may impact the clinical domain that have been associated with Native American patients. Self-disclosure and the sharing of information may be a difficult hurdle for the Native American patient. The nurse should not try to be too aggressive in attempting to get the patient to share some health history information that may be guarded by the patient. Being too aggressive may cause irreparable damage to the nurse–patient relationship. The nurse should also avoid a problem-focused approach, such as asking, "What is your problem?" Relying on a problem-oriented framework is not recommended as the Native American patients (especially if they are older) may be offended because focusing on a problem places a power differential between the patient with the problem and the nurse who has the answer to the problem. This may be difficult to remember or to do because many documentation systems are established around a problem-focused framework.

Food is an important part of Native American culture, and the traditional foods are very healthy. In recent years, because of poverty on many reservations, a reliance on the provision of foods which can be unhealthy if relied on to excess, such as cheese, lard, sugar, and white flour, has resulted. The nurse should provide nutrition guidance but be aware that the teaching must include the culturally appropriate foods of the patient's ancestors (squash, melon, corn, etc.), portions, timing of meals, as well as food-related rituals. Food is a part of social activity, and the sharing of food is an important part of the culture. The nurse should not be surprised to see a Native American patient sharing a meal tray with a visitor. It is culturally appropriate not only for the patient to offer the food to the visitor, but it would be rude for the visitor to refuse such an offer. Visitors may also bring in inappropriate foods for the patient. To avoid problems with not enough food because of sharing or access to inappropriate foods, it may be best for the nurse to encourage visiting time that avoids meal time if possible so that the patient will have access to all of the food required for the day while hospitalized.

Request permission prior to touching the patient as touching is viewed as inappropriate in some tribal cultures. Modesty and privacy are highly valued, and the utmost effort should be attempted by the nurse to ensure that this is provided and not violated in any way. The removal of clothing should only be requested if absolutely essential and if an accommodation can be made, the nurse should provide that accommodation—at a minimum, the patient should be draped if clothing must be removed. Speak quietly to not appear rude and also to maintain patient confidentiality.

If you suspect that you may be dealing with a mental health issue of some type, the nurse should proceed with caution and sensitivity. Depression, or any other mental health complaint, may not be verbalized as the chief complaint. The nurse should be on guard for somatic complaints (fatigue, tiredness), minimization of symptoms as just being a part of life, or symptoms may be expressed as a "cultural metaphor" such as "I have a heavy heart" or "I am having an issue with my esteem." The bottom line is that symptoms of this type will be minimized by both the patient and family and, often, help will not be sought out until the physical symptoms are severe. The nurse must remember that there are vast differences in beliefs, terminology, or labels utilized as well as other language differences that exist among various tribes.

Patient education should also be an important focus of the nurse. The most frequent causes of death of Native Americans are lack of patient education and that health promotion could be positively impacted through the provision of culturally competent educational programs. When providing patient education, the nurse should include demonstration whenever possible. Native Americans prefer one-on-one education rather than printed materials. Pictures and demonstrations are more effective than describing as the traditional way of teaching in Native American culture is "doing" over "talking."

Traditional Health Beliefs

Providing culturally appropriate interventions requires that the nurse assess the Native American's degree of tribal affiliation, the level or importance given to traditional health beliefs, and the degree of acceptance or acculturation to the Western biomedical model of the patient. The nurse should also keep in mind that many Native Americans have had exposure to medical care through the Indian Health Service, clinics, or from military or veteran settings, which will impact on care expectations and comfort level. There is also the possibility that the patient may be distrustful of the healthcare system because of past abuses as well as the belief that this system is based on money and greed and is not patient-centered.

Traditional Native American views of healing and wellness emphasize seeking harmony within oneself, with others, and with one's surroundings. In the traditional Native American way, medicine can consist of physical remedies, but medicine is also much more than a pill you take to cure illness or correct a physiological malfunction. Medicine is everywhere; it is the essence of their inner being that gives inner power (Garrett, 1999). The traditional Indian belief about health is that it reflects living in total harmony with nature and being able to survive even in difficult circumstances. Native Americans highly value traditional beliefs concerning relation, harmony, balance, spirituality, and wellness; as part of valuing "relation," all these beliefs are interrelated (Tsai & Alanis, 2004). Again, this may be an oversimplification because when discussing Native Americans, we are dealing with a multiplicity of cultures, so there cannot be only one belief.

Traditional healers are capable of understanding illness from a perspective that includes spirituality and symptom etiology relative to the patient's unique culture. Depending on the patient's degree of acculturation, the use of pharmacologic interventions may be culturally congruent, while with some patients, they will only respond to or permit traditional healing interventions/strategies. The degree of acceptance of Western medicine is variable. The goal is to address the patient's health concerns in a culturally appropriate manner. This is often best achieved when they are treated by both traditional and Western healers.

Native American patients may request Native American Healing (NAH). NAH has been practiced in North America for over 10,000 years. NAH is a broad term that includes healing beliefs and practices of hundreds of indigenous tribes of North America. It combines religion, spirituality, herbal medicine, and rituals that are used to treat people with medical and emotional conditions. The following concepts are associated with NAH: it takes a lot of time for healing to occur, healing takes place within the context of a relationship, achieving an energy of activation is necessary, biologic systems behave similarly across hierarchic levels, the distractions of modern life "inactivate" catalysts for change, modern culture systematically teaches us to ignore emotions and to maintain a low level of emotional awareness, physiologic change often requires a break in usual daily rhythms, and the importance of ceremony as a means of accessing help from the spiritual dimension for healing.

From the Native American perspective, medicine is more about healing the person than curing a disease. Traditional healers aim to "make whole" by restoring well-being and harmonious relationships with the community and the spirit of nature, which is sometimes called God or the Great Mystery. NAH is based on the belief that everyone and everything on Earth is interconnected, and every person, animal, and plant has a spirit or essence. Even an object, such as a river or rock, and even the earth itself, may be considered to have this kind of spirit.

Native Americans traditionally believe that illness stems from spiritual problems. They traditionally do not ascribe to germ theory as they see illness as a result from a cause and effect (not germ-related) because of an event in the past or a future event yet to pass. They also say that diseases are more likely to invade the body of a person who is imbalanced, has negative thinking, or lives an unhealthy lifestyle. Some Native American healers believe that inherited conditions, such as birth defects, are caused by the parents' immoral lifestyles and are not easily treated. Others believe that such conditions reflect a touch from the Creator and may consider them a kind of gift. NAH practices aim to find and restore balance and wholeness in a person to restore one to a healthy and spiritually pure state.

There are many types of NAH practices, and they are promoted to help with a variety of ills. Some of the most common aspects of NAH include the use of herbal remedies, purifying rituals, shamanism, and symbolic healing rituals to treat illnesses of both the body and spirit. Herbal remedies are used to treat many physical conditions. Practitioners use purifying rituals to cleanse the body and prepare the person for healing. Shamanism is based on the idea that spirits cause illness, and a Native American healer called a shaman focuses on using spiritual healing powers to treat people. Symbolic healing rituals, which can involve family and friends of the sick person, are used to invoke the spirits to help heal the sick person.

Healers may include shamans as was described above, but also herbalists, spiritual healers, and medicine men or women. Many Native Americans see their healers for spiritual reasons, such as to seek guidance, truth, balance, reassurance, and spiritual well-being, while still using conventional medicine to deal with "White man's illness." However, they believe that the spirit is an inseparable element of healing.

Healing beliefs and rituals vary a great deal since there are such a large number of tribes (over 500). Adding to the complexity is that many healing rituals and beliefs are kept secret, passed along from one healer to the next. Secrecy is considered essential because the sharing of healing information is felt exploit the culture and weaken the healer's ability to heal. This secrecy has significantly limited the amount of information that is known about these practices. Another barrier to widespread knowledge of these practices is that some of the practices were driven underground or lost completely because they were banned or illegal in parts of the United States until 1978 when the American Indian Religious Freedom Act was passed.

The American Indian Religious Freedom Act has two sections. The first section defines the policy of the United States to protect and preserve for American Indians their inherent right of freedom to believe, express, and exercise the traditional religions of the American Indian, Eskimo, Aleut, and Native Hawaiians, including but not limited to access to sites, use, and possession of sacred objects, and the freedom to worship through ceremonials and traditional rituals. The second section permits the President of the United States to direct federal departments and agencies to evaluate all policies and procedures (in concert with native traditional religious leaders) to determine appropriate changes necessary to protect and preserve Native American religious cultural rights and practices (American Indian Religious Freedom Act, 1978).

One of the most common forms of NAH involves the use of herbal remedies, which can include teas, tinctures, and salves. For example, one remedy for pain uses bark from a willow tree, which contains acetylsalicylic acid (aspirin).

Purifying and cleansing the body is also an important technique used in NAH. Sweat lodges (special, darkened enclosures heated with stones from a fire) or special teas that induce vomiting may be used by the healer for this purpose. A practice called smudging, which involves cleansing a place or person with the smoke of sacred plants, can be used to bring about an altered state of consciousness and sensitivity, making a person more open to the healing techniques. Because some illnesses are believed to come from angry spirits, healers may also invoke the healing powers of spirits. They may also use special rituals to try to appease the angered spirits.

Another practice of NAH, symbolic healing rituals, can involve the whole community. These rituals use ceremonies that can include chanting, singing, painting bodies, dancing, exorcisms, sand paintings, and even limited use of mind-altering substances (such as peyote) to persuade the spirits to heal the sick person. Rituals can last hours or even weeks. These ceremonies are a way of asking for help from the spiritual dimension. Prayer is also an essential part of all NAH techniques.

Native American treatment is usually a slow process, spread over a period of days or weeks. It may involve taking time from one's daily activities for reflection, emotional awareness, and meditation. The healer may spend a great deal of time with the person seeking help. Healing is said to take place within the context of the relationship with the healer.

Preservation of the body is an important cultural consideration. The nurse should be aware that it is not unusual for a Native American patient to request that any removed body tissue (such as organs removed during surgery and even trimmed nail clippings or hair) be returned to the patient for fear that the removed body products can be used to harm the patient or family (such as in spells). Autopsy is also frowned upon because of the cultural belief that the body must be whole in order to be able to cross over into the spirit world.

Impact of Communication

Traditionally, Native American languages have been passed down by tribe elders to the young. As Native American communities have been dispersed and moved to reservations, many languages have been lost. Of the 300 original North American languages, only approximately 150 are still spoken, and only 50 of those are widely spoken. Some of the most common Native American languages are the Navajo, Cherokee, and Choctaw. Many Native Americans today are trying to revive their native language before all of the fluent elderly pass away. It is felt that failing to preserve the unique language utilized during religious ceremonies will negatively impact the ability of children to speak with some of their elders as well as their ability to pray.

A barrier to cross-cultural communication is the fact that even a minor variation in pronunciation may change the entire meaning of the message being received or sent. Although the dominant languages differ greatly from tribe to tribe, other forms of communication (both verbal and nonverbal) are similar across tribes. This congruence is true regarding eye contact. Most Native Americans do not maintain steady eye contact. Direct eye contact is considered disrespectful and, for elders, may even be perceived as threatening. The degree of acculturation that has taken place will determine the amount of eye contact offered during an encounter as well as the amount, if any, English that is spoken. Today, many Native Americans live in homes where no English is spoken at all. It is interesting when similarities in language are discovered. It has been noted that the language spoken by an Eskimo from Alaska can be understood by an Eskimo in Greenland.

The Native American communication style tends to be circular as opposed to the American culture of a linear style. This may lead to learning difficulties if an educator or teacher is speaking in a linear style and the Native American is used to a circular style (Tsai & Alanis, 2004).

Native American languages do not make such clear distinctions between objects and actions, and North American Native American languages often collapse objects and actions into single words, such as the Eskimo word "anerquwaatit," which means, "he begs you to go out." This type of language in which elements are added to nouns to form new nouns is called an agglutinative language. When verbs are collapsed with nouns, it suggests that the culture does not think of actions as independent from the object doing the action. European languages invoke a worldview in which action can be considered a separate entity from objects.

The nurse should reciprocate eye contact and nonverbal cues from the patient during an encounter. Always ask the patient for permission to remove their clothing or to touch them for any purpose or reason. Formality when addressing the patient is recommended as most Native Americans follow the tradition of having a first, middle, and last name (i.e., the patient should be called Miss, Mister, or Missus as appropriate, followed by the last name).

Many Native American languages do not have equivalent words or concepts especially in the case of medical jargon. The nurse can impact the meaning of the communication through voice inflection so consideration of this should be made. In some Native American cultures, death and dying is not discussed because of the perceived cultural link between words and action (speaking a negative outcome can cause it to occur). In Navajo culture, speaking the name of the dead can delay the spirit's journey to the next world or keep the spirit in limbo.

The nurse should provide ample consideration time once a patient has been provided with information and expect that consultation may occur with others in the Native American community prior to any medical decisions being made.

The nurse should not rely on nonverbal cues to determine if the Native American patient is in pain. Many Native Americans were taught and socialized to withstand pain as a survival skill. The overt expression of pain (both verbal and nonverbal) is considered unacceptable, and for these reasons, the Native American patient may be extremely unlikely to request pain medication and instead rely on internal resources when coping with pain. If a request is made for a pain intervention, the nurse should respond immediately as it is not likely to be repeated. Also, the request may not come from the patient but from a family member instead. The nurse must recognize that pain is undertreated and strive to help the patient manage their pain in a culturally appropriate manner.

Impact of Time and Space

The Native American concept of time is intuitive and flexible. There is a strong belief in cause and effect, and a present time orientation and space is viewed as having no boundaries. Time is a strong factor in beliefs regarding illness as illness is viewed as being a result of something that either happened in the past or something that will happen in the future—indeed, it is viewed as the price to be paid.

Time is linked to naturally occurring phenomena such as cycles, moons, and seasons. Very little, if any, focus is placed on the future.

This is a result of the belief that many things are outside of a person's control. Time starts when the group gathers, and an event does not usually begin at a designated time. The nurse should recognize that medical appointments may not be kept, especially if something else comes up that is felt takes priority, such as helping a family member or friend.

Impact of Social Organization

The family structure varies from tribe to tribe including gender roles (some tribes are matriarchal like the Navajo while the majority of tribes are patriarchal). Despite this diversity, there are common core values and beliefs of traditional Native American culture that carries across tribal groups and geographic regions. It is these core values that will be described here. Historically, most men went to war or hunted while the women stayed home cooking and caring for the children.

Most Native American social structure is based on kinship. How highly organized each culture may be around this concept will vary, but it appears to be a universal theme to Native American cultures. Kinship-based societies are organized based on biologic relationships. There are two lines of descent: vertical and horizontal. The vertical lines, a very important concept, of descent link the relationships between ancestors and descendants. Horizontal lines describe our connection to others in our community who are not our ancestors or descendants (such as our siblings or our spouse). Native American family life is usually structured one of two ways. The first is the nuclear family which is made up of the husband and wife and their descendants. The second is the extended family, which is the most common type of family found in Native American culture, and is made up of families of two or more generations who live together as a family. Native Americans tend to view the entire world within the context of the relationship between the divine and human worlds, as a mother to her children (in a matriarchal society) or a father to his children (in a patriarchal society). This worldview is an important concept to know when attempting to understand Native American culture.

The most common political concept to Native American culture is chieftaincies. A chieftaincy included more than one kinship group and often more than one local settlement or clan. The principal role of the chief was to resolve conflicts among groups; beneath the chief are developed an entire hierarchy of decision making. The roles of the chief varied tremendously from society to society. In some, he was the chief arbiter of disputes and nothing more. In others, he was a military leader and nothing more. In others, he was a religious leader.

Authority was vested in a chief either through a descent line or through individual achievements. Some societies allowed for several chiefs of equal authority; others limited the chieftaincy to only a single individual.

Biologic Variations

Diabetes is a major health problem for Native Americans. Much work is being done in this area because of the explosion in the numbers of patients diagnosed with type 2 diabetes mellitus (DM). One explanation focuses on genetics and is the "thrifty gene hypothesis" (Neel, 1962). It is thought that evolutionary pressure selected hunter–gatherers for efficient fuel storage during times of famine. When food became plentiful and exercise less plentiful, this becomes a liability. This theory provides an explanation why the prevalence of DM is higher in some ethic groups such as Native Americans, Australian Aborigines, and Pacific Islanders. It is felt that in earlier times, people were much more physically active and ate a diet high in protein with periods of intermittent starvation present. This stress resulted in genetic selection to occur to allow for improved metabolic efficiency ("thrifty genes"). Over time, as society began and continues to modernize, further changes occurred in human diet and activity level. People are ingesting more calories, increasing dietary fat intake, and are concurrently decreasing physical activity. This has resulted in obesity, insulin resistance, and type 2 DM (Neel, 1962; Tsunehara, 1990).

The highest rate of prevalence of DM is in the Pima Indians, a tribe of Native American Indians: 70% of all Pima Indians older than the age of 35 years have type 2 DM. They have a tremendous genetic risk for the disease, and they develop diabetes at very high rates. There is an interesting "natural study" that occurred caused by the splitting off of Pima Indians from one group to two. One group resides in the state of Arizona and another group migrated to the northern part of Mexico (Sonora State). Although these two populations are genetically identical, their rates of diabetes are very different. The group in Arizona has a lot more diabetes than the group in Mexico. The reason is differing lifestyles. The Mexican groups are more physically active, they are leaner, and they have better meal planning in general (the rate of DM for those in Arizona is 4 or 5 times higher than those in Mexico).

Other Native Americans have an extremely high prevalence rate for type II DM. Among the Sioux, Chippewa, Pueblo, and Cherokee, approximately one third of adults older than age 35 have the disorder. Complication rates are also disproportionate with amputations 2–3 times and renal failure rates of 20 times the general population.

Cardiovascular disease (CVD) mortality varies among tribes but is increasing overall. The Strong Heart Study (National Institute of Health, 2001) integrated data on 13 different American Indian tribes (n = 4549) with male and female subjects aged 45–74 from American Indian communities from three different centers (Arizona, Oklahoma, and South Dakota/North Dakota). The increasing incidence of CVD among American Indians found by the Strong Heart Study is of great concern because rates of CVD are decreasing in other groups in the United States. More intensive programs to reduce CVD risk factors are needed in American Indian communities. Because the risk factors vary by tribal groups, these programs need to be tailored to each community/tribe. DM was found to be the most important contributing factor for CVD. Prevention needs to address the modifiable risk factors of DM which are increasing physical activity and decreasing weight to an acceptable body mass index. Lipid management and smoking cessation are also important preventive topics for this population. Blood pressure control, in this study, was found to be comparable or better than that of the general hypertensive population. Reduction of excessive alcohol use is also a strategy that was advocated by the authors of the Strong Heart Study (National Institute of Health, 2001).

Alcohol abuse is a big problem in this population and its excess usage has caused a corresponding problem with fetal alcohol syndrome and domestic violence. Alcohol is metabolized differently in various ethnic groups, including Native Americans. This variability causes vasomotor symptoms such as facial flushing and palpitations that are not seen in other ethnic groups. It is hypothesized (and currently under further study) that the reason for these differences is caused by alcohol metabolism. In Whites, alcohol is metabolized by the liver enzyme alcohol dehydrogenase at a level that is deemed "fairly efficient." Native Americans metabolize alcohol by acetaldehyde dehydrogenase, a "faster" metabolism, which is the reason for the vasomotor symptoms seen in the Native Americans.

Impact of Faith and Spirituality

Central to Native American spiritual traditions is the importance of "relation" as a way of existing in the world. The power of relation is symbolized by the circle of life, represented throughout the traditions, customs, and art forms of Native American people. This circle of life is believed, in many tribal traditions, to consist of the basic elements of life: fire, earth, water, and wind. Also life, from a traditional Native American perspective, is viewed as a series of concentric circles. The first circle is the inner circle, representing our spirit. The next circle is family/clan. The third circle is the natural environment and all our relations.

The fourth circle consists of the spirit world. Considering the power of relation, all life exists in an involved system of interdependence in a dynamic state of harmony and balance (Garrett & Carroll, 2000).

Among the many aspects of Native American culture is the emphasis on unity through seeking harmony and balance both inwardly and outwardly. Generally, Native American traditional values reflect the importance placed upon community contribution, sharing, cooperation, being, noninterference, community and extended family, harmony with nature, a time orientation toward living in the present, preference for explanation of natural phenomena according to the spiritual, and a deep respect for elders.

Although there is no written sacred religious book in Native American culture comparable to the Bible, some Native Americans of North America have kept written records with sacred symbols written on wooden sticks or woven into wampum belts. Religious stories and ceremonies have been transmitted through stories that have been passed down. Native American storytellers have kept alive both cultural and spiritual traditions by sharing stories about creation, morals, laws, and even survival skills.

Religion is a way of life. In many Native American languages, there is no word for "religion" because spiritual practices are believed to be an integral part of every aspect of daily life; spirituality is necessary for the harmony and balance, or wellness, of the individual, family, clan, and community.

Northeast Indians believe in a spirit world that interacts with the physical or natural world. They believe in a primary spirit that pervades all existence. This Great Spirit has different names depending on the tribe's language or dialect (Algonquians call it Kitche Manitou, which means "Great Spirit," Iroquoians call it "Orenda," and the Siouans refer to it as "Wakan" or "Wakanda"). The Great Spirit has many manifestations as it is considered present in all things, even sickness. Shamans are believed to be capable of controlling spirits, including The Great Spirit.

Burial is also a sacred and religious enterprise. In the United States in the past, tribes had been outraged by the desecration of their sacred burial grounds, which had been ransacked for skeletal remains and burial items. The fight for the return of these items was furious and long lasting. Finally, in 1990, the US government passed the Native American Graves Protection and Repatriation Act (NAGPRA). NAGPRA protects Indian gravesites from looting and sets up legal procedures for Indians to reclaim artifacts of religious or ceremonial importance. Reclaiming skeletal bones, totem poles, masks, wampum belts, medicine bundles (collections of objects believed to heal disease and ward off ghosts), and other objects from museums has inspired tribes to revive old ceremonies and tribal traditions.

For thousands of years, many Native Americans, including the Navajo, have worshipped while under the influence of peyote (from the peyote cactus). They have a polytheistic religion with one main god (or spirit) and several smaller gods. The Peyote religion, now organized as the Native American church, is a nativistic religion that began among the Kiowa and Comanche tribes during the second half of the 19th century. The religion is acceptable to many because it does not introduce new beliefs and because it incorporates the traditional native beliefs.

Finally, some Native Americans are Christians. Many missionaries have lived on reservations spreading the Christian religions, which have resulted in many conversions to Christianity.

Navajos

The largest of the American Indian tribes today are the Navajos. The first written history regarding the Navajo dates back to the 1600s. It is believed, based on archaeologic evidence, that the Navajos settled in Northwestern New Mexico by the late 1400s or early 1500s. By the early 1600s, they had migrated into northern Arizona. The proximity to Mexico and the Pueblo peoples exerted a tremendous influence on the cultural development of the Navajo despite the fact that during periods of time, the Pueblos and Navajos were enemies. At other times, they were allies (especially against the Spanish) for much more of the time than was spent as enemies or in hostility. The Navajo adopted a matrilineal clan system from the Pueblo that is still in effect today. A matrilineal lineage means that the Navajo inherits the clan from the mother and each member of the clan is considered to be a relative, each holding and carrying out unique responsibilities to each other and to the clan. Trades were also learned by the Navajo that caused the reliance on a nomadic hunting existence to be less significant. Some of the trades developed included weaving, pottery making, agriculture, and silversmithing. In fact, adopting and expanding from other cultures is considered one of the Navajos' strengths.

The Navajos have strived to stay on the sacred land of their ancestors. The Navajo nation extends into the states of Utah, Arizona, Colorado, and New Mexico covering over 27,000 miles (Navajo Nation Government, 2009). This land is located between four mountains, each of which represents the four cardinal directions of East, South, West, and North, and it is believed it was granted to them by the creator. The four mountains are Mount Blanca in Colorado, Mount Taylor in New Mexico, San Francisco Peak in Arizona, and Mount Hesperus in Colorado. According to the 2000 census data, the Navajo numbered 298,000 (US Bureau of the Census, 2000). Historians state that to fully understand the Navajo, it is important to know that the four mountains provide the boundaries for the Navajo nation. It is believed, even today, that the mountains are sacred, were a gift to the Navajo, and are extremely important in Navajo mythology and that the mountains are celebrated in prayers and songs (Navajo Nation Government, 2009).

In 1923, a tribal government was established in response to the desire of oil companies to lease Navajo land for exploration. In 1991, the government was reorganized to follow a three branch organizational structure: executive, legislative, and judiciary. Government sessions are conducted in the traditional Navajo language. It is believed that the Navajo tribal government has evolved today into the largest of all forms of American Indian government (Navajo Nation Government, 2009).

A unique difference of the Navajo is that, unlike many other Native Americans, they have been able to stay on their original tribal land. This is considered a great blessing as their sacred land (bordered by the four mountains) was a gift for them to possess and protect for the "Holy Ones" who came down from the sky. It is felt that as long as the Navajos stay on their land, the "Holy Ones" will take care of them.

The Creator of the Universe, it is believed, provided the Navajo with all they need to live and be happy between the four sacred mountains. The Creator gave Father Sun for light and energy and Mother Earth who provides all things that nurture and all things that can heal. The Navajo way of life focuses on the natural spirituality of the Earth intertwined with its physical attributes (i.e., the spiritual world is infused with the natural world that breathes life into every living thing on Earth). The Navajo take honor and delight in their ability to heal and care for Mother Earth, which they recognize is being damaged by some. It is stated that the Navajo believe that some day the people of the Earth will come to the Navajo for lessons on how to care for Earth and when that day comes, they will be ready.

The Navajo language is considered to be given by the "Holy Ones" and, as such, is considered sacred. It is felt that all answers are in the language and that it is special and very powerful. Language is a specific talent that the Navajo possess. During World War II, there were Navajo code breakers who were essential in helping the United States transmit classified information. A secret code was developed from the Navajo language that was used to transmit messages—this secret code was considered unbreakable. Today, most elderly Navajo speak only their native language and few are literate. Younger Navajo are usually bilingual and speak their tribal language in their home. There is some similarity of dialect between the Navajo and Apache and because of this, there can some limited understanding between these tribes when communicating with each other. Regional accents and the use of slang terms can result in the loss of this ability, because even a minor variation in pronunciation can change the meaning of a word or an entire sentence.

Ceremonies hold a special place in Navajo culture. There are ceremonies for many things, and they are seen as providing a link to Navajo history as well as the responsibilities that the Navajo need to carry out. During ceremonies, conversations are held with the "Holy Ones" and the Creator and are used to bless the sick and the body. Corn is very important to Navajo culture as it is a symbol of fertility and because it serves as a food source. During a Navajo wedding ceremony, the couple eats white corn (male) and yellow corn (female) mixed together with corn pollen on top to ensure a fertile marriage (Del Carlo, 2008).

Family is very important to Navajo culture. Navajo culture is matriarchal as it is built on the belief that a goddess created the Universe. Men and women are viewed as complementary equals, as one needs the other to survive. But in reality, the woman is the decision maker, especially in regard to health decisions. Traditional Navajos must obtain the permission of the leading female elder before entering a hospital or undergoing surgery (Diversity Resources, 2001). There is both the immediate and extended family. The extended family is broken into clans that were created by the "Holy Ones." The extended family can also be divided into a camp which consists of the senior married couple, their unmarried children, their married daughters, and the daughters' husbands (Diversity Resources, 2001). Today, there are 130 clans which have developed from the four original clans: Towering House, Bitterwater, Big Water, and One-Who-Walks-Around.

The Navajo are interested in sharing their culture and ways with the non-Navajo as they feel that the knowledge and skills they possess are a gift from the "Holy Ones" and are for the benefit of all human beings.

Alaska Natives/American Eskimos

There are two main groups of Eskimos: the Inuit of northern Alaska, Canada, and Greenland and the Yupik from Alaska and Russia. Terminology is problematic as the term "Eskimo" is not acceptable to those of Canada and Greenland, who prefer Inuit; however, this is not appropriate for the Yupik whose language and ethnicity is distinct from the Inuit. For purposes of this chapter, the terms Alaska Natives or American Eskimos will be used.

It is believed that the ancestors of American Eskimos came across the Bering Strait from Asia more than 30,000 years ago. The purchase of Alaska from Russia resulted in the Americanization of Alaska with the introduction of some healthcare services and through the propagation of Christianity through the work of missionaries. Unfortunately, the consequences from the mixing of people and cultures were similar to what was experienced by Native Americans. Epidemics broke out killing thousands as the natives lacked immunity to such diseases as smallpox and measles.

The plentitude of natural resources in Alaska spurred rapid settlement as miners, transportation workers, oil and gas workers, and even the military flooded into Alaska, which has caused the population of Alaska to become more diverse. According to US Census data (2002), only 15.6% of the population in Alaska is made up of Alaska Natives or American Indian. The indigenous populations are referred to as Alaska Natives. Alaska Natives can be divided into five major cultural groupings: Interior Indians (Athapascans), Aleuts, Southeast Coastal Indians (Tlingit and Haida), Northern Eskimos (Inupiat), and Southern Eskimos (Yupik). These groups have traditionally been enemies despite sharing some similarities of custom and tradition. The animosity is especially prevalent between the American Eskimo and the Indians as some American Eskimo elders caution their children to be afraid and cautious around the Indians.

The preservation of American Eskimo culture has been complicated because of acculturation into dominant American culture and the loss of young American Eskimos who leave the village to attend school, some never to return. Because the area where the American Eskimos settled is harsh and frigid, the American Eskimos are not able to rely on agriculture for survival. Instead, American Eskimos hunt, fish, trap, and gather food, which restricts the traditional diet to wild meat (caribou, seafood, and even reindeer, which was imported from Scandinavia and Russia to improve the meat supply).

Impact of Communication

Eskimoan is a difficult language to master and comprehend. Originally, the language had no written form (all American Eskimo history is recounted through storytelling, dance, and art). More recently, a written form of the American Eskimo language was developed by missionaries and is based on phonetics and is still being refined. Other complications associated with the use of the American Eskimo language is the reliance on the third person (a patient will refer to themself in the third person, for example, as someone), all language is present oriented (there are no future tenses), and one word can express an entire sentence. If a word represents an extremely important concept to the American Eskimo, it may have many different word forms to provide a more thorough description (i.e., a different word to differentiate drifting snow from falling snow). The American Eskimos also tolerate silence and may wait for several minutes before replying to even a simple statement or greeting. If the American Eskimo were to sense some intolerance from the nurse toward the use of silence, they may feel dominated and inferior so the nurse should be cautious and not try to fill any silences.

The nurse should also be aware of the importance of nonverbal communication to this cultural group. This is helpful since American Eskimos will seldom disagree in public with others. If the nurse is not certain whether an American Eskimo patient is being polite or sincere, looking for nonverbal cues may be quite helpful. Look for raised eyebrows to indicate "yes" or a wrinkled nose to indicate "no." Agreement is indicated by action, not words.

Impact of Touch

Older American Eskimos are more likely to believe in the healing touch or powers of shamans. Although the belief in shamanism exists among some American Eskimos, it is not openly discussed and it would be extremely rare for any discussion of it to occur with or around non-Eskimos.

Nursing Considerations

American Eskimos have retained many traditional beliefs despite exposure to modern American society through interaction with many settlers, missionaries, and public health workers who have come to Alaska throughout the years. Understanding that cultural differences persist will permit the nurse to provide care that is culturally responsive. Many of the adaptations that have occurred from the exposure to American culture have caused serious health consequences to the American Eskimo people. American Eskimos are developing obesity because of a change in diet and lifestyle from wild meat to mainly carbohydrates and from active physical activity to a much more sedentary lifestyle; alcoholism and tobacco abuse (smoking and chewing) has increased because of improved access and as a coping strategy caused by the stress of acculturation, and new mothers are often bottle feeding instead of breastfeeding their babies.

Impact of Social Organization

Traditional American Eskimos lived in small bands, in voluntary association under a leader recognized for his ability to provide for the group. Social status or earning a leadership position was a result of the ability to be a successful provider of food and skins. Kinship was paramount to the survival of the group in such a harsh environment. The emphasis was on group survival, not the individual. Today, strong family ties prevail. Only the most personal property was considered private; any unused equipment was reverted to those who had need for it. Honesty and sharing are highly valued traits. In the traditional American Eskimo economy, the division of labor between the sexes was strict; men constructed homes and hunted, and women took care of the homes.

Biologic Variations

The appearance and pigmentation of American Eskimos vary. Some are tall and slim, whereas others are short and stocky. The facial bone structure is similar to American Indians with eye folds similar to Asians. Pigmentation depends on the amount of ancestral sun exposure.

Impact of Faith and Spirituality

Traditional American Eskimo religion relied on magic to drive evil away, and it was felt there was a special magical connection among all things. Reincarnation was a part of the belief system and all babies were thought to be reincarnations of recently deceased relatives. The afterlife as such was a vague concept. With the migration of Christian missionaries into Alaska, many American Eskimos converted to Christianity leaving these traditional beliefs behind. Most American Eskimos adopted a Christianity that included some of their traditional beliefs (spirits and monsters) with the desire for peaceful behavior being rewarded with a positive and achievable afterlife. The major negative from the conversion was the loss of the art of dancing, which apparently was suppressed by the missionaries working in Alaska. The different Christian religions established strongholds in different parts of Alaska (Catholics in the Yukon River area, Presbyterians in the North coast, and the Moravians in the Bethel region), but despite this, Christian religious practices were fairly uniform throughout Alaska. Today, churchgoing is mainly an activity valued by the middle aged; church attendance by the young and the elderly is at a much lesser level.

In traditional Inuit culture, the angakut (or shaman) is the spiritual leader of the tribe. The angakut determines the reason for the sickness or illness and determines if there is personal or family responsibility and isolates the identified broken taboo. The angakut goes into a trance in order for his soul to leave his or her body to travel long distances, so that the cause of the illness and other community problems can be discovered.

Age of the American Eskimo seems to be the key variable related to degree of acculturation into the dominant American society. The older the American Eskimo, the more likely he or she will be to be wearing animal-skin clothing, eat seafood or caribou, speak an American Eskimo language, and to believe in spirits and ghosts. The younger the American Eskimo, the more likely he or she will be a representative of the contemporary American culture.

Summary

In spite of the enormous diversity in tribal cultures, languages, and religious beliefs, there are some shared beliefs among American Indian and Alaska Native tribes, especially related to health, illness, and health prevention. A summary of shared cultural values is in Table 8-1. All things begin with the Creator, Supreme Creator, or Great Spirit. Illness presents an opportunity to purify the soul. Disease does not just impact the patient but also the family. Health is maintained by preserving harmony among the body, mind, spirit, and the soul. Because of the interconnectedness of all of these components, spirituality and emotions are viewed as just as important as the body and mind. The spirit world exists alongside and intermingles with the physical world, and this is why death is not viewed as an enemy but as a natural part of life. It is believed that the spirit existed before it entered the physical body and that the spirit will continue on after the physical body is gone.

A reliance on traditional health beliefs seems to be more rigid when dealing with what are perceived "Indian" problems (such as pain, dysfunctional family relationships, or any sickness of the spirit such as alcoholism or mental illness). It is believed that these Indian problems should be treated with Indian medicine, whereas "White man's diseases" (such as

Table 8-1

Cultural Values

Cooperation	Silence—ability to listen and wait is valued	Present time orientation; indifference toward future planning as the future, if it comes, will take care of itself	Extended family orientation
Group harmony	Emotional control; contemplation	Work is only done if absolutely necessary; not for work's sake	Cultural pluralism with a resistance to assimilation; desire to retain Indian heritage
Modesty and humility	Patience; group decision by discussion and consensus	Time is flexible and nonlinear	Strong relationship with nature; love the creator and love the land
Noninterference	Sharing and generosity; upward mobility in non-Indian society is not sought	Strong relationship with nature	Spirituality and religion no belief in original sin or damnation; responsible for their own path

Disclaimer: This chart is comprised of the more commonly held values in Native American culture and as such is not comprehensive or representative of all Native Americans. Although many Native Americans have been taught these values, not all will exhibit or practice these values as there are many variables to consider such as tribe variation, individual experience, level of acculturation into the dominant American society, and of course particular situations.

Source: Hendrix, L. R. Health and health care of American Indian and Alaska Native elders. Retrieved May 4, 2009, from http://www.stanford.edu/group/ethnoger/americanindian.html

DM and cancer) should be treated with "White man's medicine" (Alvord & Van Pelt, 1999). Cultural considerations for the nurse and nurse practitioner are included in Table 8-2.

Native North American peoples have survived an onslaught of government policies and wars dedicated to destroying them. What sustained them

---

Table 8-2

Cultural Considerations for Nurses

Establishing Respect and Rapport	Culturally Appropriate Verbal and Nonverbal Communication	Language Assessment/Literacy Considerations
Placing an emphasis on listening versus talking may be appreciated by the Native American patient. Calmness and humility are also traits that are highly valued. Try to involve elders in all discussions. Keep in mind that personal information will not be readily shared—it will take a little time. Ideas/feelings are often conveyed through behavior rather than words. Be on the lookout for indirect criticism (such as from a family member) to let you know that the patient may have an issue with you or your care. The delivery of direct criticism is considered rude and disrespectful and will be avoided by the Native American patient. This may also be evident with requests. Be on the alert for requests to be given to the nurse by indirect routes (such as an indirect suggestion or a suggestion that comes from a family member). There may be a reliance on withdrawal as a form of communicating displeasure or disapproval with the situation. This is referred to as "voting with the feet."	Adapt your questions to the patient's level of acculturation into the dominant culture. Speak slowly—especially when communicating with the elderly. The patient will select their words very carefully and deliberately. Questions should be framed within a "caring" framework and not a "prying" one. American Indian languages have some of the longest pause times, compared to other languages and especially English. Elders frequently complain that English speakers "talk too fast." Silence is valued, so long periods of silence between speakers are commonly seen. Interruption of the person who is speaking is considered extremely rude, especially if that person is older than you. Keep body movements to a minimum and do not touch the patient beyond an introductory handshake unless absolutely necessary (and never without permission). The handshake should not be too firm. If it is a female patient, she may only touch the fingertips when returning the handshake. Maintaining a physical distance of several feet is customary. Eye contact is usually not direct or only briefly direct as a sign of respect. You may note that the Native American patient is directing their gaze over your shoulder.	Consider that your Native American patient may be monolingual (only fluent in a tribal language and not English). Always assess the patient's literacy level prior to giving the patient forms for completion of patient education paperwork. If you need to utilize an interpreter, an adult interpreter of the same gender is preferred. Be careful when providing patient education to avoid probability statements as problems with translation have frequently been noted. The probability statements often do not translate properly because of grammatical differences, which causes a probability to translate into a fact. Keep in mind that negative information may be culturally inappropriate as it may be felt that speaking of the negative may cause it to occur. There is a reliance on the spoken word (word of mouth) so the use of the Internet or other media for patient education would not be an effective intervention with this patient population. If utilizing Language Line Services for translation, the service may not be proficient in all Indian languages as there are more than 150 Indian languages still spoken in the United States. Depending on the age of the patient, and perhaps some other variables such as educational level, consider that the Native American patient may have to translate the concepts the nurse has presented into his native language to consider his response, and then back into English to provide his response to the nurse. This may take time. Try not to hurry the encounter to assure that the message you have sent is the one received and the response sent back to you is the one that the patient intended.

were traditional family and clan relationships, kinship with homelands, religious ceremonies, ancient stories connecting older and younger generations, and shared traditions that maintained each tribe's uniqueness. This should illustrate to the nurse the value that Native American culture holds for its people. Despite economic hardship and political oppression, Native Americans continue to survive and to preserve their unique and valuable culture.

Navajo American Case Study

Kai is a 58-year-old Navajo (Native American) who has been severely immobile since suffering from a cerebral vascular accident 9 months ago. She is cared for on a daily basis by a home health aid and is seen by the visiting nurse on a regular schedule. Kai has many other medical problems including some rather serious comorbidities, such as brittle DM and obesity. The nurse noticed that Kai was developing some contractures and arranged for a visiting physical therapist to come out to evaluate Kai.

When the visiting nurse returned for her next scheduled visit, Kai was not in her usual mood. When the nurse asked Kai what was wrong, she was surprised to hear that the physical therapist had mentioned hospice care as a possibility for Kai's treatment plan. Kai told the nurse that she was extremely upset by this and that she "never want to see that physical therapist again."

If you were that visiting nurse, how would you respond? In your response, make sure that you demonstrate your understanding of Navajo culture.

References

Alvord, L. A., & Van Pelt, E. (1999). *The Scalpel and the Silver Bear: The first Navajo woman surgeon combines Western medicine and traditional healing.* New York: Bantam Books.

American Indian Religious Freedom Act, Title 42, Chapter 21, Subchapter 1, USC §1996. (1978). National Park Service. Retrieved April 25, 2009, from http://www.nps.gov/history/local-law/FHPL_IndianRelFreAct.pdf.

Del Carlo, L. (2008). Between the Sacred Mountains: a cultural history of the Dineh. Retrieved May 11, 2009, from http://dc.cod.edu/cgi/viewcontent.cgi?article=1015&context=essai.

Diversity Resources, Inc. (2001). Culture sensitive health care: American Indian. Blacksburg, VA: Virginia Tech, Office of Multicultural Affairs, Diversity and Work/Life Resource Center. Retrieved July 8, 2003, from http://www.multicultural.vt.edu/divresources/indian.html.

Garrett, M. T. (1999). Understanding the 'medicine' of Native American traditional values: an integrative review. *Counseling & Values*, 43, 2, 84–98.

Garrett, M.T., & Carroll, J. J. (2000). Mending the broken circle: treatment of substance dependence among Native Americans. *Journal of Counseling & Development*, 78, 379–389.

National Park Service, US Department of the Interior. (1990). The Native American Graves Protection Repatriation Act (NAGPRA). Retrieved September 21, 2009, from http://www.nps.gov/history/nagpra.

National Institute of Health. (2001). Strong Heart Study data book: A report to American Indian communities. Retrieved April 18, 2009, from http://www.nhlbi.nih.gov/resources/docs/shs_db.pdf.

Navajo Nation Government. (2009). The Navajo Nation. Retrieved May 5, 2009, from http://www.navajo.org.

Neel, J. V. (1962). Diabetes mellitus: a "thrifty" genotype rendered detrimental by progress. *American Journal of Human Genetics*, 14, 353–362.

Ogunwole, S. U. (2002). *The American Indian and Alaska Native Population: 2000.* Washington, DC: US Department of Commerce, US Census Bureau.

Tsai, G., & Alanis, L. (2004). Journey to thinking multiculturally. The Native American culture: A historical and reflective perspective. *NASP Communique*, 32, 8. Retrieved April 24, 2009, from http://www.nasponline.org/publications/cq/cq328native.aspx.

Tsunehara, C. H. (1990). Diet of second-generation Japanese-American men with and without non-insulin-dependent diabetes. *American Journal of Clinical Nutrition*, 52, 731–738.

US Department of Commerce, Bureau of the Census. (2000). *The American Indians and Alaska Native Population, 2000 census brief.* Washington, DC: US Government Printing Office.

US Department of Commerce, Bureau of the Census. (2002). *Population profiles by age, sex, race and Hispanic origin, Summary File 3.* Washington, DC: US Government Printing Office.

US Department of Commerce, Bureau of the Census. (2005). Facts for features. American Indian and Alaska Native reports. Retrieved September 21, 2009, from http://www.census.gov/Press-Release/www/releases/archives/facts_for_features_special_editions/007489.html.

US Department of Commerce, Bureau of the Census. (2008). 2008 State-recognized tribes and American Indian and Alaska Native Organizations. Retrieved September 21, 2009, from http://factfinder.census.gov/home/aian/index.html.

Chapter 9

Whites
(Non-Hispanic)

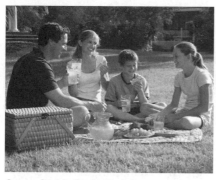

Source: © iofoto/ShutterStock, Inc.

Chapter Objectives

Upon completion of this chapter, the nurse will be able to:

1. Identify traditional health beliefs of Whites (non-Hispanics) with a European heritage.

2. Describe cultural phenomena affecting health care among Whites (non-Hispanics).

3. Plan for nursing care delivery that considers the cultural beliefs of Whites (non-Hispanic) patients.

Introduction

There are vast differences among all people. Certain cultural characteristics will be described, which may or may not be associated with individual patients. The intent is not to be stereotypical but to provide the nurse with a starting point to establish some common ground to learn about the individual patient under their care so that the patient can have nursing care that meets their unique, individual needs. A stereotype is an ending point, and no effort is then made to ascertain whether it is appropriate to apply it to the person in question. A generalization, on the other hand, serves as a starting point. Having knowledge of cultural customs and beliefs can help avoid misunderstandings and enable nurses and nurse practitioners to provide better care.

Historical Background

Over the past 4 centuries, tens of millions of immigrants have come to the "new world" to begin a new life. Immigration is a central component in the development of the United States. The constant wave of immigrants contributed to the growth and development of the United States as it developed from a new emerging nation to a country with emerging economic power and eventually into its development as a dominant world power. It is believed that the tens of millions of immigrants who have settled in the United States have significantly contributed to the country's development making the United States what it is today—a world power (Diner, 2008). Although most Americans view the United States as a White European nation, the result of continuous European migration since the 17th century, we now understand that European immigration was only one stage in the peopling of the American continent. From the 1820s through the 1990s, two thirds of the nearly 65 million immigrants to the United States came from Europe. By 1965, however, less than half of the immigrants came from Europe; by the 1990s, it was less than 10% (Katzman, 2000).

The United States was a settler society and required large waves of immigrants to settle into large areas that were undeveloped. The establishment of a settler society is not unusual as it is associated with Canada, Australia, and New Zealand, among other countries (Diner, 2008). The United States, like other settler societies, had land and capital to tap into its natural resources but lacked sufficient manpower. The reliance on the use of Native Americans, and later on African slaves who were brought here against their will, was not enough to meet the labor demands, and the call for immigration was launched.

Immigration not only led to the development of the country but also was responsible for shaping our society and national culture.

During the period when European immigration dominated, the source of immigrants changed. In the first two thirds of the 19th century, most immigrants came from Ireland, Germany, and Great Britain. In the 1880s, a permanent shift occurred. In 1882, the peak year of the "old immigration," 87% of the immigrants came from Ireland, Germany, Great Britain, Scandinavia, Switzerland, and Holland. In 1907, the peak year of the "new immigrants," 81% of immigrants came from Italy, Russia, Austria-Hungary, Greece, Rumania, and Turkey. From the 1820s to World War II, Germany provided 16% of immigrants, Ireland 12%, Italy 12%, Austria-Hungary 12%, Great Britain 11%, Russia 10%, and Scandinavia 5% (Katzman, 2000).

Historians have divided immigration to the United States into distinct time periods, each of which is associated with varying rates of immigration from differing areas of the world. All immigration, however, has contributed to shaping our national psyche.

Settlers of the New World

The first and, by far, longest of the 5 time periods extended from the 17th century through the early 19th century. Although immigrants from this time came from a variety of places, by far, the largest volume came from the British Isles (England, Scotland, Wales, and Ireland). Others came from southwest Germany (Palatinate), France, and the Netherlands as well as Jews from Poland and the Netherlands (Diner, 2008). The common denominator among these immigrants from Western and Northern Europe was the lack of ability to take advantage of the modernization of their home countries' economies and the promise of cheap land in America. Reasons for leaving their homeland included desire for personal or religious freedom, crop failure, land and job shortages, famine, and rising taxes. The goal was to come to America, which was seen as the land of economic opportunity. Because of the high travel costs associated with the journey to the United States, many of the settlers of the new world were able to come here by becoming indentured servants. A contract was signed and, in exchange for a commitment of a specific amount of time spent in hard labor, they would receive transport and, at the end of the contract, ownership of a small piece of land. The vast majority of the early immigrants were farmers who were lured here by the call of cheap land. European immigrants entered the United States through East Coast ports. The vast majority entered through New York City (more than 70%). Although many immigrants stayed close to the port of entry, some did find their way inland. Many underpopulated states would actively recruit for immigrant settlers offering jobs or land for farming.

Mass Migration of the 1820s to the 1880s

During the years of 1820–1880, 15 million immigrants came to the United States (Diner, 2008). Although many of these immigrants also came to farm in the Midwest and the Northeast, a large number settled in cities like New York, Philadelphia, and Boston. The opening of the Erie Canal in 1825 permitted the development of the Midwest for farming and agriculture, and industrial development led to the need for many textile workers in the cities.

European conditions influenced the stream of migrants. Poor harvests and famine sent millions of Irish, Swedes, and some Germans to the United States in the 1830s and after (Katzman, 2000). In the 1840s, political upheaval sent more Germans across the ocean, and a steady flow of religious dissenters came at all times. Limited economic opportunities in Europe sent tens of millions of peasants, small farmers, craftsmen, and unskilled workers, men and women alike, both as individuals and families, to America (Katzman, 2000). Ethnic and religious minorities including Jews from Eastern Europe, Poles and Germans from Russia, Macedonians from the Balkans, and Czechs and Bohemians from Austria-Hungary found freedom in the United States and formed settlements in Kansas (Katzman, 2000).

Young men from France, newly freed from the military after the fall of Napoleon, came to the United States as did others from England, Scandinavia, and central Europe in response to the changes in their home economies that resulted in great difficulty in making a living in their country of origin's new order (Diner, 2008).

Upon arrival to the United States, the newly arrived immigrants tended to cluster together in homogenous groupings. The Midwest was populated with immigrants from Sweden, Norway, Denmark, and from many regions of what would later become the country of Germany. The vast majority of these immigrants were Protestants, but during this time the first large scale wave of Irish Catholics came to the United States. The arrival of Catholics was met with hostility and a wave of nativism—a fear of Catholicism and of the Irish. The nativism movement was so sweeping that it even gave birth to a political party (the Know Nothings) which made anti-immigration and anti-Catholicism its purpose.

Also during this period, a small number of Chinese came to settle in the American West. Unfortunately, the reaction of Native Americans was extremely negative, and the government response was to pass legislation entitled the Chinese Exclusion Act of 1882, the only immigration law to specifically exclude an immigrant group.

An explosion of immigration was facilitated by improvements in technology and transportation. Ocean travel advanced from sailing to motor power. The ships also became much larger, permitting 25 million European immigrants to make the transatlantic crossing during this period. Immigrants came from Italy, Greece, Hungary, and Poland. Approximately 3 million of these immigrants were Jewish. This wave of immigrants gravitated toward the cities and sought jobs in the industrial labor pool (steel, coal, garment production, textiles, and automobiles). This influx of labor resulted in America becoming an economic strength, but there was a second wave of nativism. By the 1890s, immigration was viewed as posing a serious threat to our nation's health and security. In 1893, the Immigration Restriction League was formed and lobbying of Congress began in earnest to further restrict future immigration into the United States. Several pieces of legislation were passed over the ensuing years. In 1924, Congress passed the final version of the National Origins Act. The Act essentially gave preference to immigrants from northern and western Europe, severely limited the numbers from eastern and southern Europe, and declared all potential immigrants from Asia to be unworthy of entry into the United States. Because the Act did not apply to countries in the western hemisphere, immigration from western hemisphere countries exploded in the 1920s. Historians consider the 1920s as the penultimate era in the US immigration history. Immigrants came to America from Mexico; various countries in the Caribbean such as Haiti, Jamaica, and Barbados; and from Central and South America. The 1924 legislation was enforced until 1965. During that 40-year period, exceptions were made on a case-by-case basis for refugees (Jewish refugees from World War II, Cubans fleeing communism and Fidel Castro, and defectors from behind the Iron Curtain), but the law remained intact and enforced.

A consequence of the civil rights revolution in the United States during the 1960s was the passage of the Hart–Cellar Act in 1965, which eliminated the racially-based quota system. Preference was given to potential immigrants with family already in the United States and to the applicants who had skills or occupations that were deemed critical by the US Department of Labor. Immigrants came from Europe but also from Korea, China, India, the Philippines, Pakistan, and from some African countries. By the year 2000, immigration had returned to the levels of 1900. No matter where they come from or the timing of when they come, immigrants bring to the United States languages, cultures, and religions that over time contribute to the nation as a whole. European immigrants have a positive and negative legacy. On the negative side, there has been little respect for the indigenous population of the United States (Native Americans) with a history of ethnic and religious intolerance (Katzman, 2000). The positive contributions include language from the English, the Irish gave personalized politics, and the Germans contributed to the culture of US cities (Katzman). The United States has evolved into an industrial, modern, and multicultural nation.

Projections

In the history of the United States, the majority population has been White (non-Hispanic). Although this majority status is still true with 6% of the US population projected to be White in the year 2010, it is changing. Those numbers will start to decline around the 2030s as White deaths begin to outpace White births (US Census Bureau, 2008a). By the year 2042, a White majority will no longer be the reality (US Census Bureau, 2008a). By the year 2023, more than half of the country's children will be present-day minorities. By the mid-century mark, when the United States is projected to have a population of 439 million people, 54% of the population will consist of present-day racial minorities. Whites will be outnumbered by Americans who call themselves Hispanic, African American/Black, Asian, American Indian, Native Hawaiian, and Pacific Islander. In some geographic areas (such as New York, Los Angeles, Chicago, Houston, Philadelphia, and Detroit, as well as the states of California and Texas), the change in status for Whites to a minority group has already occurred (US Census Bureau, 2008b). Earlier projections said this change in majority status to minority status for Whites would not happen until the year 2050. There will also be an explosion of population growth in the United States during this same time period. It is estimated that we will reach the 400 million people milestone in the United States by the year 2039 and that more than 130 million additional people will be added to the population by the year 2050 (raising the US population to over 439 million people) (US Census Bureau, 2008a). All US Census Bureau projections are based on actual Census 2000 results and assumptions about future childbearing, mortality, and net international migration.

In addition to declining birth rates, another contributing factor are the declining immigration rates from European countries to the United States. In the year 2005, 15.7% of immigrants entering the United States self-identified as being from Europe. See Table 9-1 for a listing provided by the Office of Homeland Security identifying the top 20 countries of birth for immigrants admitted into the United States in the year 2005. The first European country on the listing is the Ukraine and that is in tenth place (Office of Homeland Security, 2005).

Table 9-1

Immigrants Admitted by Region and Top 20 Countries of Birth for the Year 2005

Region and Country of Birth	Number	Percent
Africa	85,102	7.6
Asia	400,135	35.7
Europe	176,569	15.7
North America	345,575	30.8
Caribbean	108,598	9.7
Central America	53,470	4.8
Other North America	183,507	16.3
Oceania	6546	0.6
South America	103,143	9.2
Unknown Country	5303	0.5
1. Mexico	161,445	14.4
2. India	84,681	7.5
3. China, People's Republic	69,967	6.2
4. Philippines	60,748	5.4
5. Cuba	36,261	3.2
6. Vietnam	32,784	2.9
7. Dominican Republic	27,504	2.5
8. Korea	26,562	2.4
9. Colombia	25,571	2.3
10. Ukraine	22,761	2.0
11. Canada	21,878	1.9
12. El Salvador	21,359	1.9
13. United Kingdom	19,800	1.8
14. Jamaica	18,346	1.6
15. Russia	18,083	1.6
16. Guatemala	16,825	1.5
17. Brazil	16,664	1.5
18. Peru	15,676	1.4
19. Poland	15,352	1.4
20. Pakistan	14,926	1.3
Other	**395,180**	**35.2**
All countries	**1,122,373**	**100.0**

Source: Office of Homeland Security (2005).

Statistics

According to the most recently available census data from July 1, 2007, the White non-Hispanic population of the United States is 199,091,567. The median age for both genders is 40.8 years of age. The majority of this population are female (101,346,238 compared to 97,745,329 males). The White population has seen only a minor increase of slightly over 3 million people from 195,575,485 (based on 2000 census data from the US Census Bureau). This pace is significantly less than the growth rate seen in other racial/ethnic groups.

Beginning in 1980, the US Census began to include a question regarding a person's ancestry self-identification. Ancestry is a broad concept that can mean different things to different people. The Census Bureau defines ancestry as a person's ethnic origin, heritage, descent, or "roots," which may reflect their place of birth, place of birth of parents or ancestors, and ethnic identities that have evolved within the United States. The top 10 most common self-identified ancestries listed in descending order from the 2000 census were: German, Irish, African American, English, American, Mexican, Italian, Polish, French, and American Indian. See Table 9-2 for the top 10 self-identified European-only ancestries from the 2000 census. See Table 9-3 for the top 10 countries of birth of the foreign-born population for the years of 1850–2000 from the US Census Bureau.

Several White ethnic groups will be described in this chapter with a focus on common cultural beliefs related to traditional health beliefs, disease management, and interactions with the healthcare delivery system to help the nurse plan for and deliver culturally appropriate care.

Table 9-2

Top 10 Most Common Self-Identified European Ancestries from the 2000 US Census

2000 Ranking Among All Ancestries	European Ancestry Group	Number	Percentage
1	German	42,841,569	15.2
2	Irish	30,524,799	10.8
3	English	24,509,692	8.7
4	Italian	15,638,348	5.6
5	Polish	8,977,235	3.2
6	French	8,309,666	3.0
7	Scottish	4,890,581	1.7
8	Dutch	4,541,770	1.6
9	Norwegian	4,477,725	1.6
10	Scotch–Irish	4,319,232	1.5

The ancestry groups listed on this table were self-identified. Many respondents listed more than one area of ancestry. Overall, about 500 different ancestries were reported during the 2000 census.

Source: US Census Bureau. (2004). Ancestry 2000. Retrieved August 28, 2009, from http://www.census.gov/prod/2004pubs/c2kbr-35.pdf.

Table 9-3

Top 10 Countries of Birth of the Foreign-Born Population of the United States, 1850–2000

Ten Leading Countries by Rank	1850	1880	1900	1930	1960
1.	Ireland 962,000	Germany 1,967,000	Germany 2,663,000	Italy 1,790,000	Italy 1,257,000
2.	Germany 584,000	Ireland 1,855,000	Ireland 1,615,000	Germany 1,609,000	Germany 990,000
3.	Great Britain 379,000	Great Britain 918,000	Canada 1,180,000	United Kingdom 1,403,000	Canada 953,000
4.	Canada 148,000	Canada 717,000	Great Britain 1,168,000	Canada 1,310,000	United Kingdom 833,000
5.	France 54,000	Sweden 194,000	Sweden 582,000	Poland 1,269,000	Poland 748,000
6.	Switzerland 13,000	Norway 182,000	Italy 484,000	Soviet Union 1,154,000	Soviet Union 691,000
7.	Mexico 13,000	France 107,000	Russia 424,000	Ireland 745,000	Mexico 576,000
8.	Norway 13,000	China 104,000	Poland 383,000	Mexico 641,000	Ireland 339,000
9.	Holland 10,000	Switzerland 89,000	Norway 336,000	Sweden 595,000	Austria 305,000
10.	Italy 4,000	Bohemia 85,000	Austria 276,000	Czechoslovakia 492,000	Hungary 245,000

Ten Leading Countries by Rank*	1970	1980	1990	2000
1.	Italy 1,009,000	Mexico 2,199,000	Mexico 4,298,000	Mexico 7,841,000
2.	Germany 833,000	Germany 849,000	China 921,000	China 1,391,000
3.	Canada 812,000	Canada 843,000	Philippines 913,000	Philippines 1,222,000
4.	Mexico 760,000	Italy 832,000	Canada 745,000	India 1,007,000
5.	United Kingdom 686,000	United Kingdom 669,000	Cuba 737,000	Cuba 952,000
6.	Poland 548,000	Cuba 608,000	Germany 712,000	Vietnam 863,000
7.	Soviet Union 463,000	Philippines 501,000	United Kingdom 640,000	El Salvador 765,000
8.	Cuba 439,000	Poland 418,000	Italy 581,000	Korea 701,000
9.	Ireland 251,000	Soviet Union 406,000	Korea 568,000	Dominican Republic 692,000
10.	Austria 214,000	Korea 290,000	Vietnam 543,000	Canada 678,000

*Data are not totally comparable over time because of changes in boundaries for some countries. Great Britain excludes Ireland. United Kingdom includes Northern Ireland. China in 1990 includes Hong Kong and Taiwan.

Source: US Census Bureau. (2001). Profile of the Foreign-Born Population in the United States: 2000. Retrieved August 28, 2009, from http://www.census.gov/prod/2002pubs/p23–206.pdf.

Irish Americans

Historical Background

Ireland comprises 26 counties and became a free state in 1921. The Republic of Ireland was proclaimed in 1948, when Ireland withdrew from the British Commonwealth. The British government reasserted its claim to Northern Ireland, a claim that was not recognized by the Republic of Ireland. Since that time, warfare has been present with repeated on and off cease-fires negotiated. Today, the unrest continues and many Irish Americans send money to support the Irish Republican Army. Today, the population of Ireland is 4,062,235 (World Almanac, 2006). Ireland is bordered on the northeast by Northern Ireland (province of Ulster), which remains a part of the United Kingdom. It is bordered by the Atlantic Ocean to the South and West. The ocean separates Ireland from Great Britain by an average of 50 miles. Ireland was colonized by European settlers from Great Britain with the Celtic influence remaining dominant today.

Throughout the history of the United States, immigrants have made their way from Ireland. During colonial times, the early Irish immigrants were Presbyterian Protestants from Ulster, now known as Northern Ireland. The motivation to come to America was to seek financial gain and a better life. The majority of the Ulster-born Irish immigrants were tenant farmers or skilled artisans. The Irish who came later were motivated not to seek a better life but to simply survive. The famine in Ireland, as a result of a blight that struck the potato crop between the years 1845–1854, left death and destruction in its wake. Tenant farmers were left with no crop and therefore no money. Although some landlords were initially compassionate, the passage of the Poor Law Extension Act of 1847 by Parliament changed that. Because of that law, a landlord became financially responsible for the cost of care for their tenants—an expense that many landlords were just not able to financially handle so evictions became extremely common. Once evicted, the tenant farmer was left with few options: move into a disease-infested workhouse or starve while searching for food and shelter. Many chose to flee their native land—to America—with the goal and hope of survival. These Irish immigrants were different than the Ulster Irish in many ways. The Ulster Irish were Protestant and the newer Irish immigrants were Catholics. The penal laws in Ireland had long placed Irish Catholics at a distinct disadvantage. They were poor farmers who were uneducated and totally dependent on their rocky plot of land (that was owned by the landlord) for survival. The potato crop was the sole food source. They came from large families with a lifestyle that favored close social interaction. Although they possessed little, they shared readily and enjoyed celebrating their beliefs with tradition, song, dance, and religious rituals. When their land was lost, they felt there was no place left for them in Ireland. Between 1840 and 1860, more than 1.5 million Irish came to the United States. Where they settled was determined by their financial situation. Although a large contingent settled in New Orleans and other cities, the Irish who immigrated to escape the famine stayed in the Eastern port cities of New York or Boston simply because they had no money or marketable skills to move on. Some were forced to move westward to Chicago in search of employment. The vast majority were poor and Catholic and were the first wave of non–Anglo-Saxon immigrants to the United States, and because of this difference, they were often met with hostility. Another unique difference was that many of the immigrants were unaccompanied women. Many women took jobs as domestic servants in the homes of the wealthy. The uneducated men took jobs of hard labor digging ditches or building canals or bridges. Both worked and saved with the goal to bring additional family members to America. Although they were on the lowest rung of American society, over time they began to dare to dream their own version of the "American Dream."

Table 9-4

Cultural Values of Euro-Americans (White Non-Hispanics)

Competition	Strong Expression of Opinion	Saving for the Future (Retirement)	Mastery over Nature
Individual achievement	Action valued over inaction; direct confrontation	Puritan work ethic; work for work's sake Rigid schedule	Judeo-Christian beliefs; emphasis on a second coming and the need for salvation
Overt identification of accomplishments; pride	Rapid responses and decision making valued	Euro centric obsession with money (i.e., time is money)	Nuclear family orientation; measure of successful child rearing is the child being able to leave home and thrive
Advice giving, directness	Individual ownership; upward social mobility	Future orientation—ability to delay gratification to the future	Follow the rules of dominant society, which is to work to get ahead; one who has developed social and economic mobility.

Source: Hendrix, L. R. Health and health care of American Indian and Alaska Native elders. Retrieved May 4, 2009, from http://www.stanford.edu/group/ethnoger/americanindian.html.

Today, approximately 40 million people of Irish descent live in the United States (US Census Bureau, 2002). Irish ranks as the second largest ancestry group in the United States, second only to German.

Traditional Health Beliefs

Some Irish Americans follow folk medicine beliefs. These practices are considered safe as they have been determined to be "neutral" (do not cause benefit or harm) (Giger & Davidhizar, 2003). These activities include blessing of the throat, tying a bag of camphor around the neck to prevent flu, keeping closet doors closed to block evil spirits, not looking in a mirror at night, keeping a strong and loving family, and the wearing of holy medals.

Irish Americans often have a reactive rather than a proactive approach to illness as they often delay seeking medical attention until the situation is quite serious. The first line of treatment will often be home remedies. Some folk medicine practices are deemed beneficial: getting plenty of rest, maintaining a positive attitude, eating a balanced diet and taking vitamins (Spector, 2004).

Impact of Communication

The official language of Ireland is Irish (Irish Gaelic). English is the second recognized language and is universally spoken in Ireland. An understanding of the Celtic language is necessary. The Celtic language was initially an oral one, so the culture was passed on orally most notably through poetry. Although a modern day Irish language persists today, it was almost wiped out because of the onslaught of the English language in the 19th century. Because many Irish immigrants arriving in the United States spoke English, they had an easier time with assimilation into the dominant American society than other immigrants.

Impact of Social Organization

The parish church was the center of social activity. Because many of these Irish immigrants were viewed as different because they were Catholic, they began to face hostility in society. The result was the formation of tightly knit social circle. As time passed, the children of these immigrants began to see possibilities for a better future because of their large numbers and ambition. They began to explore politics, which was a natural progression from the organizational structure of the parish system (Bankston & Hidalgo, 2006). In many cities, precinct by precinct, the Irish began to embrace the political system of the United States as not only a tool to improve their personal situation, but as an outlet for social change (Bankston & Hidalgo, 2006). The Irish political machine was particularly powerful and effective in New York (where Alfred E. "Al" Smith became Governor of New York in 1918), Kansas City, and Chicago. Political expansion was difficult outside these strong enclaves caused by fear and distrust of the Irish and the fear of involvement or interference of the Pope in government that existed within the larger American society. These factors contributed to the defeat of Governor Smith when he ran for President of the United States in 1928. These factors were not overcome until the election of President John F. Kennedy (a descendant of peasant Irish Catholic stock) in 1960—a feat that has not been repeated to date.

Labor unions were also a social organizing force for Irish Americans. Political activity and the church were seen as the best means for upward mobility. The Catholic Church also established Catholic Universities such as Notre Dame, Fordham, and Boston College to provide higher education opportunities for Irish Americans.

The family unit is extremely significant to Irish Americans. The nurse should include the family when planning care for it is felt that nursing interventions will only be successful if the family is included. Family roles tend to be gender based with the Irish American women viewing her role as primary caretaker. If the primary caretaker is ill, the nurse must help the family cope with the role strain and to help the family develop strategies to meet the family's needs in the absence of the caretaker.

Impact of Faith and Spirituality

The Ulster Irish were Protestant, and the majority of famine Irish were Catholic. The Irish Catholics were isolated by their religious beliefs and set up parishes within their neighborhoods. The Catholic parishes evolved into social and educational centers for the community. The parish priest served as a role model and counselor for the community. The church cared for the immigrants' spiritual, social, educational, medical, and emotional needs. As the number of immigrants increased, parishes and religious orders built schools, hospitals, and orphanages to meet the needs of the communities (Bankston & Hidalgo, 2006).

Biologic Variations

Some genetic variations have been identified in Irish Americans. Some are only associated with some identified Irish subgroups such as the Travellers of Ireland. These genetic variations include neural tube defects, sarcoidosis, cystic fibrosis, Tay-Sachs disease, bimaxillary dental protrusion, abdominal aortic aneurysm, and alcoholism.

Among all American ethnic groups, Irish Americans have either been ranked the highest or near highest for alcoholism rates (Butler, 1996). The nurse should remember that for Irish Americans, alcoholism is influenced by a variety of factors, including patterns and characteristics of the family, social and economic conditions, and psychologic orientation, rather than a biologic variation. Because some Irish drink for reassurance and to escape what is perceived as an intolerable burden, the nurse must develop strategies to teach such individuals more positive ways to alleviate stress and tension. Such individuals should be taught to verbally communicate feelings and anxiety rather than repressing or denying such feelings. The client must be taught the value of verbal expression to communicate needs. In addition, it is important to assist these clients in developing positive outlooks on life that may be perceived as positive coping strategies. The nurse also must remember the value of working not only with the client but also with the family because of the perception of family relationships as being paramount to a healthful existence.

Table 9-5

Nursing Considerations for the White Non-Hispanic Patient (Euro-American)

Appropriate Ways to Show Respect and Establish Rapport	Culturally Appropriate Verbal and Nonverbal Communication	Language Assessment/ Literacy Level
Utilize a firm handshake as it denotes power and authority. Self-disclosure is valued. Strive for an open and honest communication style. Expect directness in all patient interactions: Direct criticism will be utilized to alter behavior; disapproval will be directly expressed; and request will be made directly.	Use direct eye contact as it is viewed as a sign of honesty and sincerity. Rely on the verbal expression of ideas/feelings (the speech is more important than the behavior). Speaking is emphasized over listening. The expression of one's opinion is highly valued. Verbal and written communicated valued over nonverbal communication.	Consider the use of alternative methods for patient education such as media and Internet as this type of information passing is culturally appropriate.

Source: Hendrix, L. R. Health and health care of American Indian and Alaska Native elders. Retrieved May 4, 2009, from http://www.stanford.edu/group/ethnoger/americanindian.html.

Case Study 9-1

Irish American Case Study

This case demonstrates what can occur during a cross-cultural encounter (the culture of the patient and the provider are different).

A middle-aged Irish woman was hospitalized and scheduled to have bowel resection surgery once her condition had been stabilized. After a few days, the patient suddenly started complaining of severe abdominal pain to her family but said nothing to her physician. Her physician was unaware of the cultural manifestations of pain in Irish Americans, that is, the Irish, as a group, tend to minimize expressions of pain. When the patient's family spoke to the physician about the patient's pain, the physician expressed little concern because in the physician's country, women having serious pain are much more vocal than this patient was being. The physician did not listen to the patient's family and also did not follow up with the patient to see if the pain complaint was legitimate. The physician ignored the family's request that the surgery be done sooner, deeming it unnecessary. The surgeon had placed his cultural beliefs onto the patient which impacted his medical judgment.

By the time the patient went to surgery, her condition had worsened, and she died from the surgery. The family felt that had the surgeon operated when they first complained about the patient's pain, she might have lived, and they filed a malpractice case against the surgeon.

Rationale: In this case, the surgeon made the mistake of stereotyping the patient—she was a woman, and in the physician's experience, women complained loudly when in pain. Therefore, the physician exercised poor and negligent medical judgment when he failed to re-examine the patient. If the physician had been aware of the generalization about Irish people in pain, the patient's complaints may have been taken more seriously, which may have led to an earlier surgical intervention.

From: Galanti, G. A. (2000). An introduction to cultural differences. *Western Journal of Medicine, 172*, 5, 335–336.

Italian Americans

Historical Background

Italian Americans are actual immigrants or descendants from mainland Italy, Sicily, Sardinia, and other Mediterranean islands that make up Italy. Most of these immigrants came to the United States during the "Great Migration" between 1880 and 1922. Today, the descendants of those early immigrants number nearly 16 million; making them the fifth largest ethnic group in the United States (US Census Bureau, 2000). The frequency of intermarriage has resulted in the number of Americans who have at least one Italian grandparent to be estimated at 26 million.

Traditional Health Beliefs

Italian Americans have several traditional health beliefs including the belief that the cause of illness is a result of a contagion or contamination caused by heredity related to a supernatural or human cause, related to wind currents that bear diseases, or psychosomatic causes. First-generation immigrants are more likely to ascribe to these traditional health beliefs.

It is important to make the distinction between "fresh air" and drafts. Fresh air is considered healthy and vital for health maintenance while drafts, on the other hand, are a cause of illness. Ventilation of the home and workplace is valued, but avoidance of drafts is essential.

Supernatural causes of illness include the "evil eye" (malocchio) and curses (castiga). The severity of the illness is related to the supernatural causes with curses resulting in the most serious or even fatal medical problems. Curses are the result of either God or sent by an evil person, and they may be seen as a punishment for sinning or other bad behavior.

Emotions need to be released, which is one explanation for the animation associated with the Italian culture. Keeping emotions bottled up is unhealthy, and if an outlet for release of these emotions is not found, serious consequences will result.

Impact of Communication

According to data from the 2000 US Census, there are 1 million speakers of Italian in the United States, which ranked sixth on the top 10 list of languages spoken in the home excluding English and Spanish (Box 9-1). Many scholars have attributed the loss of the Italian language to Italian Americans during World War II. The American government had a strong propaganda campaign telling Americans not to speak the enemy's language. Also during the war, some Italian Americans (as well as Japanese Americans) were placed in internment camps—this was more likely to occur if Italian was spoken.

Box 9-1

Ten Languages Most Frequently Spoken at Home Other Than English and Spanish: 2000

Population Aged 5 Years and Older	Number in Millions
Chinese	2.0
French	1.6
German	1.4
Tagalog	1.2
Italian*	1.0
Vietnamese*	1.0
Korean	0.9
Russian	0.7
Polish	0.7
Arabic	0.6

*The number of Vietnamese speakers and the number of Italian speakers were not statistically different from one another.

Source: US Census Bureau. (2000). United States Census 2000. Retrieved September 21, 2009, from http://www.census.gov/main/www/cen2000.html.

The Italian language of today (what is taught in schools/colleges) is different than traditional Italian. Over 80% of Italian Americans are of Southern Italian descent where the Neapolitan or Sicilian dialects were spoken. Today, this Italian is anachronistic and demonstrates Southern Italy dialects of the past and not the language of the present (Italian Standard). The language situation is even more pronounced for Italian Americans of Northern descent, as their language is even more linguistically different than Southern Italian dialects. Because of this, Italian Americans who wish to learn Italian are learning a language that does not include many of the phrases they may have learned from their families.

Language problems can face the nurse when the elderly or a new Italian immigrant seeks medical care. Modesty may impact the ability to get adequate or complete answers to medical questions, even when an interpreter is used. Italian Americans tend to overreport symptoms or report their symptoms in a very dramatic manner. Because of this, physicians tend to diagnose more emotional problems more often for Italian American patients than for any other ethnic group (Giordano & McGoldrick, 1996).

The nurse should recognize that Italian Americans are motivated to seek full and complete explanations regarding their health status and the proposed treatment plan. If the instructions are clear, cooperation is enhanced. It is recommended to provide thorough oral patient education followed up with the provision of written instructions to ensure safety and adherence.

Impact of Social Organization

The family is the main organizing framework in Italian American culture. The family provides strength, helps with coping with stresses, and provides a sense of continuity. Italian Americans take pride in their family and their home. The man is the head of the household, and the female is considered to provide the heart of the family. The church is also an important focus of Italian American life. Italian feasts are commonplace and provide the opportunity for proliferation of the culture's love of food and its devotion to God and to patron saints.

Often, the care of illness is managed in the home with all family members contributing to patient care and management of household responsibilities. Intermarriage is common with more than 80% of Italian Americans marrying people from a different ethnic group (Giordano & McGoldrick, 1996).

Impact of Faith and Spirituality

Most Italian Americans are Catholic, and it has been reported that many immigrants become even more devoutly Catholic once they arrive in America. There are some who, despite possessing a Catholic background, have chosen to leave the church to practice Protestant Christianity for various reasons. Some worship in non-Catholic churches but continue to enroll their children in parochial schools. Some have become disenchanted with the leadership in the Catholic Church, abhor lack of agreement with certain church rituals, and believe that the Catholics have misinterpreted certain important Christian doctrines.

Biologic Variations

There are two genetic diseases commonly seen in Italian Americans, both of which are anemia disorders. The first is favism, which is a severe hemolytic anemia that results from a deficiency of the X-linked enzyme glucose-6-phosphate dehydrogenase that is triggered when the patient eats fava beans. The second type of anemia disorder is the thalassemia syndromes of which there are two subgroupings. Beta-thalassemia, which is also referred to as Cooley's anemia or thalassemia major, is a serious form of the disease, and alpha-thalassemia. The thalassemias are a diverse group of hereditary blood diseases that result in reduced or flawed production of hemoglobin. Some cases of thalassemia can be quite debilitating, requiring extensive medical intervention, whereas others require little or no medical intervention.

Appalachians

Historical Background

Appalachians are people who were either born in or live in the Appalachian Mountain region of the United States. This large area crosses 13 states and is considered a rural, nonfarming area. Although there is diversity among Appalachians, there are some commonalities. The majority of the population is White (approximately 96%), primarily of Scottish-Irish or British descent, and predominately follow the fundamentalist Protestant religion. Others trace their ancestry to Germany and France. Most Appalachians also share a genetic link to Native Americans who lived in the area prior to European settlement. The ruggedness of the terrain has resulted in a deep-rooted work ethic, loyalty, family-oriented, religious, and resourceful people (Marger & Obermiller, 1987).

Traditional Health Beliefs

There is a general distrust of all outsiders, which includes nurses and other healthcare professionals. There is an acceptance of a wide variety of healers. Because of the isolation, these folk healers are often the primary providers of health care available. One of these is the "granny midwife." Granny midwives are usually older women who may be responsible for all of the births in their region of the Appalachians.

The traditional healer's goal is the restoration of harmony. Products from nature are utilized, including poultices and teas. A strong belief in folk medicine is a strong part of the culture, and these practices are followed by all persons from all socioeconomic and educational levels. It is essential that the nurse become familiar and knowledgeable about these herbs because their use is so prevalent. Some of the ingredients can have serious side effects and may interact with prescribed pharmacologic therapies. The nurse must ascertain if the patient intends to use folk medicines at the same time as any prescription medications so that the treatment plan can be modified and essential education imparted to the patient to prevent untoward or adverse events. See Table 9-6 for information about herbal remedies.

Impact of Communication

Although the dominant language is English, there are some words from the 16th century Gaelic and Saxon languages that persist. Also, some areas have perpetuated Elizabethan English that can cause communication difficulties during health encounters if the nurse is not

Table 9-6

Appalachian Traditional Herbal Therapies

Medical Condition	Herbal Therapy
Arthritis	1. Ginseng tea—ingested orally or rubbed onto affected joints. Nursing implication: Ginseng can prolong bleeding; use caution with heparin, warfarin, aspirin, and nonsteroidal anti-inflammatory drugs. Interacts with monoamine oxidase inhibitors. Use in combination with stimulants (caffeine) can elevate blood pressure. Concomitant use with furosemide, nifedipine, and estrogen may increase risk of side effects. 2. Tea made from alfalfa seeds or stems, or tea from the stems of the barbell plant. 3. Drinking a combination of liquor with the roots of ginseng and goldenseal, or tea from rhubarb and whiskey. 4. Drink a mixture of honey, vinegar, and liquor.
Asthma	1. Drink tea from the bark of wild yellow plum trees, mullein leaves, and alum twice a day. 2. Combine gin and the heartwood of a pine tree twice a day. 3. Drink a mixture of honey, lemon juice, and whiskey.
Boils/Sores	1. Apply a poultice of walnut leaves or the green hulls with salt. 2. Apply a poultice of the house leek plant. 3. Apply a poultice of flaxseed meal.
Fever	1. Drink water from wild ginger. Nursing implication: Ginger may inhibit platelet aggregation/decrease thromboxane production theoretically, increasing bleeding risk. There is evidence that ginger may increase stomach acid production, which may be of significance in patients with peptic ulcer disease or who are prescribed antacids, H2 receptor antagonists, or proton pump inhibitors. Other studies indicate that ginger may act to protect the stomach. Ginger may interfere with medications affecting heart contraction (including beta-blockers and digoxin among others). Ginger may also interact with drugs taken for nausea/vomiting, arthritis, blood disorders, high cholesterol, high/low blood pressure, allergies (antihistamines), cancer, inflammation, vasodilators, or weight loss. Caution is advised when taking ginger with drugs that weaken the immune system, because of a possible interaction. 2. Drink tea made from butterly weed, wild horsemint, or feverwood.
Headache	1. Drink tea made of lady's slipper plants. Nursing implications: Lady's slipper contains quinines, which may have an additive effect when taken concomitantly with other quinine-containing agents, often used to treat malaria. Lady's slipper is thought to contain tannins, glycosides, resins, and quinines. Patients taking cardiac glycosides or digoxin should use with caution. Based on traditional use, lady's slipper may have additive effects when used with other sedatives. 2. Rub camphor and whiskey on the head.
Hypertension	1. Drink sarsaparilla tea. 2. Drink a half cup of vinegar
Heart Disease	1. Drink tea made from heartleaf leaves or bleeding heart. 2. Eat garlic.
Kidney Disease	1. Drink tea made from peach leaves or mullein roots. 2. Drink tea made from corn silk or arbutus leaves.
Sore Throat	1. Gargle with the sap from a red oak tree. 2. Eat honey and molasses. 3. Drink honey and whiskey. 4. Apply a poultice of cottonseed to the throat.
Warts	1. Apply milkweed juice to the affected area.

Source: Purnell, L. D., & Paulanka, B. J. (1998). *Transcultural health care: A culturally competent approach.* Philadelphia: F. A. Davis.

familiar with the characteristics of that speech. The best policy when confronted with an unfamiliar word is to request clarification from the patient.

Impact of Social Organization

The traditional household is male led with the women responsible for childrearing. Women usually marry young (by age 20), whereas men marry by the age of 28 (McNeil, 1989). Because of a loss of welfare benefits/services upon marriage, some Appalachians are deciding not to marry. Women are also relied upon for their emotional strength. Older women are responsible to perpetuate the culture and to care for the ill through the preparation of remedies. Grandparents are often called upon to be caregivers to the children of the family. The elders arc rewarded for this commitment to the family as the physical structures of many Appalachian homes are designed to permit function in aging persons. Nursing home placement is not culturally acceptable as it is considered the equivalent of a death sentence (Halperin, 1994). The rough mountainous terrain makes travel difficult in the Appalachians. The result of this has been the formation of informal social networks that also serves to meet the need for worship. Difficulty with travel makes attendance at organized churches difficult, although Fundamentalist Protestant religion is important to the community. Difficulty with access and the lack of public transportation and insufficient and inadequate roads are responsible for the continued geographic and social isolation. Isolation has also resulted in a dichotomous population divided by educational level: poorly educated or well educated.

Acceptance is an important characteristic of Appalachian culture. Alternative lifestyles (divorce, homosexuality) are accepted, but not usually discussed. This acceptance is linked to the Appalachians need for privacy and the desire not to interfere with other's lives through the avoidance of arguments and seeking common ground.

Biologic Variations

The Appalachians are predominately a White population that has incurred little variation over time. Some can trace their genetic background to include a mixture of White European ancestry with either Cherokee or Apache Native American blood. This mixture has resulted in a darker pigmentation than would exist without the genetic Native American influence. There is a very small minority of Blacks who self-identify as Appalachians. There are no reported studies that have found variations in drug metabolism specific to this population.

Mortality/Morbidity

The environmental factors associated with geographic location and occupations of Appalachians have resulted in serious health problems. Appalachians are at a higher risk for respiratory diseases such as black lung disease, emphysema, and tuberculosis. Parasitic infections are common because many Appalachians live without electricity or access to plumbing. The incidence of type II diabetes is 400–600% greater than the national average (Brown & Obermiller, 1994). Cancer, myocardial infarction, cerebral vascular accident, mental illness, accidental injury, and suicide rates are significantly higher in the Appalachian versus the general population ranging from 150 to 400% greater (Brown & Obermiller, 1994; Edwards, Lenz, & East-Odom, 1993).

Impact of Nurses and Nurse Practitioners in Appalachia

Lay midwives (often referred to as granny midwives) have been practicing in Appalachia for many decades but it was not until 1927, when Mary Breckenridge founded the Frontier Nursing Service, that the people of Appalachia had access to formally trained nurse–midwives and nurses for healthcare delivery. Since then, access has expanded to include the provision of primary care in nurse-managed centers throughout the large geographic area making up Appalachia. Often, it is a struggle to earn the trust of the community as it is a slow process to earn the trust when viewed as an outsider. The nurse providing care in the home is usually a more successful approach. Asking the patient what they consider the problem to be prior to designing the treatment plan is also an effective strategy (Helton, Barnes, & Borman, 1994).

The Amish

Background

The Amish are linked to the Anabaptists of 16th century Europe. This group broke off from the Catholic Church because they felt the scriptures did not support infant baptism and that only believers should be baptized. The Anabaptists term came from the practice of adults being rebaptized. There were other differences such as a desire for separation of church and states, pacifism, and a commitment to live peaceably. The Anabaptists became a persecuted group throughout the next century in Western Europe. The Anabaptists, despite this persecution, gave birth to three religious movements that still exist today. These three groups are the Mennonites, the Hutterites, and the Swiss Brethren (Hostetler, 1993). The Amish are a branch of the Swiss Brethren and derived its name from their leader Jakob Ammann, who was a Swiss

Brethren bishop from Alsace (Christian Light Publications, Inc.; Gross, 1997). The most well-known descendants of the Anabaptists are the Mennonites and the Amish. According to Christian Light Publications, Inc., the Amish, a smaller body of Swiss Brethren, settled in Pennsylvania in Berks County in 1736. The motivation for German migration to the American colonies was the impact of many wars on Germany and the desire for religious freedom. Taxes were high to pay for the wars, famine spread over the land, and the armies had trampled farmland and burned down farmsteads (Christian Light Publications, Inc). In Europe, the rulers determined the religion of the land and many pious Germans found this difficult to accept. The Colonies and especially Pennsylvania offered the opportunity for religious freedom.

A break occurred between the Swiss Brethren and the Amish under Ammann's leadership in 1693. The Amish then refused to have anything to do with their former brethren or any excommunicated members, a tradition that is referred to as "shunning."

Today, the Amish live in rural areas in over 28 states. The vast majority of the Amish (about 75%) live in Pennsylvania, Ohio, and Indiana (Kraybill, 1993). Recently, the Amish have been expanding their presence in search of affordable farm land in response to a doubling of population over the past 16 years. Reasons given for the increase in population include large families, increase in marriages within the community, a lower than average child mortality rate, and longer life spans. Amish couples typically have five or more children. With more than four out of every five deciding in young adulthood to remain within the church, their population has grown steadily. More than half the population is under 21. A small portion of the increase is also caused by conversions to the faith. In Ontario, Canada, the only Amish community outside the United States is also growing. It consists of about 4500 people, up from 2300 in 1992 (Kraybill, Nolt, & Johnson-Weiner, 2008).

The Amish are attracted to areas with relatively cheap farms, a rural lifestyle, and nonfarming jobs such as construction or cabinet making that fit their values and allow them to remain independent. In some cases, they have migrated to resolve leadership problems or escape church-related disputes.

The most important concept that the nurse needs to know in an attempt to understand Amish culture is that the reason for the departure from contemporary American culture is caused by the Amish people's perceived biblical mandate to live a life separated from a world they see as sinful (Kraybill, 2003; Hostetler, 1993). The old-fashioned appearance can be misunderstood. Although the eschewing of modern technological conveniences is present (i.e., reliance on the use of horse and buggy for transportation and the lack of electricity in the home), this does not mean the Amish will not be open to the use of state-of-the-art medical technology if it is deemed necessary to health promotion (Huntington, 1993).

Traditional Health Beliefs

The Amish wish to be born at home and to die at home. God's will is absolute as it determines all and their belief is to accept God's will as it is. This belief is associated with a deep fear of disability—it is feared much more than death. If disability can result from the refusal of treatment, it is essential that the patient and family be educated about this risk. However, a child with birth defects or other disabilities is readily accepted as a child of God and the parents will not be deterred from having additional children. As was stated earlier, the use of modern medicine and medical technology is not forbidden. Prior to accepting medical care, the patient and/or family will ask for the blessing of the church. The reason for this is that the community will need to come together to help pay the medical bills as the Amish do not have medical insurance because it is viewed as a "worldly product" and therefore reflects a lack of faith in God. If deemed necessary, the Amish will permit surgery, anesthesia, dental work, and even blood transfusions and transplantation. The only exception is for heart transplantation, as the heart is viewed as the soul of the body. The Amish do not want to be seen by or have student practitioners participate in their care. Because they are paying cash for their medical care, they only want to be seen by experienced and licensed medical professionals. All medical decisions will be jointly made by both the husband and the wife because of the belief that they are true partners in family life (Lee, 2005).

The Amish are unlikely to seek medical attention for minor complaints. Instead, they are more likely to rely on folk or herbal remedies. They like to use healing aids such as vitamins, homeopathic remedies, health foods, reflexology, and chiropractors.

Traditional health beliefs are shaped by their conservative rural values, a preference for natural remedies, a lack of information, unfamiliarity with technology, difficulties with access, and a strong reliance on God with an associated willingness to suffer if it is God's will (Kraybill, 1993).

Impact of Communication

The Amish speak English and a hybrid language of German and Dutch referred to as "Pennsylvania German" or "Pennsylvania Dutch." It is a Germanic language with a large amount of English mixed in. The Pennsylvania Dutch language is an oral one. Writing done by the Amish is in English. Many Amish are trilingual as they also speak "high German," which is the language of their bibles and the language used during church services.

Impact of Social Organization

The social organization of the Amish is guided by the desire to avoid assimilation and acculturation into dominant American culture. The Amish have been able to maintain a distinctive ethnic subculture by successfully resisting acculturation and assimilation. The Amish try to maintain cultural customs that preserve their identity. They have resisted assimilation into American culture by emphasizing separation from the world, rejecting higher education, selectively using technology, and restricting interaction with outsiders.

The Amish church prescribes dress regulations for its members, but the unwritten standards vary considerably by settlement. Men are expected to wear a wide brim hat and a vest when they appear in public. In winter months and at church services, they wear a black suit coat that is typically fastened with hooks and eyes rather than with buttons. Men use suspenders instead of belts.

Amish women are expected to wear a prayer covering and a bonnet when they appear in public settings. Most women wear a cape over their dresses as well as an apron. The three parts of the dress are often fastened together with straight pins. Various colors, including green, brown, blue, and lavender, are permitted for men's shirts and women's dresses, but designs and figures in the material are taboo. Although young girls do not wear a prayer covering, Amish children are typically dressed similar to their parents.

Although some holidays are celebrated, such as Thanksgiving, Christmas, Easter, and New Years Day, they are free from commercial trappings. The Amish, as conscientious objectors, do not celebrate holidays that are military based such as Memorial Day, Veterans Day, and the Fourth of July.

Cultural ties to the outside world are curbed by speaking the dialect, marrying within the group, spurning television, prohibiting higher education, and limiting social interaction with outsiders. Parochial schools insulate Amish youth from outside influences and threatening ideas. From birth to death, members are embedded in a web of ethnicity. These cultural defenses fortify Amish identity.

Biologic Variations

As a result of the inbreeding associated with a closed community like the Amish, genetic abnormalities are common because of the "founder effect." Almost all Amish are descended from about 200 founders. These genetic disorders, such as dwarfism, unusual blood typing, and metabolic disorders, are accepted as God's will.

Roma (Gypsies)

Historical Background

The Roma most likely originated in India around the year 1000 AD. The Roma are travelers and have settled in many different European countries since then. The population has experienced many divisions over the years, which makes the placement of the Roma into one ethnic group impossible. Today, there are approximately 12 million Roma living in the world. The term Roma is preferred as the more well-known terminology of Gypsy, which has negative connotations. There is no census data on the Roma but estimates range from 100,000–300,000 members of several diverse groups in the United States.

Traditional Health Beliefs

There is a general lack of knowledge about access to health services and how to provide them appropriately to the Roma population. The Roma people possess a strongly held set of health-related beliefs in which some diseases are seen as belonging to the Roma (to that group), therefore requiring treatment by their own traditional healers, whereas other diseases are seen as a result of contact with the outside world and as such require medical care from the American healthcare delivery system. The majority of Roma are governed by a series of rules about what is considered pure or impure. There are also a range of specific rituals dealing with birth, death, and caring for the ill. These beliefs and reliance on rituals can result in the Roma people accepting some aspects of medical care and rejecting other aspects. This behavior can be labeled as nonadherent and can be viewed as irresponsible for not fitting in with the norms of dominant American society.

Impact of Communication

The Roma speak many different dialects of the Roma language. Those from Western Europe and the majority in the United States speak Romany (also known as Romanes or Romani). Romany is a Sanskrit-based language that belongs to the Indo-Aryan branch of Indo-European languages. All of the dialects have traces of other languages in them because of the influence of the many different countries in which Roma have lived. All Roma speak a second or even a third language from the countries in which they have lived or travelled. The Romany language is a principal factor of Roma ethnic identity. It is primarily a spoken rather than written language. Until recent years, most Roma were illiterate, and illiteracy rates remain very high in most Roma communities. In light of this, the nurse should not rely on written materials when providing patient education to Roma patients and families.

Impact of Social Organization

Roma families have settled throughout the United States. Family consists of extended members who may or may not be related by blood. The family is a strong, tightly knit unit, known as a clan or "kumpania." The clan often live, work, and celebrate together. The elder members are the authority figures and decision makers in all situations. Clan leaders sometimes adopt the title of "King" or "Queen." These titles denote respect and not the possession of an actual political position. The nurse should always speak to the elders if any healthcare decisions are required.

Marriages are often arranged and at a very young age. Until marriage at the age of 12 or 13 for most Roma girls, strict morality is upheld through the use of chaperones. Marriage creates an alliance between a family or clan. The payment of a "bride price" (dowry) is common. This payment from the groom's family is meant to compensate the bride's family for the loss of their daughter and to ensure that she will be well treated as a member of her new family.

Disputes are settled within the community itself. An informal Romani court called the kris decides matters of common law and custom and determines penalty. A kris-determined penalty can be as severe as exclusion from the community.

Most Roma currently living in this country were born here and have since adopted to many of the dominant American society cultural norms. This goes against traditional Roma beliefs which include that society is "dirty" and potentially polluting, and in traditional clans, children are often removed from school at puberty (Sutherland, 2004).

Today, some have a less nomadic lifestyle that is contradictory to traditional Roma lifestyle, which holds that isolation away from the dominant society is crucial to maintaining Roma culture (Rundle, Carvalho, & Robinson, 1999). There are a number of diverse Roma groups and not all of them have the same cultural practices.

Impact of Faith and Spirituality

Some Roma still practice the religion of their homelands, most commonly Christianity or Islam. Some are Born Again Christians and follow the main Protestant Holy Days (Hancock, 1987). Most practice a religion similar to Wicca which believes in both Satan and God, while placing an emphasis on luck and the supernatural (Rundle et al., 1999). There is resistance to the emergence of Christianity by those who seek to uphold the older traditions such as arranged marriages, dowries, and fortune telling (Hancock, 1987).

Biologic Variations

There is little research on the Roma population. There is evidence that the life expectancy is 10 years less than that of their non-Roma neighbors and that infant mortality is up to four times higher (Braham, 1993). Two studies conducted in Spain found a high prevalence for the antibody to hepatitis A (a nine times greater prevalence) and for lead poisoning in children (McKee, 1997). Some Roma groups have a high incidence of inherited congenital abnormalities, which may be a result of a closed community and a reluctance to mix with outsiders.

Jewish Americans

Historical Background

The inclusion of Jewish Americans is important because, unlike followers of other religions, being Jewish is not only following a religions but a culture and a way of life, although it is not a race. Terms to describe Jewish people throughout history include Hebrew, Israelite, and Jew. The terms can also be used interchangeable as the people are called Jewish, the faith is Judaism, the land is Israel, and the language spoken is Hebrew. The United States is home to the largest number of Jews in the world second only to Israel. There are several different types of Judaism that range on a continuum from the most extreme or conservative which is strict Orthodox, to the most liberal which is liberal Reform. Although there is no formal social hierarchy within the Jewish American community, in the case of ultra-Orthodox followers, decisions may be made in concert with their rabbi. According to US Census Bureau data (2007), 1.7% of the adult American population is Jewish, which converts to 5,128,000 people. This number is very close to the number of Jews living in Israel, which has been estimated by Israel's Central Bureau of Statistics as 5,435,800 people in the year 2007. See Box 9-2 to see how this compares to other religious organizations in the United States.

The Jewish community of the United States is varied. It consists mainly of Ashkenazi Jews who immigrated to the United States from Eastern and Central Europe and their descendants (who were US-born citizens). There are other Jewish ethnic divisions as well, including Sephardics and Mizrahis. There are also some Jewish Americans who were converts to the religion as well. This variability has resulted in a wide range of Jewish cultural traditions with an associated wide range of religious observance (from extremely religious to those living a secular lifestyle).

Jews have been present in the United States for some time, perhaps even earlier than the 17th century. The early immigrants were almost

Box 9-2

Religious Composition of the United States of America in Descending Order

Religion	Percentage of Adult Population
Protestant—all types	51.3
Catholic	23.9
Unaffiliated (includes atheist, agnostic, and nothing in particular)	16.1
Mormon (also includes Church of Jesus Christ of Latter Day Saints)	3.3
Do not know	0.8
Jehovah's Witness	0.7
Unitarians and other liberal faiths	0.7
Buddhist	0.7
Muslim	0.6
Orthodox	0.6
Hindu	0.4
New Age (includes Wiccan, Pagan, and other New Age groups)	0.4

From the Religious Landscape Survey, a survey conducted in the summer of 2007 among a representative sample of 35,556 adults (over age 18) living in the continental United States. (US The Pew Forum on Religion & Public Life. Religious Landscape Survey. Retrieved August 28, 2009, from http://www.census.gov/compendia/statab/tables/09s0074.pdf.)

exclusively Sephardic Jews of Spanish and Portuguese descent. Large scale Jewish immigration began in earnest in the 19th century with the arrival of many secular Ashkenazi Jews from Germany.

Over 2,000,000 Jews arrived between the late 19th century and 1924, when the Immigration Act of 1924 and the National Origins Quota of 1924 restricted immigration. Most settled in the city of New York and its immediate surrounding areas, establishing what is today one of the world's major concentrations of the Jewish population. Today, the top three states with the highest proportion of Jews are New York, New Jersey, and Florida.

During the early 20th century, assimilation was encouraged and Jews became a part of American life. Half of all Jewish adult males aged 18 to 50 served in World War II (500,000 men), and after the war ended were part of the suburban sprawl that occurred in the United States. Further assimilation and high intermarriage rates further contributed to secularization. As a group, American Jews have been very active in civil rights and fighting prejudice and discrimination. Some Jewish scholars attribute this to the history of the Jews beginning in slavery and the yearning for freedom.

Although Jewish Americans are included in this chapter on White non-Hispanic cultures, do not conclude that there are no African American Jews. Estimates range from a low of 20,000 to a high of 200,000 African American Jews in the United States. These Jews, who are not of European descent, are sometimes referred to as "Black Jews" to differentiate them from Jews who are directly descended from the Israelites of the Torah. Despite this distinction being made, the relations between the two groups are apparently amicable.

Traditional Health Beliefs

Jewish Americans are health conscious and believe in keeping both the mind and body healthy. They practice preventative health care and will participate in routine screenings and complete all recommended immunizations. It is believed that illness requires early and prompt treatment. All branches of Judaism believe that religious requirements (if a conflict were to exist) may be disregarded if a life is at stake or if the person is suffering with a potentially life-threatening illness.

Ancient Jews followed good hygiene and sanitation practices, which have provided the basic principles for public health care. It was Lillian Wald, a Jewish nurse, who established the prototype for public health nursing when she established the Henry Street Settlement in Manhattan, New York City, in 1893. Physicians and nurses are held in high regard by Jews. There is the belief that once standard therapy has failed and there is no further treatment available, the physician must be willing to change hats from "curer" to "carer" (Rosner, 1993).

Impact of Communication

American Jews speak English and a large number are bilingual speaking Modern Hebrew as well. Modern Hebrew is the official state language of Israel and is the language used for prayers. Hebrew is read from right to left and books are opened from the opposite side compared to books written in English. Recent immigrants from Israel may only speak Modern Hebrew. A number of other languages may also be spoken depending on the type of Jew the patient is. Many Hasidic Jews (of Ashkenazi descent) speak Yiddish. Yiddish was the primary language spoken by many European Jewish immigrants to the United States and is a Judeo-German dialect. Some Yiddish terms have become a part of American English (some examples are schmuck for fool and nosh for snack).

The Persian Jewish community (mainly centered in Los Angeles and Beverly Hills, California, and eastern parts of New York including Great Neck, Long Island) speak Persian during religious services, in the home, and even publish Persian language newspapers.

Russian Jews may speak Russian, often as the primary language in the home. American Bukhori Jews speak Bukhori (a Persian dialect) as well as Russian.

Although Modern Hebrew is primarily spoken today, Classical Hebrew is the language of Jewish religious literature including the Tanakh (Bible) and Siddur (prayer book).

There is also a contingent of Hispanic Jews who descended from immigrants from Latin America who speak Spanish in the home.

Impact of Time, Space, and Touch

Jewish Americans have a time orientation that encompasses the past, the present, and the future all at once. Although the emphasis is on living for today and plan for and worry about tomorrow, they cannot escape the past for fear that if the past, and that includes the Holocaust, is forgotten, it can be repeated. This unique time orientation focus is a dominant part of the culture.

Modesty and humility are important Jewish values. Modesty is expressed not only by dress but by actions. Jews do not like to call attention to self or appreciate when someone tries to call attention to self or impress others. This is tied to the belief that people are judged by their actions.

Hasidic American males consider women to be seductive and may not look directly upon a female's face or talk with them. Touching of the female is also an issue. They may even keep their hands in their pockets to avoid touching a female as they are not permitted to touch a woman who is not their wife. The female nurse should not offer her hand in greeting to the male Hasidic Jew and if it is done the nurse should not consider the patient rude if the patient refuses to accept the offered hand. Non-Hasidic Jews may be more informal maintaining a shorter spatial distance during communication and may use touch.

Impact of Social Organization

The family is the heart and soul of Jewish society with an emphasis placed on making sure all family members' needs are met and respected. Today, because of assimilation, there is little difference in gender roles between Jewish American and other White American families as both parents share the home and family responsibilities. Parents are honored and that means the adult children will care for them in old age. Providing respect to the elderly is essential even if the elderly is senile or acts inappropriately, respect is still essential. Marriage is considered the ideal state since it is stated in the Bible that man should not be alone. Marriage is viewed as being of benefit for procreation but also for procreation. Sexuality is deemed an important part of marriage and nonprocreative sexual intercourse is acceptable but only in marriage. Premarital sexual activity goes against Jewish values.

Biologic Variations

The skin complexion associated with a Jewish American is dependent on the type of Jew they have descended from. Ashkenazi Jews have the same skin coloring as other White Americans. Darker complexioned Jews, similar to people from the Mediterranean areas, are Sephardic Jews. There are also Jews from throughout Africa whose pigmentation of skin is considered black.

Just as skin color is dependent on the type of Jew the patient is, so are the biologic variations the nurse should consider or assess for. Most genetic conditions are seen in descendents of immigrants from Eastern Europe (Ashkenazi Jews). The majority of genetic conditions result from autosomal-recessive disorders (the gene is carried by both parents) and as such most of the resulting genetic conditions result in death in infancy or early childhood. These genetic disorders include Tay-Sachs disease, Bloom's syndrome, cystic fibrosis, familial dysautonomia, and Gauchers disease (Fares et al., 2008). Unlike with Tay-Sachs disease, there is no simple biochemical or enzymatic test to detect for carriers of these autosomal recessive disorders (Vallance & Ford, 2003). Tay-Sachs disease, arguably the most widely known of these disorders, results in progressive neurologic degeneration and has a carrier frequency of around 1 in 25 or 30 people of Ashkenazi Jewish origin, which is a likelihood 10 times higher than is found in other groups.

There are a few adult disorders associated with Jews of Ashkenazi descent. Kaposi's sarcoma is most commonly seen in these males who are over 50 years of age. The nurse should expect the manifestation to be malignant tumors of the endothelium that are slow-growing and confined to the skin, and the condition should not be confused with the Kaposi tumors seen in patients with acquired immunodeficiency syndrome (AIDS). The tumors in AIDS patients are much more aggressive, and they also affect internal organs as well as the skin. In one study by Engels, Clark, Aledort, Goedert, and Whitby (2002), it was found that the Kaposi sarcoma herpes virus seroprevalence rate (this virus is the Kaposi sarcoma agent) in elderly US Jews was 8.8% (which is similar to other studies rates which ranged between 5–10%).

An important nursing implication is the higher incidence of a serious adverse drug reaction in persons of Ashkenazi descent with the use of clozapine (an antipsychotic drug especially used to treat schizophrenia). In the general population, the side effect rate for agranulocytosis is about 1%, but in this Jewish population the incidence significantly increases up to 20% (Lieberman, 1990). A genetic reason has been identified to account for this difference. The nurse should remind the provider that adequate laboratory testing is provided for the Jewish patient on clozapine to monitor for agranulocytosis.

Impact of Faith and Spirituality

Judaism is one of the world's oldest religions dating back more than 3000 years. It is a monotheistic faith (the belief in one God as the Creator of the Universe). The history and the laws of Judaism are chronicled and described in the Old Testament of the Bible. The first five books of the Bible are handwritten in the Hebrew language on scrolls made of parchment. This is called the Torah. The Torah is kept in a "Holy Ark: under an eternal light within each synagogue" (Project Genesis, Inc). These are the Jewish laws, and they guide the Jews on every aspect of how they should live their lives. The spiritual leader is the Rabbi (which literally translates to teacher in English), and the Rabbi serves as the interpreter of Jewish law. It is not believed that a Rabbi is any closer to God than any other Jew, and a Jew can pray directly to God. Unlike in other religions, including different types of Christianity, the spiritual leader is not needed to intercede on the person's behalf with God, does not grant atonement, and do not hear confession. The Sabbath is the holiest day, and it begins 18 minutes before sunset on Friday and ends 42 minutes after sunset or when three stars can be seen on Saturday evening. If at all possible, elective or nonemergent procedures should not be performed on the Sabbath but the nurse should be aware that illness is considered a valid reason to keep the Jew from the synagogue on the Sabbath.

Although there is only one Jewish religion, the religion has three main branches: Orthodox (most traditional), Conservative (less strict as the branch make concessions to modern life), and Reform (considered a liberal or progressive denomination). According to a 1990 nation-wide survey, 7% of American Jews consider themselves Orthodox Jews and 42% reform Jews (Anonymous). There are also multiple smaller groups of ultra-Orthodox Jews—one of the most widely known of these are the Hasidic Jews as they wear full beards, dark clothing, and fully covered extremities. A newer denomination of Judaism is the Reconstructionists which is an amalgamation of the three main branches, and views the Jewish religion in evolution as its followers seek to adapt to and reside in a more modern world than is described in the Old Testament or the Torah.

The nurse should be careful not to assume that a deep faith or even a belief in God exists in all patients. This is also true of the Jewish American patient. Jewish religious practice is quite varied ranging from the highly devout to the atheist. It appears that American Jews are more likely to be atheist or agnostic than most Americans, especially so compared with Protestants or Catholics. A 2003 Harris poll found that while

79% of Americans believe in God, only 48% of American Jews do, compared with 79% and 90% for Catholics and Protestants, respectively. While 66% of Americans said they were "absolutely certain" of God's existence, 24% of American Jews said the same. And though 9% of Americans believe there is no God (8% Catholic and 4% Protestant), 19% of American Jews believe God does not exist (Harris Poll, 2003).

Traditional Judaism believes in an afterlife in which the soul continues to thrive. In the afterlife, things that were not understood in life will become known and clear. Although not much thought is given to life after death on a daily or even regular basis, it is believed that the righteous will be rewarded with a place in the afterlife.

The nurse needs to be aware that for an actively religious Jew, the provision of active euthanasia is forbidden. Active euthanasia is considered murder, which is in direct violation with one of the Ten Commandments. Even a dying patient with a terminal prognosis is considered a living being and, as such, active euthanasia (when something is given or done to cause or have the result of death) is not permitted. Suicide is also not permitted. Suicide is so frowned upon that it is considered both a criminal act and a moral violation. It is believed that the act of suicide prevents any repentance. In cases of adult suicide, full burial rights are not provided (unless the patient is deemed mentally incompetent) as the person will be buried in the outer perimeters of the Jewish cemetery and mourning will not be conducted. Children are the exception, as suicide in the case of children is never viewed as a voluntary act.

Passive euthanasia is a grayer area as it may be permitted depending on the situation and interpretation of that situation. Anything that artificially prevents death (i.e., cardiopulmonary resuscitation, mechanical ventilation) may possibly be withheld depending on the patient and family's wishes, as well as their specific and individual religious views. The nurse should consider this information fully prior to initiating any do not resuscitate discussions with the patient and or his family.

Russian Americans

Historical Background

The former Soviet Union was made up of 15 republics, of which Russia is the largest. Russia is also referred to as The Russian Federation. Russia is the largest country in the world as it extends to both the continents of Europe and Asia and is approximately two times the size of the United States. There are Russian-born nonethnic Russians living inside and outside of Russia, over 100 nationalities in total from Russia, and it is important to distinguish their separate identities. By far, the largest number are Russian at approximately 81.5% (Central Intelligence Agency, 2009).

There is a huge unemployment problem as well as extensive poverty in Russia. Forty percent of the population of Russia falls below the poverty line. Both of these financial issues have resulted in life today in Russia being very difficult, and crime is on the rise. Health indicators in the country are very poor. Low birthrates and high death rates have contributed to a population decline of more than 500,000 people annually. Life expectancy is significantly less for males—it is believed that men die much sooner than women because of cardiovascular disease, accidents, alcoholism, and suicide (Aslund, 2001). As of 2001, life expectancy at birth for Russians is 57.4 years for men and 72.8 years for women (Central Intelligence Agency, 2001). Infectious disease also has resulted in a public health crisis. The rate of tuberculosis (TB) is astronomical, killing more than 100,000 people in just a few years, while 2 million more Russians have been exposed to TB. Human immunodeficiency virus (HIV) is also believed to be a growing problem, but the extent of the problem is not as well-known as the TB issue. Access to effective treatments, including pharmaceuticals, also makes treatment difficult. Since the financial collapse of Russia in 1998, there are only a few pharmaceutical companies left. The Russian healthcare system is publicly supported but has problems with inefficiency, corruption, and very low salaries for both physicians and nurses.

All of these factors have spurred the desire to emigrate from Russia to come to the United States. A significant increase in immigration rates have been noted recently in response to these factors but immigration to the United States has been ongoing since 1917; this coincides with the end of the Russian Revolution.

The first Russian immigrants were very intelligent and educated and left Russia after the Russian Revolution. Conflict spurred the second wave of immigration, which occurred at the end of World War II. Anti-Semitism after World War II became a significant issue and many Russian Jews who were well-educated entered the United States as refugees. Immigration restrictions limiting US immigration based on family presence has resulted in new Russian immigrants being related to earlier Russian immigrants. This has resulted in a close-knit circle grouping of Russian Americans.

During the waning years of the Soviet Union, the United States encouraged free immigration among Soviet Jews. As a direct result of a 1973 law, a large wave of Soviet Jews arrived in the United States— 66,480 people in one 5-year period between 1975 and 1980. Policy in the Soviet Union during these waves of immigration was quite strict. If one family member wanted to leave (and this was usually the younger ones), the entire family also had to leave. This means that there are a significant number of Russian Americans who did not wish to immigrate and leave their homeland. The amount of time required for immigration has decreased over time. It is not uncommon to find an older immigrant who arrived in the 1980s sharing they experienced a 10-year wait to be able to immigrate while today the wait is often closer to only 1 year in length. This has caused some frustration and bitterness between newer and older immigrants. Toward the end of the Soviet Union, the numbers of immigrants from Russia to the United States dramatically increased. In the final year of the Soviet Unio, that country was number one in providing immigrants to the United States.

Another factor impacting immigration is the rise in international adoption rates. There are a growing number of Russian children who have been adopted by citizens of the United States; in fact, the number is so significant that Russia has become the number one source for adopted foreign children in the United States.

The nurse should recognize you may be called upon to care for Russian Americans of all ages—the very young who may be newly adopted, and the elderly who may be here reluctantly. More than half of the arriving Russian immigrants are over age 50 years old, which may impact assimilation. It is important to consider the reasons for immigration or presence in the United States when planning for nursing care delivery. You may encounter Russian immigrants (someone who wishes to live in another country) or Russian American Jews who are refugees. Refugees come to the United States because of declared political problems—in this case, Anti-Semitism and a need for safety. Refugees are entitled to numerous services to assist with the transition that can include financial help, access to training programs, and the granting of permanent resident status.

Statistics

US Census figures show that there are more than 3 million people of Russian ancestry in the country or 1% of the total population in the United States (US Census Bureau, 2007b). Almost a million more (0.3% of the total US population) is of Ukrainian heritage and nearly as many others indicate Slavic origins. All of them could have recognizable ties to history and culture associated with Russian-speaking peoples.

Ukraine

Ukraine is the second largest country in Europe. After the breakup of the Soviet Union, the Ukraine got its independence in 1991. Since this time, the economy has been suffering a crisis in spite of the Ukraine being a highly industrialized country. Agricultural issues, such as inadequate harvests and fuel shortage, have further compounded the economic problems and many are experiencing malnourishment in the Ukraine. Another complicating factor is the nuclear power plant accident that occurred at Chernobyl in 1986, which caused an explosion and contamination. Approximately 100,000 people were exposed to radiation prior to evacuation. These factors have impacted the desire for many Ukrainians to leave their country of origin and immigrate to other countries, including the United States.

Traditional Health Practices
Preventive health care is practiced and health screening is seen as the key to good health. The exception to this is that routine mammograms and routine breast examinations are seen as being of little value, as are cholesterol screening tests. In fact, a criticism made by many Russian Americans is the US healthcare system not placing enough emphasis on prevention and instead placing the reliance on pharmaceuticals. Russians instead prefer to utilize alternative therapies such as cupping, massage therapy, and acupressure/acupuncture.

Some Russian immigrants, especially the elderly, like to utilize homeopathic or folk medicines. Amber can be ground into a powder and, when added to hot water, becomes a medicine. Herbs are also utilized in either enema or drink form. Hot steam baths are also utilized as is drinking mineral water.

Health is seen as a goal to strive for and a gift to possess. Illness is seen as a disharmony in the body. Spirituality holds an important place in end of life care. Russians do not believe that a poor prognosis should be given to a terminally ill patient because it will only result in anxiety, lessen hope, and perhaps even hasten death.

In the Ukraine, herbal and folk medicines are used along with Western pharmaceuticals. In rural areas where access is an issue, the use of folk medicines is higher. An example of a commonly used medication is "zelenka" which is a mercurochrome-based green ointment for skin problems. Overall, folk medicines are believed to be less harmful than pharmaceuticals or "chemical medicine" by Ukrainians (Bologova, 1996).

Trust is essential to the doctor–patient or nurse–patient relationship. If the Ukrainian American patient does not trust the provider, the treatment plan will not be followed. Ukrainian Americans prefer a one-on-one relationship and value dialogue in health care. There is a general belief that Western physicians rely too much on fancy diagnostics and not enough on history taking. There is also a preference for the Ukrainian view of medical care, which is to reveal the cause of the disease. Ukrainian Americans feel that in the United States, the physician has little concern with the cause of disease and the main focus is on treatment. The nurse should be aware that it is culturally appropriate for a Ukrainian to offer a gift to ensure cooperation. This may result in an uncomfortable situation because in the Ukraine it is not uncommon for people to offer their district doctor a "bribe" to maintain a good relationship.

Chiropractors are gaining respect within the Ukrainian American population and the use of a chiropractor in certain situations is preferred (Bologova, 1996). Unfortunately, mental problems are considered taboo and the discussion of this does not occur even within the affected family. In the Ukraine, mental illness was considered shameful, and could even be dangerous to the family if it became known that a family member had mental health issues.

The nurse should recognize the prevalence of alternative therapy use in this population. If the use is nonharmful or neutral, the nurse should remain open to usage. The nurse should ask the patient about the use of any alternative healthcare practices as part of the initial data gathering.

Impact of Communication

Because of increased exposure to English-speaking media by most Russians, English is becoming widely used. Some may have even studied English in school; although, in that case, they most probably studied British English and not American English. Some elderly Russian Americans may also speak Yiddish. In the former Soviet Union, the speaking of Yiddish was discouraged and considered to be an antistate activity (Petersen, 2001). The official language of Russia is Russian. Russia is a Slavic language consisting of a 33-character alphabet; approximately one sixth of the world's population speaks Russian. There are geographic variances associated with the language. Tone, inflection, speed, and pauses as well as nonverbal cues are important when communicating in the Russian language as it denotes the value being placed on the words that are being said. Russian Americans may use an increased voice volume when attempting to have their needs met. The nurse should not feel that the Russian American patient is being rude if even normal conversation appears to be loud and boisterous. The nurse should also consider the distinction about the importance of nonverbal and subtle meanings underscores the importance of using professional interpreters when working with Russian Americans who are not fluent in American English. The use of family members as interpreters is especially problematic with this population. The close-knit community of Russian Americans breeds a high level of familiarity, which can make confidentiality impossible to maintain or ensure.

Impact of Communication for Ukrainian Americans

The Ukrainian language was different than other Slavic languages, including Russian since the 12th century. The language continued to develop independently until Russia seized the Ukraine at the end of the

17th century. By the beginning of the 19th century, the Russian Czars began to ban the use of the Ukrainian language and, because of this, the language fell into decay. In the western Ukraine, the language was exposed and absorbed influences from Polish, Hungarian, German, and Romanian. Ukrainian was restored as the official language of the Ukraine in 1917.

Most Ukrainian Pentecostals (many of whom are refugees who came to the Unites States because of religious oppression) speak only Ukrainian, but can often understand Polish and Russian. Ukrainian Jews, on the other hand, are often bilingual and speak both Ukrainian and Russian. A few may also speak or understand Yiddish as well.

Impact of Touch, Space, and Time

Touch is freely shared among close or intimate friends. Affection is readily demonstrated as women will kiss women and men will kiss men. They may also exchange three kisses on each cheek, which appears to be a cultural trait carried over from the Middle East. A handshake is particularly significant and is often viewed as more binding than a signed document.

A consequence of the many years of communist rule in Russia is that many Russian Americans still try to act in a neutral manner—eye contact is avoided, maintaining a flat affect and slouchy posture. Once exposed to a society that values personal freedom, such as the United States, some will be able to loosen up, but others may maintain the stance of neutrality. Great warmth will be expressed in private when dealing with close friends and family and unannounced or unplanned visits are common. The nurse should expect many visitors when caring for a Russian American patient.

The expectation is that the nurse will remain professional and caring at all times. A robotic approach to healthcare delivery will result in the loss of trust. Formality is also expected and the nurse should greet the patient as Mr. or Mrs. followed by the surname. To address a Russian American patient by their first name only is a major faux pas. It is also considered inappropriate to use terms of endearment in place of the patient's formal name (e.g., "honey" or "sweetie") (Smith, 1996). It is considered appropriate for the nurse to enter the patient's personal space within a professional capacity—this space is usually reserved for the spouse and children. It would be wise for the nurse to fully communicate the need to enter the patient's personal space or if any violation of modesty is required in advance.

Russian American patients place a high premium on a nurse being very friendly, warm, and caring and to be there to help the patient and family cope with physical and psychosocial consequences of illness. The nurse can best communicate friendliness by maintaining an open body posture, smiling frequently, and speaking in a calm, pleasant tone of voice. It has also been noted, interestingly enough, that Russian American patients prefer to be cared for by a nurse from any other cultural group than Russia. It had been reported anecdotally that for some Russian Americans, it is felt they will experience more compassion and their needs will be better met by a non-Russian provider (Lester, 1998).

Impact of Social Organization

Family is an important concept and in America, like in Russia, extended family members often live together and rely on each other to make life easier. If the Russian American has family still in Russia, those family members who are with the patient in the United States become even more significant to them. Within the family structure, the father exerts the greatest influence. The female role is to care for the child or children. Women's liberation is not a part of the traditional Russian family structure. If she is well-educated, her husband may consult her on some decision making. Arguments within the family, when they occur, can be quite loud and dramatic and objects may be thrown.

Social events are often framed around the arts. The arts, such as ballet, theatre, music, and museums, are highly valued in Russian culture. The family often strives to keep the arts alive by exposing the children to this early in life.

The elderly, who were usually cared for in exchange for child care, may be a reminder of the old ways once immigration by the Russian family has occurred. It is not unusual for the elderly Russian immigrant to lose their authority and status within a short time after immigration to the United States (Aroian, Balsam, & Conway, 2000).

Within a few years of immigration to the United States, children become completely assimilated into American culture. Children are very important in Russian culture as they are seen as symbols of innocence and the family's hopes for the future. Children grow up often overprotected and cared for by elderly family members. One child families are very common and extended family members, such as cousins, are treated as substitute siblings. If a child becomes ill, the family will fight vehemently for the child's rights and may request unnecessary diagnostic testing or prolonged hospital stays. Russians may be accustomed to longer lengths of stay than are typical today in the United States as the average in-patient stay in Russia is 3 weeks (Rundle et al., 1999). The nurse should assure the family that the primary concern is the child's welfare, which may ease the worry. In addition, helping both patients and families understand the differences between the Russian and US healthcare systems and how to navigate the US healthcare system is time well spent by the nurse.

Impact of Social Organization on Ukrainian Americans

Ukrainians often have very large families, and the older family members help to care for the children. Because of limited housing and cost, it is not uncommon to have three generations of a Ukrainian family all living together in a small living space. Pentecostal Ukrainians, by virtue of their refugee status, are able to receive refugee benefits and services from refugee organizations in their new communities.

Impact of Faith and Spirituality

In Russia, as a consequence of communism, the nonreligious may make up the majority of the population. The nonreligious constitutes anywhere between 24%–48% of the population, according to a study by Zuckerman (2005). Russia ranks third on the listing of top 20 Atheist countries in the world (Zuckerman, 2005). Russian Orthodox has a following of 45% of Russians, although the vast majorities are not churchgoers. In a poll conducted in 2007 by the Russian Public Opinion Research Center, about 75% of Russia's people affirm the Orthodox faith, and only 10% are regular churchgoers. In a post-Soviet Union Russia, Orthodoxy has become the national faith. It is difficult to gauge the actual number of followers because many Russians, although they may never attend church services, identify and consider themselves Russian Orthodox. The Central Intelligence Agency (2006) estimated the number of practicing worshippers of Orthodoxy in Russia as being between 15% and 20%, with Muslims making up 10–15%, and other Christians making up 2%. The Central Intelligence Agency states that post-Soviet rule Russia was left with a large population of nonpracticing believers and nonbelievers. The remaining Russians are made up of Tatars (an Islamic religion) and Jews. Despite these varying statistics, there can be no doubt that the fall of communism has brought a resurgence of the Christian religion in Russia.

Impact of Faith and Spirituality on Ukrainian Americans

The largest religion in the Ukraine, just as in Russia, is Eastern Orthodox, a branch of Christianity. Prior to 1990, the Ukrainian Orthodox Church was forced to become a part of the Russian Orthodox Church. After Ukrainian independence, the Ukrainian Orthodox Church was restored. The second largest Christian religion in the Ukraine is the Greek Catholic Church. In the past, Pentecostal and Baptist churches were active in western Ukraine. Persecution resulted when Ukraine was under Russian control, prompting many Pentecostal to become refugees from the former Soviet Union. This is another example of people being forced to leave their homeland for the United States in search of religious freedom. Indeed, the primary reason for leaving the Ukraine is religious oppression (Bologova, 1996). Ukrainian Pentecostals value hard work and the family, and they have strict rules against drugs and alcohol usage. The rejection of birth control usage, which is supported by the religion, often results in very large families.

Biologic Variations

There is a significant genetic mutation problem in the Russian population. It is felt that because of chronic exposure to environmental toxins from pesticides, cigarette smoking, and even the Chernobyl nuclear power plant accident, the genetic mutation rates are higher with an associated higher risk for health consequences caused by accumulated genetic damage. It has been estimated that the rate of accumulated genetic damage is 250% higher in Russians than Americans (Vadlamani et al., 2001). This genetic damage seems to be implicated in higher colorectal neoplasm rates in this population, which should highlight for the nurse the need for vigilant cancer screenings in this population.

The foods that are preferred in Russian culture have contributed to an obesity problem in this population, especially among elderly women. Many foods are high in fat and salt, which also has resulted in a significant problem with hypertension and coronary heart disease. There has been a trend in decreasing life expectancy in Russia since 1990. It is felt that this decrease is a result of a tremendous increase in coronary heart disease mortality among men, which increased by about 30% in Russia between 1990 and 2000 (Landsbergis & Klumbiene, 2003). Poor diet, excessive alcohol intake, and tobacco usage have been implicated in the high coronary heart disease numbers. Hyperlipidemia and hypercholesterolemia are also problematic in this population since most Russians, although compliant with most health screening; do not see the value or accuracy of cholesterol screening tests. Cholesterol levels among Russian Americans are generally well above normal limits (Mehler et al., 2001).

TB also has higher rates in this population. The reasons for this are many and include problems with the Russian healthcare system, significant number of HIV/AIDS patients, increased prison population, as well as indifference. The nurse should consider TB in this population and provide for infection control practices as needed.

Although alcoholism and excessive alcohol usage is a tremendous public health issue in Russia, the incidence of alcohol abuse in Russian immigrants to the United States is very low. The nurse should not assume that the Russian American will have an alcohol issue. Russian alcoholics have lost hope and would not be motivated to emigrate from Russia in search of a new life. Immigrants from Russia to the United States, on the other hand, are extremely motivated in changing their lives for the better and want to survive here in America. Those immigrants who are religious also will be unlikely to drink alcohol because of the religious sanctions against its use/abuse among Jewish and Pentecostal affiliates.

Summary

As we have seen the White non-Hispanic population is extremely diverse and is unified by a similarity of skin pigmentation. The White population has diverse and multiple places of origin within Europe. Since presently, the majority of the American population is considered White non-Hispanic, it is important to also understand the differences among various these ethnic groups. An overview of the historical background, statistics, traditional health beliefs, and barriers to care were presented. As with all patients, it is important to question the patient to determine what their health and illness beliefs are so that a culturally competent plan of care can be developed that incorporates the similarities and the differences between all human beings.

Related Web Sites

Diner, H. (2008). Immigration and U.S. History. Retrieved May 11, 2009, from http://www.america.gov/st/diversityenglish/2008/February/20080307112004ebyessedo0.1716272.html.

Christian Light Publications, Inc. The Germans come to North America. Retrieved August 28, 2009, from http://www.anabaptists.org/history/ss8001.html.

References

Anonymous. Judaism. Retrieved August 28, 2009, from http://www.religionfacts.com/judaism/.

Bankston, C. L., & Hidalgo, D. (2006). *Immigration in U.S. history: Irish immigrants.* Pasadena, CA: Salem Press.

Bologova, N. (1996). Voices of the Ukrainian community. Retrieved August 28, 2009, from http://www.ethnomed.org/ethnomed/voices/ukraine.html

Braham, M. (1993). The untouchables: A survey of the Roma people of central and eastern Europe. Geneva: UNHCR.

Brown, K. M., & Obermiller, P. J. (1994). The health status of children living in urban Appalachian neighborhoods. In K. M. Borman & P. J. Obermiller (Eds.), *From mountains to metropolis: Appalachian migrants in American cities* (pp. 70–82). Westport, CT: Greenwood Publishing Company.

Butler, S. (1996). Substance misuse and the social work ethos. *Justice for Substance Misuse for Nursing Health and Social Care,* 1, 3, 149–154.

Central Intelligence Agency. (2006). The World Factbook. Retrieved May 23, 2009, from https://www.cia.gov/library/publications/the-world-factbook/fields/2122.html.

Central Intelligence Agency. (2009). The World Factbook. Retrieved September 21, 2009, from https://www.cia.gov/library/publications/the-world-factbook/geos/us.html.

Christian Light Publications, Inc. The Germans come to North America. Retrieved August 28, 2009, from http://www.anabaptists.org/history/ss8001.html.

Diner, H. (2008). Immigration and U.S. History. Retrieved September 21, 2009, from http://www.america.gov/st/diversityenglish/2008/February/20080307112004ebyessedo0.1716272.html.

Edwards, J. B., Lenz, C. L., & East-Odom, J. C. (1993). Nurse-managed primary care: Serving a rural Appalachian population. *Family and Community Health,* 16, 2, 50–56.

Engels, E. A., Clark, E., Aledort, L. M., Goedert, J. J., & Whitby, D. (2002). Kaposi's sarcoma-associated herpesvirus infection in elderly Jews and non-Jews from New York City. *International Journal of Epidemiology,* 31, 946–950.

Fares, F., Badarneh, K., Abosaleh, M., Harrari-Shaham, A., Diukman, R., et al. (2008). Carrier frequency of autosomal-recessive disorders in the Ashkenazi Jewish population: should the rationale for mutation choice for screening be reevaluated? *Prenatal Diagnosis,* 28, 3, 236–241.

Galanti, G. A. (2000). An introduction to cultural differences. *Western Journal of Medicine,* 172, 5, 335–336.

Giger, J. N., & Davidhizar, R. E. (2003). *Transcultural Assessment: Assessment & Intervention.* 4th ed. St. Louis: Mosby.

Giordano, J., & McGoldrick, M. (1996). Italian Families. In M. McGoldrick, J. Giordano, & J. K. Pearce (Eds.), *Ethnicity and family therapy* (2nd ed.). New York: Guilford.

Gross, L. (1997). Background dynamics of the Amish movement: The Dutch Mennonites vis-á-vis the Swiss Brethren: pivotal individuals within the Swiss Brethren division of the 1690s, and the question of Reformed (Calvinist) influence. Retrieved January 20, 2009, from http://www.goshen.edu/facultypubs/GROSS.html.

Halperin, R. H. (1994). Appalachians in cities: Issues and challenges for research. In K. M. Borman, & P. J. Obermiller (Eds.), *From mountains to metropolis: Appalachian migrants in American cities* (pp. 70–82). Westport, CT: Greenwood Publishing Company.

Hancock, I. F. (1987). *The pariah syndrome: An account of gypsy slavery and persecution.* Ann Arbor, MI: Karoma.

Harris Poll. (2003). While most Americans believe in God, only 36% attend a religious service once a month or more often. The Harris Poll #59, October 15, 2003. Retrieved May 19, 2009, from http://www.harrisinteractive.com/harris_poll/index.asp?PID408.

Helton, L. R., Barnes, E. C., & Borman, K. M. (1994). Urban Appalachia and professional intervention: A model for education and social service providers. In K. M. Borman & P. J. Obermiller (Eds.), *From mountains to metropolis: Appalachian migrants in American cities* (pp. 106–120). Westport, CT: Greenwood Publishing Company.

Hostetler, J. A. (1993). *Amish society* (4th ed.). Baltimore: John Hopkins University Press.

Huntington, G. E. (1993). Health care. In D. B. Kraybill (Ed.), *The Amish and the state.* Baltimore: The John Hopkins University Press.

Katzman, D. M. (2000). European immigrants leave mark on continent. *The Brown Quarterly*, 4, 1. Retrieved May 11, 2009, from http://brownvboard.org/brwnqurt/04-1/04-1b.htm.

Kraybill, D. B. (2003). *The Amish and the state* (2nd ed.). Baltimore: The Johns Hopkins University Press.

Kraybill, D. B., Nolt, S. M., & Weaver-Zercher, D. L. (2007). *Amish grace: How forgiveness transcended tragedy.* Hoboken, NJ: Jossey-Bass.

Landsbergis, P., & Klumbiene, J. (2003). Coronary heart disease mortality in Russia and Eastern Europe. *American Journal of Public Health*, 93, 11, 1793.

Lee, D. (2005) Our Amish neighbors: providing culturally competent care. *Multicultural Health Series.* Videotape and handout available from the UMHS, PMCH, Cultural Competency Division.

Lester, N. (1998). CE credit: Cultural competence: a nursing dialogue. *The American Journal of Nursing*, 98, 9, 36–43.

Lieberman, J. A. (1990). HLA-B38, DR4, DQw3 and clozapine-induced agranulocytosis in Jewish patients with schizophrenia. *Archives General Psychiatry*, 47, 10, 945–948.

Marger, M. N., & Obermiller, P. J. (1987). Urban Appalachians and Canadian Maritime migrants: Comparative study of emergent ethnicity. In P. J. Obermiller & W. W. Philliber (Eds.), *Too few tomorrow: Urban Appalachians in the 1980s* (pp. 23–34). Boone, NC: Appalachian Consortium Press.

McKee, M. (1997). The health of gypsies. *British Medical Journal*, 315, 7117, 1172.

McNeil, W. K. (1989). *Appalachian images in folk and popular culture.* Ann Arbor, MI: University of Michigan Press.

Mehler, P. S., Scott, J. Y., Pines, L., Gifford, N., Biggerstaff, S., & Hiatt, W. R. (2001). Russian immigrant cardiovascular risk assessment. *Journal of Health Care for the Poor and Underserved*, 12, 2, 224–235.

Office of Homeland Security. (2005). *2005 yearbook of immigration statistics.* Washington, DC: US Department of Homeland Security: Office of Immigration Statistics.

Petersen, R. D. (2001). *Resistance and rebellion: Lessons from Eastern Europe.* New York: Cambridge University Press.

Project Genesis, Inc. torah.org. Retrieved August 28, 2009, from http://www.torah.org/

Purnell, L. D., & Paulanka, B. J. (1998). *Transcultural health care: A culturally competent approach.* Philadelphia: F. A. Davis.

Rosner, F. (1993). Hospice, medical ethics and Jewish customs. *American Journal of Hospice and Palliative Care,* 10, 4, 6–10.

Rundle, A., Carvalho, M., & Robinson, M. (1999). *Cultural competence in health care: A practical guide.* San Francisco: Jossey-Bass.

Russian Public Opinion Research Center. (2007). Retrieved September 21, 2009, from http://wciocm.com.

Smith, L. S. (1996). New Russian Immigrants health problems, practices and values. *Journal of Cultural Diversity,* 3, 3, 68–73.

Spector, R. (2004). *Cultural diversity in health and illness.* New York: Appleton-Century-Crofts.

Sutherland, A. H. (2004). Roma of the United States and Europe. In C. R. Ember, & M. Ember (Eds.), *Encyclopedia of medical anthropology: Health and illness in the world's cultures.* New York: Springer Publishing.

US Census Bureau. (2000). United States Census 2000. Retrieved September 21, 2009, from http://www.census.gov/main/www/cen2000.html.

US Census Bureau. (2002). Population profiles by age, sex, race and Hispanic origin. Summary File 3, Washington, DC: US Government Printing Office.

US Census Bureau. (2007a). Religious composition of US population: 2007. Retrieved May 19, 2009, from http://www.census.gov/compendia/statab/tables/09s0074.pdf.

US Census Bureau. (2007b). Selected social characteristics in the United States: 2007. Retrieved May 21, 2009, from http://factfinder.census.gov/servlet/ADPTable?_bmy&-contextadp&-qr_nameACS_2007_1YR_G00_DP2&-ds_nameACS_2007_1YR_G00.

US Census Bureau. (2008a). An older and more diverse nation by midcentury. Retrieved May 13, 2009, from http://www.census.gov/Press-Release/www/releases/archives/population/012496.html.

US Census Bureau. (2008b). Table 4: annual estimates of the Black or African American alone or in combination population by sex and age for the United States: April 1, 2000, to July 1, 2007. Source: Population Division, US Census Bureau. Release Date: May 1, 2008.

Vadlamani, A., Maher, J. F., Shaete, M., Smirnoff, A., Cameron, D. G., Winkelmann, J. C., et al. (2001). Colorectal cancer in Russian-speaking Jewish emigrés: Community-based screening. *American Journal of Gastroenterology,* 96, 9, 2755–2760.

Vallance, H. & Ford, J. (2003). Carrier testing for autosomal-recessive disorders. *Critical Reviews in Clinical Laboratory Sciences,* 40, 4, 473–497.

World Almanac. (2006). New York: World Almanac Books.

Zuckerman, P. (2005). Atheism: Contemporary rates and patterns. In M. Martin (Ed.), *The Cambridge companion to atheism.* Cambridge, UK: Cambridge University Press.

Glossary of Additional Cultural Terms

Acculturation—becoming a competent participant in the dominant culture. In the United States, it is assumed that the usual course of acculturation takes three generations for completion (i.e., the grandchildren of an immigrant would be considered fully acculturated or Americanized) (Spector, 2004).

Assimilation—becoming in all ways like the members of the dominant culture; the process by which an individual develops a new cultural identity (Spector, 2004).

Bicultural—a person may self-identify with more than one cultural group and that bicultural person sees both sides and can function in two worlds (McGrath, 1998).

Biopsychosocial Model—incorporates social, psychologic, and emotional factors in diagnosis and treatment. It recognizes that illness cannot be studied or treated in isolation from the social and cultural environment. Whereas the biomedical model prioritizes professional knowledge, the biopsychosocial model expects health careers and doctors to acknowledge and take into account individual patient circumstances.

Campinha-Bacote's The Process of Cultural Competency in the Delivery of Health Care Services—consists of five constructs: cultural awareness, cultural knowledge, cultural skill, cultural encounters, and cultural desire.

Collectivism—"Collectivism means the subjugation of the individual to a group—whether to a race, class or state does not matter. Collectivism holds that man must be chained to collective action and collective thought for the sake of what is called 'the common good'" (Rand, 1944). "Collectivism is the political theory that states that the will of the people is omnipotent, an individual must obey; that society as a whole, not the individual, is the unit of moral value" (Bernstein, 2005).

Cultural awareness—an appreciation of the objective, external signs of diversity, such as the arts, music, dress, and physical characteristics (Lattanzi & Purnell, 2006).

Cultural competency—no single definition of cultural competency is universally accepted yet all of the definitions share the requirement that healthcare professionals adjust and recognize their own culture in order to understand the culture of the patient (Johnson, Saha, Arbelaez, Beach, & Cooper, 2004).

Cultural diversity—interacting with persons from a culture different from your own (Purnell & Paulanka, 1998). It refers to diversity in race, color, ethnicity, national origin, religion, age, gender, sexual orientation, ability/disability, social and economic status or class, education, occupation, religious orientation, marital and parental status, and other related attributes of groups of people in society (Giger et al., 2007).

Cultural humility—incorporates a lifelong commitment to self-evaluation and self-critique, to redress the power imbalances in the patient clinician dynamic, and to develop mutually beneficial and advocacy partnerships with communities on behalf of individuals and defined populations. Cultural humility is proposed as a goal in healthcare education (Tervalon & Murray-Garcia, 1998).

Cultural mismatch—when the healthcare provider has a personal style of interaction that does not match the patients. It is essential that this cultural mismatch be recognized or else the healthcare provider risks the consequences that result when a therapeutic alliance is not established with the patient (Leininger, 1991).

Cultural sensitivity—experienced when neutral language, both verbal and not verbal, is used in a way that reflects sensitivity and appreciation for the diversity of another. Cultural sensitivity may be conveyed through words, phrases, and categorizations that are intentionally avoided, especially when referring to any individual who may be interpreted as impolite or offensive (Giger et al., 2007).

Culturally competent care—the provision of appropriate, sensitive care to people from ethnic backgrounds different from that of the provider (Giger & Davidhizar, 2004). Cultural discordant care—arises from unaddressed cultural differences between healthcare providers and their patients (Assemi, Cullender, & Hudmon, 2004; Saha, Komaromy, Koepsell & Bindman, 1999).

Culture—the totality of socially transmitted behavioral patterns, arts, beliefs, values, customs, life ways, and all other products of human work and thought characteristics of a population of people that guide their world view and decision making (Purnell & Paulanka, 1998). A learned, patterned behavioral response acquired over time that includes explicit and implicit beliefs, attitudes, values, customs, norms, taboos, arts, habits, and life ways accepted by a community of individuals. Culture is primarily learned and transmitted within the family and other social organizations, is shared by the majority of the group, includes an individualized world view, guides decision making, and facilitates self-worth and self-esteem (Giger et al., 2007). Culture influences beliefs about what causes illness and how it should be treated. These cultural beliefs may guide patient actions in health maintenance and during times of illness in patients, their families, and the community.

Diversity—the concept of diversity encompasses acceptance and respect. It means understanding that each individual is unique, and recognizing our individual differences. These can be along the dimensions of race, ethnicity, gender, sexual orientation, socioeconomic status, age, physical abilities, religious beliefs, political beliefs, or other ideologies. It is the exploration of these differences in a safe, positive, and nurturing environment. It is about understanding each other and moving beyond simple tolerance to embracing and celebrating the rich dimensions of diversity contained within each individual. The range of human variation, including age, race, gender, disability, ethnicity, nationality, religious and spiritual beliefs, sexual orientation, political beliefs, economic status, native language, and geographical background.

Ethnic group—a group of people whose members have different experiences and backgrounds from the dominant culture by status, background, residence, religion, education, or other factors that functionally unify the group and act collectively on each other (Giger et al., 2007).

Ethnicity—the condition of belonging to a particular ethnic group. According to the Office of Minority Health (2001), ethnic is a group of people that share a common and distinctive racial, national, religious, linguistic, or cultural heritage.

Ethnocentrism—the universal tendency of human beings to think that their ways of thinking, acting, and believing are the only right, proper, and natural ways can be a major barrier to providing culturally conscious care. Ethnocentrism perpetuates an attitude that beliefs that differ greatly from one's own are strange, bizarre, or unenlightened, and therefore wrong (Purnell & Paulanka, 1998). Ethnocentrism is a belief in the superiority of one's own ethnic group.

Giger and Davidhizar Transcultural Assessment Model—provides a framework to systematically assess the role of culture on health and illness and has been used extensively in a variety of settings and by diverse disciplines. The model postulates that every individual is culturally unique and should be assessed according to the six phenomena (Giger & Davidhizar, 2004). It is important to emphasize that the model does not presuppose that every person within an ethnic or cultural group will act or behave in a similar manner (Giger & Davidhizar, 2004). In fact, Giger and Davidhizar (2004) inform that a culturally appropriate model must recognize differences in groups while avoiding stereotypical approaches to client care.

Healing—According to Spector (2004) there are four types of healing: spiritual healing, inner healing, physical healing, and deliverance or exorcism. Healing should consider the impact of religion and/or spirituality to the patient. A healing focus would be on the removal of evil which has originated inside or outside the body.

Health—defined by Florence Nightingale (1860) as "being well and using one's powers to the fullest extent." It is defined by the World Health Organization (1946) as "Health is not only the absence of infirmity and disease but also a state of physical, mental and social well-being."

Health Illness Belief Model—based on the constructs of perceived susceptibility, severity, benefits, barriers, and cues to action. The health belief model suggests that patients are more likely to comply with doctor's orders when they feel susceptibility to illness, believe the illness has the potential to have serious consequences for health or daily functioning, and do not anticipate major obstacles, such as side effects or costs (Conrad, 2009).

Health disparities—differences in the incidence, prevalence, mortality, and burden of diseases and other adverse health conditions that exist among specific population groups in the United States (National Institutes of Health, 1999).

Health literacy—the degree to which individuals have the capacity to obtain, process, and understand basic health information and services needed to make appropriate health decisions (US Department of Health and Human Services, 2000).

Illness—a highly personal state in which the person feels unhealthy or ill; may or may not be related to disease (Kozier, Erb, Berman, & Burke, 2000).

Interdisciplinary health care—implies the existence of a team. It is an integrated approach to patient care in which all team members actively coordinate care across all health care disciplines.

LEARN (Berlin & Fowkes, 1983)—some pneumonics have been developed to help the nurse navigate a cross-cultural encounter. L, listen to the patient's explanation of the problem; E, explain your perception of the problem; A, acknowledge similarities and differences; R, recommend suggest an intervention or treatment; and N, negotiate to find a mutually acceptable plan.

Leininger's Sunrise Model—illustrates the major components and interrelationships of Leininger's Culture Care, Diversity, and Universality Theory. Nurses can use the Sunrise Model when caring for patients to ensure that nursing actions are culture specific. The Culture Care, Diversity, and Universality Theory states that nurses must take into account the cultural beliefs, caring behaviors, and values of individuals, families, and groups to provide effective, satisfying, and culturally congruent nursing care (Leininger, 1991).

Multidisciplinary health care—involves membership in a clinical group, practicing with an awareness of and toleration for other disciplines. Groups of professionals provide discipline-specific care, independently of one another. The patient's problems are subdivided and treated in parallel. Each provider conducts his or her practice in a parallel relationship with that of other group members.

National Standards for Culturally and Linguistically Appropriate Services in Health Care (CLAS)—Fourteen standards established in 1997 by the Office of Minority Health (within the Department of Health and Human Services) that must be met by most health-care related agencies. Accreditation and credentialing agencies can access and compare providers who say they provide culturally competent services and assure quality care for diverse populations, including the Joint Commission on Accreditation of Healthcare Organizations (JCAHO), the National Committee on Quality Assurance, American Medical Association (AMA), American Nurses Association (ANA), and Peer Review Organization. (The standards are listed in Box 4-1.)

Patient-centered health care—health care the patient needs, provided when they need it and in the manner that they want. It is care that is informed by both scientific evidence and the patient's values.

Purnell and Paulanka Model of Cultural Competence—to provide a framework for all healthcare providers to learn inherent concepts and characteristics of culture; define circumstances that affect one's cultural world view in the context of historical perspectives; provide a model that links the most central relationships of culture; interrelate characteristics of culture to promote congruence and facilitate the delivery of consciously competent care; provide a framework that reflects human characteristics such as motivation, intentionality, and meaning; provide a structure for analyzing cultural data; and view the individual, family, or group within a unique ethnocultural environment (Purnell & Paulanka, 1998).

Race—a viable term that relates to biology but has sociologic implications. Members of a particular race share distinguishing physical features such as skin color, bone structure, or blood group. Race is a social construct, which limits or increases opportunities depending on the setting (Giger et al., 2007).

Sick role—In our society, a person is expected to have the symptoms viewed as an illness confirmed by a member of the health care profession. Parsons (1951) described four main components of the sick role: (1) The sick person is exempted from the performance of certain normal social obligations. (2) The sick person is also exempted from a certain type of responsibility for their own state. (3) The legitimization of the sick role is only partial. This means that the sick role is only considered acceptable if it falls within a reasonable time frame as determined by health care and society. (4) Being sick, except in the mildest of cases, is being in need of help (Parsons, 1951).

Stereotyping—the assumption that all people in a similar cultural, racial, or ethnic group are alike and share the same values and beliefs (Giger & Davidhizar, 2004).

Unidisciplinary practice—care delivery where a healthcare professional functions in isolation from members of other healthcare disciplines.

US Biomedical Model Health Belief Model—tenets are dichotomization of mind and body, the belief that individuals can control their environment, and the value of taking responsibility for one's own health (Reiser, 1985). There is a strong emphasis on disease prevention in this model, but disease prevention in many cultures is a foreign concept. This is especially so in the areas of childbirth preparation, the care of newborns, the taking of medications, or to the death or dying process. Inquiring about the patient's preferences and practices with the goal to incorporate and negotiate acceptable approaches to healthcare delivery will serve the patient and provider best. How long one has been living in the United States also is an important variable as it may greatly impact their attitude toward health care.

Vulnerable Populations—social groups with increased relative risk (i.e., exposure to risk factors) or susceptibility to health-related problems. The vulnerability is evidenced in higher comparative mortality rates, lower life expectancy, reduced access to care, and diminished quality of life (Center for Vulnerable Populations Research, UCLA School of Nursing, 2008).

Western Biomedical Model—the focus is on objective, measurable phenomena, and technology can be used to achieve diagnoses. Advances in medical technology led to a greater ability to localize disease processes within the body so that sites of pathology could be pinpointed with greater accuracy (Helman, 2001).

References

Assemi, M., Cullender, C., & Hudmon, K. S. (2004). Implementation and evaluation of cultural competency training for pharmacy students. *Annals of Pharmacotherapy*, 38, 5, 781–786.

Berlin, E. A., & Fowkes, Jr., W. C. (1983). A teaching framework for cross-cultural health care. Application in family practice. *The Western Journal of Medicine*, 139, 934–938.

Bernstein, A. (2005). Villainy: an analysis of the nature of evil (part five of five). *Capitalism Magazine*. Retrieved April 2, 2009, from http://www.capmag.com/article.asp?ID=4433.

Center for Vulnerable Populations Research, UCLA School of Nursing. (2008). Retrieved November 24, 2009, from http://www.nursing.ucla.edu/orgs/cvpr/default.asp. 2008

Conrad, P. (2009). *The sociology of health and illness.* 8th ed. New York: Macmillan

Giger, J. N., & Davidhizar, R. E. (2004). *Transcultural nursing: Assessment and intervention* (4th ed.). Philadelphia: Mosby.

Giger, J., Davidhizar, R. E., Purnell, L., Harden, J. T., Phillips, J., Strickland, O., et al. (2007). American Academy of Nursing Expert Panel Report: Developing cultural competence to eliminate health disparities in ethnic minorities and other vulnerable populations. *Journal of Transcultural Nursing*, 18, 2, 95–102.

Helman, C. G. (2001). Health beliefs about diabetes: patients versus doctors. *Western Journal of Medicine*, 175, 5, 312–313.

Johnson, R. L., Saha., S., Arbelaez, J. J., Beach, M. C., & Cooper, L. A. (2004). Racial and ethnic differences in patient perceptions of bias and cultural competence in health care. *Journal of General Internal Medicine*, 19, 2, 101–110.

Kozier, B., Erb, G., Berman, A. J., & Burke, K. (2000). *Fundamentals of nursing, concepts, process, and practice.* Upper Saddle River, NJ: Prentice-Hall Health.

Lattanzi, J. B., & Purnell, L. D. (2006). *Developing cultural competence in physical therapy practice.* Philadelphia: F. A. Davis.

Leininger, M. M. (1991). *Culture care diversity and universality: A theory of nursing.* New York: National League for Nursing.

McGrath, B. (1998). Illness as a problem of meaning: Moving culture from the classroom to the clinic. *Advanced Nursing Science*, 21, 2, 17–29.

National Institutes of Health. (1999). Retrieved October 9, 2009, from http://crchd.cancer.gov/disparities/defined.html.

Nightingale, F. (1860). *Notes on nursing: What it is and what it is not.* New York: D. Appleton and Company (first American Edition). Retrieved October 9, 2009, from http://digital.library.upenn.edu/women/nightingale/nursing/nursing.htm.

Office of Minority Health. (2001). OMB standards for data on race and ethnicity. Retrieved October 9, 2009, from http://www.omhrc.gov/templates/browse.aspx?lvl=2&dlvlid=172.

Parsons, T. (1951). *The social system.* Glencoe, IL: The Free Press.

Purnell, L., & Paulanka, B. (1998). *Transcultural health care: a culturally competent approach.* Philadelphia: F. A. Davis.

Rand, A. (1944). The only path to tomorrow. *Readers Digest*, 88–90.

Reiser, S. J. (1985). Responsibility for personal health: A historical perspective. *Medical Philosophy*, 10, 7–17.

Saha, S., Komaromy, M., Koepsell, T. D., & Bindman, A. B. (1999). Patient-physician racial concordance and the perceived quality and use of health care. *Archives of Internal Medicine, 159*, 9, 997–1004.

Spector, R. E. (2004). *Cultural diversity in health and illness.* 6th ed. Upper Saddle River, NJ: Pearson-Prentice-Hall.

Tervalon, M. & Murray-Garcia, J. (1998). Cultural humility versus cultural competence: A critical distinction in defining physician training outcomes in multicultural education. *Journal of Health Care for the Poor & Underserved*, 9, 2, 117–125.

US Department of Health and Human Services. (2000). Quick guide to health literacy. Fact Sheet. Retrieved October 9, 2009, from http://www.health.gov/communication/literacy/quickguide/factsbasic.htm.

World Health Organization. (1946). Retrieved October 9, 2009, from http://www.who.int/en.

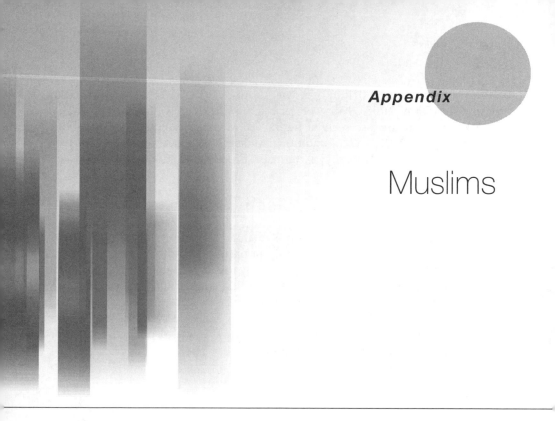

Muslims

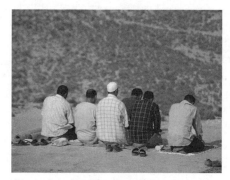

Source: © Jaroslaw Grudzinski/ShutterStock, Inc.

Background

Not all Muslims share all of the same health beliefs. The health beliefs, values, and practices of Muslims are influenced by geographical, cultural, and ethnic factors in addition to the individual degree of faith and spirituality a Muslim may possess. There are differences in health belief practices among Arab, Asian, African, and African American Muslims. Islam is the second largest and fastest growing religion in the world. While the perception in the United States that Islam is a Middle Eastern religion, in fact, only about 25% of Muslims are Arab; the majority of Muslims are either African or Asian. About 30% of US Muslims are African American (Ohm, 2003). Followers of Islam are known as Muslims, Moslems, or Islamic. There are also sects of traditional Muslims. Sunnis represent about 90% and Shiites 10%–15% of traditional Muslims. There are also several smaller sects, including Sufi, Ahmadiyya, Wahhabi, Ismaili, and Dawoodi Bohra.

Principles of the Muslim Faith

The supreme being of Islam is Allah and the religion's founder is the Prophet Muhammad. The holy book is called the Koran or Qur'an. Daily living of Muslims is guided by the Koran and also by additional teachings from Muhammad, the Hadith, and the Sunna. Some Muslims use prayer beads and prayer rugs and may pin amulets and charms to their clothing. The use of idolatry is forbidden and the use of statues, figurines, or other likenesses that attempt to personify Allah or Muhammad are considered idol worship.

Muslim Health Beliefs

Muslims view illness as an atonement for sins. Illness is dealt with by both the patient and family by praying. They are open to receiving medical treatment, but if it is felt it is time for death, they will view it as an opportunity to begin their journey to meet their Lord. The major tenet of Islam is peace and submission to the will of God (Allah). Cleanliness is an important concept to Muslims as maintaining cleanliness is viewed as being "half of the faith" (Athar). The Qur'an, the holy book, prohibits eating pork or pork products, meat of dead animals, blood, and encourages the avoidance of all intoxicants. The practice of fasting, which occurs from dawn to dusk daily for 1 month a year during Ramadan, is considered restorative and is viewed as restful to the body.

Important Nursing Implications

There are certain health practices which are generally acceptable and others which are not acceptable to the Muslim patient. As with any other cultural group, it is essential that the nurse question the patient to determine what beliefs and practices are of significant to each individual Muslim patient. Generally, the following healthcare practices are permitted by the Muslim patient: circumcision, blood transfusions (after proper screening), transplantation (with some restrictions), reproductive technology (but only within an intact marriage), living wills, and genetic engineering (but not cloning). The following healthcare practices are

---

Table A-1

Cultural Implications when Providing Nursing Care to Muslim Patients

Physical Examination/ Assessment	If an examination can be performed over a gown, it should be done that way. Provide for modesty/privacy. Always examine a female patient in the presence of another female patient (this is mandatory if the nurse or physician is male). It is best to provide same sex health care if at all possible. Preferably no males in the delivery room during labor (except the husband).
Nutrition/Diet	Offer Muslim or Kosher meals. Permit the family to bring in food if there are no dietary restrictions. If restrictions are necessary, request that the dietitian work with the family to incorporate foods from home if possible.
Faith/Spirituality	Allow for uninterrupted prayer and for the patient to read the Koran. Allow their Imam to visit. Do not insist on autopsy or organ donation. In the event of patient death, allow the family and Imam to follow Islamic guidelines for preparing the dead body for an Islamic funeral. After death, the female body should be given the same respect and privacy as if she was still living.
Communication	Inform them of their patient rights and encourage living wills. Take time to explain diagnostic tests, treatments, and procedures. Many Muslims are new immigrants and there may be a language barrier. Identify the patient clearly as Muslim on the patient chart and ID bracelet.

Source: Athar, S. Information for health care providers when dealing with a Muslim patient. Retrieved October 29, 2009, from http://www.islam-usa.com/index.php?option=com_content&view=article&id =169:information-for-health-care-providers-when-dealing-with-a-muslim-patient&catid=68:health— medicine&Itemid=137.

---

generally not acceptable to the Muslim patient: assisted suicide/euthanasia, autopsy (unless required by law), maintaining a terminal patient on life support for a prolonged period in a vegetative state, abortion (unless it is to save the mother's life), cloning.

Table A-1 describes what nurses can and should do for the Muslim patient.

al-Shahri, M. Z., & al-Khenaizan, A. (2005). Palliative care for Muslim patients. *Journal*

References

Supportive Oncology, 3, 6, 432–436.

Andrews, C. S. (2006) Modesty and healthcare for women: understanding cultural sensitivities. *Community Oncology*, 3, 7, 443–446.

Athar, S. (2009). Information for health care providers when dealing with a Muslim patient. Retrieved October 29, 2009, from http://www.islam-usa.com/index.php?option=com_content&view=article&id=169:information-for-health-care-providers-when-dealing-with-a-muslim-patient&catid=68:health—medicine&Itemid=137.

Bahar, Z. (2005). The effects of Islam and traditional practices on women's health and reproduction. *Nursing Ethics*, 12, 6, 557–570.

Carter, D. J., & Rashidi, A. R. (2004). East meets west: integrating psychotherapy approaches for Muslim Women. *Holistic Nursing Practice*, 18, 3, 152–159.

Gatrad, A. R., & Sheikh, A. (2004). Risk factors for HIV/AIDS in Muslim communities. *Diversity Health Soc Care*, 1, 1, 65–69.

Giaramazidou, T. (2005). A study of dietary knowledge and its religious relationship in patients receiving hemodialysis. *Journal Renal Care*, 31, 4, 199–202.

Mirghani, H. M. (2006). The effect of maternal diet restriction on pregnancy outcome. *American Journal of Perinatology*, 23, 1, 21–24.

Ohm, R. (2003). The African American experience in the Islamic faith. *Public Health Nursing*, 20, 6, 478–486.

Suwaidi, AJ., Bener, A., & Gehani, A. A., Behair, S., Mohanadi, H. D., et al. (2006). Does the circadian pattern for acute cardiac events presentation vary with fasting? *J Postgraduate Medicine*, 52, 1, 30–33.

Topacoglu, H., Karcioglu, O., & Yuruktumen, A. (2005). Impact of Ramadan on demographics and frequencies of disease-related visits in the emergency department. *International Journal of Clinical Practice*, 59, 8, 900–905.

Ypinazar, V. A., & Margolis, S. A. (2006). Delivering culturally sensitive care: the perceptions if older Arabian Gulf Arabs concerning religion, health, and disease. *Qualitative Health Research*, 16, 6, 773–787.

Index

A

AAN. *See* American Academy of Nursing
AAPIs. *See* Asian/Pacific Islander
    Americans
Acculturation, 13, 55, 250
Acupuncture, 207–208, 211
African Americans. *See* Black Americans
AIDS
    Black Americans, 149, 154
    Hispanic Americans, 184
    white (non-Hispanic) Americans,
        304–305, 314
Aiken, L. H., 120
Alaska Natives
    acculturation, 265–267
    background, 264–265
    biological variations, 267
    communication, 265–266
    faith, spirituality, 267
    Giger Davidhizar transcultural
        assessment model,
        265–267

language, 265–266
nonverbal communication, 266
nursing considerations, 266
nursing implications, 51
obesity, 266
shamanism, 266
social organization, 266–267
touch, 266
vs. American Eskimos, 264
vs. Inuit, 264
Alcohol
    Native Americans, 260, 266
    white (non-Hispanic) Americans,
        286, 314–315
American Academy of Nursing,
        cultural competence
        recommendations, 11
American Academy of Nursing (AAN),
        10, 11, 17
American Association of Colleges of
        Nursing, 17, 122
American Diabetes Association, 35, 183